HIV/AIDS in China and India

HIV/AIDS IN CHINA AND INDIA

Governing Health Security

Catherine Yuk-ping Lo

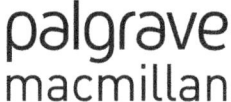

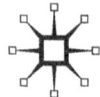

HIV/AIDS IN CHINA AND INDIA
Copyright © Catherine Yuk-ping Lo, 2015.

All rights reserved.

First published in 2015 by
PALGRAVE MACMILLAN®
in the United States—a division of St. Martin's Press LLC,
175 Fifth Avenue, New York, NY 10010.

Where this book is distributed in the UK, Europe and the rest of the world, this is by Palgrave Macmillan, a division of Macmillan Publishers Limited, registered in England, company number 785998, of Houndmills, Basingstoke, Hampshire RG21 6XS.

Palgrave Macmillan is the global academic imprint of the above companies and has companies and representatives throughout the world.

Palgrave® and Macmillan® are registered trademarks in the United States, the United Kingdom, Europe and other countries.

ISBN: 978–1–137–50419–7

Library of Congress Cataloging-in-Publication Data

Lo, Catherine Yuk-ping, 1984–, author.
    HIV/AIDS in China and India : governing health security / Catherine Yuk-ping Lo.
        p. ; cm.
    Includes bibliographical references and index.
    ISBN 978–1–137–50419–7 (hardcover)
    I. Title.
    [DNLM: 1. HIV Infections—China—Comparative Study.
2. HIV Infections—India—Comparative Study. 3. Security Measures—China—Comparative Study. 4. Security Measures—India—Comparative Study. 5. Health Policy—China—Comparative Study. 6. Health Policy—India—Comparative Study. 7. International Cooperation—China—Comparative Study. 8. International Cooperation—India—Comparative Study. WC 503]

RA643.7.C6
362.19697'9200951—dc23   2014049650

A catalogue record of the book is available from the British Library.

Design by Newgen Knowledge Works (P) Ltd., Chennai, India.

First edition: June 2015

10 9 8 7 6 5 4 3 2 1

This book is dedicated to Abraham Lam for his endless support

Contents

List of Illustrations		ix
Acknowledgments		xi
List of Abbreviations		xiii
1	Introduction	1
2	Security: A Revised Framework for Analysis	15
3	Health Security and HIV/AIDS	45
4	The Changing Face of Public Health Care Systems in China and India	65
5	Securitizing HIV/AIDS in China	79
6	Audience Acceptance in China: Case Studies in Beijing, Shanghai, and Kunming	97
7	Securitizing HIV/AIDS in India	123
8	Audience Acceptance in India: Case Studies in New Delhi, Mumbai, and Imphal	139
9	Conclusion: Reconsidering HIV/AIDS Securitization	161
Notes		177
Bibliography		237
Index		265

Illustrations

Figure

2.1	A Revised Securitization Framework for Health	28

Tables

2.1	A Matrix of Securitizing Moves	32
3.1	Public Spending on Health, Education, and Military in Developed and Developing Countries	50
6.1	Proliferation of HIV/AIDS-Focused NGOs in China	114
7.1	Health Budget Allocated to the NRHM and HIV/AIDS (2005–2011)	134
7.2	Summary of the Financial Expenditures of the Indian Government and External Agencies on NACPs	137

Acknowledgments

I would like to express my sincere gratitude to those who helped me in this long journey. I could not have completed this book without the support of many individuals. I would like to thank Professor Ian Holliday and Dr. Nicholas Thomas for accepting me as a PhD student. As the old saying goes, "Once a teacher, for life a father-figure." With patience and encouragement, Ian skillfully guided me throughout this intellectual journey from which I learned life lessons.

I would also like to thank Nick for his knowledgeable and thorough comments regarding this book. Had I not been employed by Nick at the Centre of Asian Studies (now renamed Hong Kong Institute for the Humanities and Social Sciences) as a research assistant in summer 2007, I might never have applied for the postgraduate research program. Nick's support and belief in my abilities have been an important stepping stone in my academic endeavors. Nick inspired me as a teacher and researcher, in addition to his contributions to my PhD studies. He helped me realize that I can use my interests as motivation to develop my career. Nick has also provided unwavering support and inspiration during my years in teaching at City University of Hong Kong. Nick remains an important supervisor and adviser.

I am grateful to my colleagues at the Department of Asian and International Studies, City University of Hong Kong, for providing a supportive and friendly environment of teaching and research. I would like to extend my special gratitude to my colleague Brad Williams for reading and commenting on the earlier draft of this work.

I presented a paper based on chapters 5 and 7 of this book at the British International Studies Association Annual Conference and received a highly useful feedback from Simon Rushton to whom I also owe my gratitude.

I want to express my heartfelt gratitude to all the individuals who shared their ideas regarding HIV/AIDS in China and India. I would also like to thank my friends in China and India for providing support, assistance, and encouragement during my fieldwork.

My gratitude goes to commissioning editor Rachel Krause for accepting this project. I also thank Veronica Goldstein, our editorial assistant, for patiently replying to my emails. Furthermore, I appreciate the help extended by the anonymous reviewers in reviewing my work.

Most importantly, I would like to thank Auntie Sui-lin for being a reliable friend and prayer partner; she is one of the kindest and most generous people I know because she has always been there for me not only in good times but also in tough times. She always reminds me that everything is possible with God. I would also like to express my gratitude to my sister Eunice for her research assistance. Furthermore, I would like to give my sincerest thanks to my partner, Abraham Lam, to whom this book is dedicated.

This book was supported by a University Research Grant, General Research Fund award, Asian Diseases in International Affairs, #9041938.

Abbreviations

AIDS	Acquired Immune Deficiency Syndrome
ANC	Antenatal Clinic
ANM	Auxiliary Nurse Midwife
ART	Antiretroviral therapy
ARV	Antiretroviral
AZT	Azidothymidine, Zidovudine, and Retrovir
BMGF	Bill and Melinda Gates Foundation
BSS	Behavioral Surveillance Survey
CBO	Community-Based Organization
CCM	Country Coordinating Mechanism
CDC	Centers for Disease Control and Prevention
CHC	Community health centers
CMP	Common Minimum Program
CMS	Cooperative Medical Scheme
COPRI	Copenhagen Peace Research Institute
CRF	circulating recombinant forms
CROI	Conference on Retrovirus and Opportunistic Infection
CSWs	commercial sex workers
DAPCU	District AIDS Prevention and Control Unit
DFID	Department for International Development
DNA	deoxyribonucleic acid
ERIDs	Emerging and Re-emerging Infectious Diseases
FPP	Family Planning Programs
FSWs	female sex workers
GDP	gross domestic product
GFATM	Global Fund to Fight AIDS, Tuberculosis, and Malaria
GIPA	greater involvement of people living with or affected by HIV/AIDS
GRID	Gay Related Immunodeficiency Disease
HAART	*highly active antiretroviral therapy*
HIV	Human Immunodeficiency Virus
HRG	high risk group

HTLV-I	Human T cell lymphotropic virus
IBBA	Integrated Biological Behavioral Assessments
ICMR	Indian Council for Medical Research
ICTC	Integrating Counselling and Testing Centre
IDA	International Development Association
IDUs	intravenous/injecting drug users
IEC	information, education, and communication
IMF	International Monetary Fund
IPC	Indian Penal Code
IR	International Relations
KS	Kaposi's sarcoma
LAV	lymph-associated virus
LFA	local fund agent
MDGs	Millennium Development Goals
MHLW	Ministry of Health, Labour and Welfare
MMT	Methadone Maintenance Treatment
MOCA	Ministry of Civil Affairs
MOIC	Ministry of Industry and Commerce
MRSA	methicillin-resistant Staphylococcus aureus
MSM	men having sex with men
MTCT	mother-to-child transmission
NACO	National AIDS Control Organization
NACP	National AIDS Control Program
NCAIDS	National Center for AIDS/STD Control and Prevention
NFHS	National Family Health Survey
NGOs	nongovernmental organizations
NIAID	National Institute of Allergy and Infectious Diseases
NIC	National Intelligence Council
NNRTIs	*non-nucleoside reverse transcriptase inhibitors*
NPC	National People's Congress
NRHM	National Rural Health Mission Program
NSP	Needle Syringe Program
OIs	Opportunistic Infections
PCP	*Pneumocystis carinii* pneumonia
PEPFAR	President Emergency Plan for AIDS Relief
PHC	primary health centers
PHFI	Public Health Foundation of India
PIs	protease inhibitors
PLHA/PLWHA	people living with HIV and AIDS
PR	Principal Recipient
PRC	People's Republic of China

RCH	Reproductive and Child Health
RNA	ribonucleic acid
RRE	Red Ribbon Express
SACS	State AIDS Control Society
SAPs	structural adjustment programs
SC	subcenter
SCAWC	State Council AIDS Working Committee
SIV	Simian Immunodeficiency Virus
STD	Sexually Transmitted Disease
STI	Sexually Transmitted Infection
TG	transgender
TI	Targeted Intervention
TRIPS	Trade-Related Aspects of Intellectual Property Rights Agreement
UNAIDS	Joint United Nations Program on HIV and AIDS
UNDP	United Nations Development Report
UNGASS	United Nations General Assembly Special Session
UNSC	United Nations Security Council
UPA	United Progressive Alliance
USAID	United States Agency for International Development
WHO	World Health Organization

Chapter 1

Introduction

On June 6, 1985, at the Peking Union College Hospital in Beijing, an Argentine tourist from the United States died of Human Immunodeficiency Virus/Acquired Immune Deficiency Syndrome (HIV/AIDS).[1] It was a death of a foreigner caused by the so-called Western disease. This was the first case of HIV/AIDS to be documented in China. In India, the first reported case of HIV/AIDS death was that of a businessman in Mumbai the following year.[2] Indian officials claimed the man was believed to have contracted the disease in Europe or the United States.[3] Before the end of the decade this misperception would be shattered as more and more indigenous cases emerged.

In China, the first indigenous HIV/AIDS infections were recorded among 146 injecting drug users (IDUs) in Dehong in Yunnan Province in late 1989,[4] while a group of Indian female sex workers (FSWs) was confirmed as HIV-positive in Chennai and Mumbai in late 1986.[5] Since the Chinese and Indian governments and societies hold a relatively hostile view on FSWs and IDUs and their associated behaviors, HIV/AIDS was conceived as "a disease of the poor, the illiterate, the prostitutes and the deviants."[6] Thus, FSWs and IDUs living with HIV/AIDS face double stigma in China and India. The disease had not been localized due to the misconception that as long as people were good and virtuous, they had nothing to worry about.

Misperceptions of HIV/AIDS in the early years were not confined to the Chinese and Indian communities. Prior to 1982, the disease was named Gay Related Immunodeficiency Disease (GRID) in the United States, since most HIV/AIDS cases were found among homosexual men in the country. So long as people abstained from a homosexual lifestyle, again, they had nothing to worry about. However, what started as GRID was soon identified among the population irrespective of social, economic, or sexual markers. The multiple syndromes appearing on the host were attributed to the collapse of the human immune system with a low number of white blood cells. Thus, the disease was renamed as AIDS.

In both China and India, such moves into the social mainstream take longer. Both are conservative societies with anticolonized legacies that continue to shape their worldviews. Nonetheless, by the end of the 1980s, China and India came to recognize that HIV/AIDS was not a Western or marginalized population disease. By 1995, an estimated 10,000[7] and 1.75 million[8] people were infected with HIV/AIDS in China and India, respectively.

Since the beginning of the HIV/AIDS epidemic, more than 60 million people have been infected with the disease globally. The top three largest populations with HIV/AIDS are in South Africa (6.1 million), Nigeria (3.4 million), and India (2.1 million).[9] The latest estimate of people living with HIV/AIDS in the world is 35.3 million.[10] Of the 35.3 million, 4.78 million people live in Asia.[11] Louise Garrett, senior fellow of global health in the Council on Foreign Relations, debated that "the scale and geographical scope of the HIV/AIDS pandemic has only two parallels in recorded history: the 1918 flu pandemic and the Black Death in the fourteenth century."[12] Why is HIV so destructive in the human body?

In the host body, HIV basically attacks and destroys the T cells (a kind of white blood cell) in the human immune system. The infected individual becomes extremely vulnerable to all kinds of bacterial and viral infections due to the depletion of the number of T cells. AIDS thus refers to the multiple syndromes appearing in the infected individual that result in a total collapse of the immune system in the later stages of infection. Apart from its destructive nature, HIV is deemed to be the smartest virus in human history. HIV knows its limits. It cannot reproduce on its own without the host. More importantly, the virus is neither infectious nor can it survive for more than a few hours outside the human body.[13] In order to survive and reproduce itself, the virus hides itself inside the host without the host's awareness and tactically conquers the host's immune system by integrating itself directly into the DNA of the T cell. Eliminating the virus thus results in the unavoidable destruction of the white blood cells. By replacing the DNA of T cells with the viral ones, HIV makes use of the infected T cells as its virus producing factory to reproduce as many of itself as possible—about 10 billion of its copies daily.[14]

After knowing all these facts about HIV/AIDS, the next question is how can we understand and deal with the problem? Medical practitioners argue that HIV/AIDS is purely a medical problem that requires medical solutions, for example, the development of antiretroviral (ARV) drugs and vaccines. Sadly, HIV/AIDS is still an incurable disease. There is only one documented case of someone being successfully cured of HIV/AIDS in the world. Timothy Brown, also known as the Berlin patient, was cured of HIV/AIDS after he had a bone marrow transplant that replaced his infected blood with healthy blood from a person who had a rare natural resistance to HIV/AIDS.[15] After the Berlin patient, the "Mississippi baby" was once counted as the second successful case.[16] However, the four-year-old child relapsed in 2014 despite being "functionally cured" of HIV/AIDS after the doctor gave her an aggressive cocktail therapy, consisting of AZT, Neviripine, and Lamivudine, when she was just 29 hours old.[17] It is predicted that the "California baby" could likely become the next successful case of being cured of HIV/AIDS.[18] However, these two cases are considered very rare and provide no treatment protocol for the millions of others infected by the disease.

Public health scholars and practitioners argue that HIV/AIDS is a public health problem that requires public health responses: surveillance, testing, condom distribution, methadone maintenance treatment, and needle exchange programs. Perceiving HIV/AIDS as a public health problem, some scholars recommend a further integration of HIV/AIDS-related interventions into the primary health care system. Interviews with respondents working in HIV/AIDS-related non-governmental organizations (NGOs) in Asia indicate a pessimism that HIV/AIDS could be fully resolved in public health systems where the disease is considered to be a stigma.[19]

Some lawyers and human rights advocates strongly argue that HIV/AIDS is a social and human rights issue. Stigmatization and discrimination of people living with HIV/AIDS are obvious in many Asian countries. The reason is that the general population and even the health workers have an inaccurate understanding of how HIV/AIDS is transmitted. They perceived that causal contacts such as shaking hands and sharing toilets with an infected individual will result in the transmission of the disease. Because of the positive status, infected individuals are barred from working as civil servants and teachers, fired by employers, or refused operations by doctors. In particular societies, the HIV/AIDS stigma is often layered on top of many other stigmas associated with commercial sex workers, homosexual men, IDUs, and their related behaviors such as sex outside marriage and illegal drug injection. Such stigma cannot be fully addressed if we consider HIV/AIDS only as a medical or public health problem. Linking HIV/AIDS and human rights is feasible; however, it may do more harm than good in authoritarian or totalitarian regimes in which human rights are notably sensitive issues.

A different perspective is held by some political leaders and security scholars who robustly debate that HIV/AIDS is a security issue. In the

UN Security Council meeting in January 2000, then US vice president Al Gore claimed that HIV/AIDS is a security issue as "it threatens not just individual citizens, but the very institutions that define and defend the character of a society. The disease weakens workforces and saps economic strength. HIV/AIDS strikes at teachers, and denies education to their students. It strikes at the military, and subverts the forces of order and peacekeeping."[20] In July 2000, the UN Security Council passed Resolution 1308 acknowledging the urgent need to address HIV/AIDS, which threatens the stability and security of the nation if left unchecked.[21] These events are significant as it was the first time the UN Security Council devoted an entire session to a disease. It was also the first time that the international political authorities framed HIV/AIDS as a global health threat to national and international security rather than solely as a developmental or public health problem. In this sense, HIV/AIDS has been prioritized by the international community. Using the terminology of securitization theory, we can say HIV/AIDS has been "securitized" since 2000.

What is securitization? Securitization here does not refer to the practice in the financial sector. Securitization in International Relations (IR) is a concept that describes the process by which an issue becomes a security issue. Framing HIV/AIDS as a security issue, HIV/AIDS is securitized (prioritized). Emergency measures (redirection of existing resources, new policies or practices) are implemented to address the issue following the security-threat claim.

The Concept of Securitization Theory

> Speech has power. Words do not fade. What starts out as a sound, ends in a deed.[22]

What constitutes a theory? A theory is based on hypotheses and assumptions and is backed by evidence. A theory possesses the predictive power (testability) to explain a phenomenon or a set of phenomena in real-world situations. For example, Darwin's theory of evolution is a theory because it helps us understand the evolution of animals and plants with the idea of natural selection. Securitization theory is similar. It attempts to explain how an issue becomes a security issue.

Securitization theory is a constructivist theory that originated from the Copenhagen School of security studies in 1998, led by the theorists Barry Buzan, Ole Wæver, and Jaap de Wilde.[23] Grounded in constructivist perspectives, the theory outlines the process of defining or framing an issue as a security threat and as a reaction to policy, to block the adverse development of the perceived threat.

How are threats framed in a securitization process? A securitizing actor initiates the process by declaring a particular referent object as an existential threat to security. This threat identification is declaratory in nature (speech acts), and is followed by acceptance of the issue by a target audience convinced of its potential to be an existential threat (audience acceptance). A discourse that presents "X" as an existential threat to a referent object does not itself create securitization—this is merely a *securitizing move*; the issue is securitized only when it is accepted by the target audience as such, based on their knowledge of the issue.[24] Gaining such acceptance leads to a shift in political measures from normal to emergency mode; extraordinary measures (emergency measures) are adopted in the latter mode, thereby breaking the normal democratic rules and regulations of policy making in handling the threat.[25]

The concept of security in securitization theory is illustrated here as "a self-referential practice, because it is through this practice that an issue becomes a security issue—not necessarily because a real existential threat exists but because the issue is presented as such a threat."[26] From the constructivist perspective, the concept of security does not bear any fixed, rigid, or closed definition. Instead, the concept is subject to be framed and reframed in accordance with the actor's contextual understanding or historical experience of "security."[27] In short, instead of discovering the "real" threat, securitization theory focuses on addressing the "truth" effect of the power of language in transforming an issue into a security threat via speech acts uttered by the securitizing actors.[28]

Despite its self-referential characteristic, the success of securitization is not determined by the securitizing agents but by the audience (the citizens).[29] Without audience acceptance, the issue is not securitized, and is only considered a securitizing move,[30] which connotes an incomplete securitization. A theoretical assumption such as this corresponds to the idea of intersubjectivity embedded in the constructivist paradigm, in which the meaning of security is constructed through interactions and sharing with other actors.[31] In short, intersubjectivity is another characteristic of securitization theory.

Given the self-referential definition of security, its scope can be expanded to issues other than traditional military problems, whereas the referents of security can be deepened from the state to the more specific individual levels. More importantly, the theory addresses concerns of security scholars that the concept of security is not widened or deepened to an extent that it loses its analytical value and power; security is deemed successfully constructed only when the audience regards the existential threat, that is, intersubjectivity, with the same value ascribed by the securitizer.

These theoretical strengths have caused securitization theory to become one of the most flourishing and influential theories developed within security studies in the last two decades.[32] The theory has provided a security perspective in investigating a broad range of issues, such as transnational crime[33] and human and drug trafficking,[34] religion,[35] migration,[36] environmental deterioration,[37] and infectious diseases[38] such as HIV/AIDS[39] and H5N1.[40]

Despite being a key approach to security studies, securitization theory is not without conceptual and methodological weaknesses. Having examined the various debates on securitization theory, its major weaknesses are underscored in this book. Shortcomings raised by security scholars are primarily: lack of operationalization and differentiation, together with the presence of Eurocentrism of securitization theory in general, and the three core elements, namely "speech acts," "emergency measures," and "audience acceptance" in particular.[41] In addressing the weaknesses of the securitization framework, this book proposes a revised securitization model that offers an alternative framework for studying the HIV/AIDS securitization process in China and India.

HIV/AIDS: China and India

Historically, the 1918 Spanish flu and the Black Death were two of the worst global pandemics that threatened the survival of mankind. The Spanish flu claimed between 20 and 40 million lives between 1918 and 1919,[42] whereas the Black Death (1348–1351) killed 40 million people,[43] eliminating more than one third of the population in Europe in a mere 18 months.[44]

Among the infectious diseases that prevailed in the contemporary era, none dramatically affected human population in world history until the emergence of HIV/AIDS.[45] Peter Lamptey, president of the Family Health International AIDS Institute in the United States, declared that 40 million people would die due to HIV/AIDS-related diseases without access to ARV drugs; thus, "HIV/AIDS is likely to surpass the Black Death as the worst pandemic ever."[46] Given that many of the most severely affected sites for the disease are in the Third World, access to ARV drugs is limited—making this a conservative estimate.

Considering its devastating impact on the survival of mankind, HIV/AIDS is the first infectious disease to be framed as a security threat by international organizations and national governments.[47] The pandemic was declared as a security issue in the 2000 UN Security Council Resolution

1308, citing that HIV/AIDS may pose a risk to international stability and security if left unchecked.[48] McInnes and Rushton argued that the HIV/AIDS securitization in 2000 was merely a securitizing move instead of a successful (full) securitization.[49] However, other scholars contended that HIV/AIDS has been successfully securitized at the international level since 2000, because the Resolution was unanimously adopted by 15 member-states of the Security Council.[50]

This book is not intended to discover whether the international HIV/AIDS securitizing move has been fully accepted by the target audience. It is intended to explore how the two largest countries in the world (by population) have responded to HIV/AIDS to date, and what this might mean for the future. However, at least one point can be ascertained: The move to securitize HIV/AIDS has been generated at the international level since 2000. Indeed, despite these momentous moves by the UN at the state level, HIV/AIDS is not a problem that can be easily securitized. Gauri and Lieberman have suggested that some issues, such as HIV/AIDS, which traditionally are not highly prioritized, tend to be neglected by national authorities.[51] Although HIV/AIDS is a long-wave event,[52] the epidemic is commonly perceived as "a silent and largely invisible problem,"[53] or an indirect or "soft" security threat;[54] thus, it is frequently ignored, especially when the government agenda is laden with "a multitude of more visible priorities."[55]

Societal structures and accompanying cultures and norms likewise play vital roles in the conceptualization of threats. Gauri and Lieberman asserted that political leaders and the general public are less likely to view HIV/AIDS as a universal threat in ethnically divergent and polarized communities.[56] Given its association with behaviors considered socially and culturally unacceptable in some countries, HIV/AIDS is widely downplayed in a society's culture and norm. Ignorance of the HIV/AIDS problem has thwarted the implementation of even the most effective prevention methods. State leaders are thus discouraged from acknowledging or taking timely reactions against the threat posed by HIV/AIDS.[57]

The full securitization of HIV/AIDS has become more difficult to achieve in developing countries. Generally, public health expenditures of developing countries are comparatively lower than that in developed countries. For example, Norway, Canada, and Japan allocated over 9 percent of GDP to health, whereas the health expenditures in Bangladesh, Azerbaijan, and Pakistan were below 1.5 percent.[58] The two largest developing countries, China and India, spent 2.7 percent and 1.2 percent of their GDPs, respectively, on public health.[59] Kapila argued that health care provision is one of the most neglected concerns in India.[60] Additionally, the issue has rarely been an important topic in election campaigns except in 2004 when the United Progressive Alliance (UPA) government promised to raise health care expenditures to 3 percent of its GDP.[61]

In addition to the lower priority placed on health, national governments may inevitably forego long-term disease prevention and instead pursue short-term economic development.[62] As an authoritarian regime, the Chinese government needs to pursue economic growth to maintain its legitimacy as a one-party dominant regime. India, as a democratic regime, suffers from a similar problem: namely that the short-term nature of the electoral cycle restricts the ability of governments to reallocate resources to a potential threat and away from economic and development priorities. In other words, to secure a post in the next elections, legislators may choose to enact policies that yield short-term rather than long-term outcomes.

China and India were selected as test sites in this book to investigate the HIV/AIDS securitization process. The rationale for choosing China and India is threefold. As emphasized by Curley and Herington, one criticism of the Eurocentric securitization framework is that few empirical studies have been conducted in a non-Western, nondemocratic, or even Asian context.[63] In contrast, one can examine any country in Europe and apply the results to other European countries. In studying the applicability of the theory among Asian countries, one should carefully consider the sociopolitical variation across different Asian states. A comprehensive study of socialist China and democratic India sheds light on the application of securitization theory in the Asian context.

China and India have much in common. Both countries rank among the world's largest developing nations, the most populous states, the fastest growing economies, and the greatest ancient civilizations, together they form the foremost rising powers in Asia.[64] In the past quarter of the century, the productive forces and overall national strengths of both countries have been constantly enhanced, leading to images of "the rise of China" and "emerging India."[65] Most notably, the US government has acknowledged China and India as new major global players in its 2005 report entitled *Mapping the Global Future: Report of the National Intelligence Council's 2020 Project*; the report proposes that "in the same way that commentators refer to the 1900s as the 'American Century,' the 21st century may be seen as a time when Asia, led by China and India, comes into its own."[66]

Taking their economic development into consideration, these two Asian countries have experienced unprecedented economic growth in the last decade as they have integrated more with the market economy since the 1980s. Their growth is more than 200 times greater than that experienced thus far by the United Kingdom and the United States, and is unprecedented in world history.[67] The World Bank has predicted that both countries will almost triple their economic strength in the next ten years.[68]

Despite their remarkable economic development, China and India possess the largest populations infected with HIV/AIDS in Asia: 780,000 in China, and 2.1 million in India, in 2012.[69] The HIV/AIDS problem could seriously affect economic prospects if left unchecked,[70] because financial resources would have to be diverted from economic and infrastructure development to programs related to the control and prevention of HIV/AIDS.[71]

Both Chinese and Indian governments have started addressing the HIV/AIDS problem after years of denial. The central governments of both countries now have full-fledged national plans or programs on HIV/AIDS interventions.[72] Using the revised framework of the current study, the change in the political stance of these countries' national governments toward HIV/AIDS is depicted chronologically. In addition, the perception of the audience (individuals working in HIV/AIDS-related NGOs) with regard to framing HIV/AIDS as a threat, and the engagement of related programs in their countries will be illustrated at length.

The comparative study of HIV/AIDS securitization in China and India is a novel research area that remains unexplored, at least in the social sciences. According to Walt, the basic objective of social sciences is to offer valuable knowledge, which provides an accurate and relevant accounting of past human behavior, or a description of certain groups or incidents in society.[73] In that sense, this book attempts to investigate HIV/AIDS in China and India through a social science perspective, as opposed to a primarily medical perspective.

Research Program

Given the enormous size of China and India and the diverse societal situations in different parts of these countries, the book adopts the core–periphery differential in case studies. For both China and India, the division is based on the geographical location of a province or state within the country. In this sense, provinces in the eastern/coastal region in China[74] and the states located in mainland India[75] fall into the core category. To fully represent the situations in the core part, a two-tiered structure—political and economic capital—is established within the core category. Political capital is characterized by the authority of the central government, whereas economic capital represents the trade and international/globalized node of the country. With regard to the peripheral category, provinces in the central and western regions of China[76] and states in the northeastern region of India[77] belong to the peripheral areas of the country. Following this strategy, six cities were selected to represent the level of audience acceptance in different areas of these countries: Beijing, Shanghai, and Kunming in China; and New Delhi, Mumbai, and Imphal in India.

With respect to the human behaviors leading to HIV/AIDS infections in core and peripheral cities, sexual contact (either FSWs or MSMs—men having sex with men) and IDUs constitute two of the most common transmission modes in both the core and peripheral areas of China and India.[78] However, there is a trend that the principal transmission route in the core part of the countries is sexual contact, whereas it is the IDUs in the outlying areas.[79] These generalized patterns can be attributed to the rapid economic development and migration in the core areas, and weak economic development and political control, coupled with geographical proximity to the Golden Triangle—one of Asia's two main illicit opium-trading areas—in the outer areas.

Modernization is one of the hallmarks of the core part of the two countries. In the urbanized areas, sophisticated development plans and adequate infrastructures and resources result in faster and higher economic growth, coupled with a large floating population. People originating from the rural areas migrate to the urban areas because of better employment opportunities.[80] Given the high standard of living in the cities, migrant workers usually leave their parents, partners, and children behind and stay in the cities for a long time without returning home. In this sense, migrants leave their social environment and the usual normative constraints. When they do, they are more likely to engage in some nontraditional activities[81] such as engaging in unsafe sex with one or multipartners, becoming FSWs, or MSMs.

In comparison, peripheral areas (provinces in the western part of China and states in the northeastern part of India) are relatively impoverished and less developed. Developing countries usually have inadequate resources for distribution, or tend to concentrate their efforts on developing the core part by extracting the resources from the peripheral region. Hence, core–peripheral disparity can be observed within the countries.

Aside from the economic backwardness in the rural areas, these regions in China and India are usually located at the periphery of the country that is geographically far from the economically well-developed and politically stable areas. This circumstance can be precisely captured by a conventional Chinese proverb: "The mountain is high and the emperor is far away." In other words, the political influence and control of the ruling government in the peripheral areas is debilitated. Together with the destitute economic conditions plus weakened political control of the central government, geographical proximity to the infamous Golden Triangle is a striking contributor to the entry and spread of drugs in the outlying districts of China and India.

Individuals working in HIV/AIDS-related NGOs and officials working in government agencies in these cities and other relevant places are the target interviewees. At the end of the data collection process, a total of 58 NGOs respondents (30 in China and 28 in India) had been successfully interviewed. Apart from the NGOs respondents in the selected cities, the research interviewed NGOs in Hong Kong and government officials in both countries, since they "are 'richer' than others and that these people are more likely to provide insight and understanding for the researcher."[82] Thus, ten government officials working on HIV/AIDS interventions in China and India, plus four respondents from Hong Kong, were interviewed. Primary data from fieldwork helped supplement and verify the existing secondary data, and determined the level of audience acceptance toward the current securitizing move of HIV/AIDS in the respective countries.

In terms of securitization analysis, Buzan et al. found that "the obvious method is discourse analysis, since we are interested in when and how something is established by whom as a security threat."[83] The authors also cited the use of discourse analysis in securitization as one that involves "read [ing], looking for arguments that take the rhetorical and logical form defined here as security."[84] In addition to comments made in interview sessions, an array of sources was collected to identify and analyze security acts on HIV/AIDS expressed by top-level political leaders in Chinese or English print media, including newspapers, press, official documents, and archival materials.

Organization of the Book

The remainder of this book is divided into eight chapters. Chapter 2 describes securitization theory in detail. An enhanced theoretical framework, which is a typology with eight branches of securitization, is proposed based on the theory's shortcomings as discussed in the chapter. The types of securitization are illustrated using real-world examples of HIV/AIDS securitization in different countries.

Chapter 3 addresses the securitization of HIV/AIDS in the Asian context. A succinct discussion on HIV/AIDS—in terms of historical, virological, and social perspectives—is offered prior to describing HIV/AIDS securitization. Despite possible negative outcomes, securitizing HIV/AIDS is still a worthy pursuit because its benefits far outweigh its costs, especially in developing countries. These benefits include (1) reducing the HIV/AIDS stigma and discrimination and (2) maintaining a sustainable budget in relation to the HIV/AIDS epidemic. As noted earlier, the low priority traditionally placed on health and the scarcity of resources hinders political leaders' commitment to HIV/AIDS securitization, despite recognizing its possible benefits to developing countries. Thus, the chapter identifies the international institutions and funding agencies, particularly the United Nations and the Global Fund to Fight AIDS, Tuberculosis, and Malaria (GFATM), which provide normative and technical support to this endeavor.

After exploring the theory and its main points, chapter 4 offers a backdrop of health governance in China and India, with a particular focus on the evolution of the public health care system in the countries and the implications of the changes toward the emergence and spread of HIV/AIDS problems in both countries. Illustrating the changes of public health care systems in China and India during the economic reforms, it is argued that the urban–rural disparity and ineffective public health care system, to a certain extent, results in the widespread of HIV/AIDS in both countries.

The HIV/AIDS-related policy-making process (in terms of securitization) in China and India is discussed in chapters 5 and 7, respectively. An overview of the historical and current HIV/AIDS situation in these countries is provided at the beginning of each chapter. National policies related to HIV/AIDS that have been generated throughout the years are analyzed chronologically. In explaining the chronological path, the shift from a failed to a full HIV/AIDS securitizing move by the Chinese and Indian governments can be clearly demonstrated.

Specifically, chapter 5 is on China and reveals that a full HIV/AIDS securitizing move has been achieved by the Chinese government since 2004, and continues to prevail over the country. This chapter highlights the local bureaucratic resistance that exists alongside positive, proactive political measures on HIV/AIDS, which may impede the constructive influence of full securitizing moves in China.

Chapter 7 shows that a full HIV/AIDS securitizing move has been likewise attained in India since 2004. However, unlike China, India's full HIV/AIDS securitizing move has sapped since 2010. The forthcoming HIV/AIDS program (NACP-IV) in India is predicted to exist as a standalone program, yet is better integrated with the country's primary health care program, the National Rural Health Mission (NRHM). However, future HIV/AIDS programs will be largely formulated as infectious disease programs under the NRHM umbrella. The chapter offers an explanation for such change in priority assigned to HIV/AIDS; namely a massive reliance on foreign funds that has prompted the Indian government to alter its securitization and strategies to match those of dominant international funding agencies on primary health care, thereby assuring continued support for its programs on HIV/AIDS.

Identifying the type of securitizing move generated by the national government only comprises the first half of the study of securitization. As securitization theory suggests, whether the securitizing move initiated by policy makers turns to securitization is decided by the acceptance of the target audience. Chapters 6 and 8 of this book examine the acceptance, in terms of moral and technical support toward particular HIV/AIDS securitizing moves, of individuals in Chinese and Indian NGOs involved in HIV/AIDS policy evaluation.

A comparison among the selected cities in China and India, in terms of the level of audience acceptance of the HIV/AIDS securitizing move, is also presented in chapters 6 and 8, respectively. Each case study first provides an overview of the HIV/AIDS situation in the city. A section concerning local understanding of the HIV/AIDS securitizing moves follows. This section aims to discover the audience's actual understanding of the political stance on HIV/AIDS, to ascertain whether the respondents accept or reject what they know about the issue. The level of audience acceptance is then analyzed through interview materials obtained from fieldwork. In determining the overall level of audience acceptance, the type of HIV/AIDS securitization in each country is thus identified.

The concluding chapter summarizes the major findings included in this book. In response to the inadequacies of the original framework as raised by security scholars, this book develops a revised securitization model for security studies in public policy. To demonstrate the analytical ability of this new model in the public policy, this book investigates the process of HIV/AIDS securitization in China and India. The book contributes to existing knowledge on general security studies and public policy theory, particularly to security and policy issues on HIV/AIDS. The finding from this final chapter also identifies further areas for research in health security in Asia and beyond.

Chapter 2

Security: A Revised Framework for Analysis

Introduction

What is security? The *Oxford English Dictionary* defines it as "the condition of being secure"; "freedom from doubt; confidence, assurance"; "freedom from care, anxiety or apprehension; [and] a feeling of safety or freedom from, or absence of, danger."[1] Simply put, security involves (1) describing the physical condition of being protected from, or not exposed to danger, and (2) delineating the psychological condition of feeling secure. These definitions relate to the general meaning of security, but are different from the concept used by IR theorists and experts when referring to national security or security policies.[2]

In the IR field, the notion of security is based on the realist precept: states threaten each other to defend their sovereignty as an independent entity. Modification of this concept was suggested by constructivists in the 1990s so as not to refer simply to objective military and power competition, but to focus on the subjective meaning of security as constructed by states, societies, or individuals, based on their historical, cultural, or psychological experiences of threat and security.

Despite the popular usage of this concept in IR debates, scholars readily admit that the term "security" is "an underdeveloped concept,"[3] with comparatively few conceptual reflections on the subject prior to the 1980s.[4] This gap gave rise to the security debate between "wideners" and "traditionalists" on the reconceptualization and broadening of security. Wideners suggested that the inclusion of issues other than the traditional military issue could enhance the analytical value of the concept. In contrast, traditionalists argued that the value could be preserved by narrowly confining security to military problems. Nevertheless, neither view caters well to the contemporary security agenda. Wideners treat security as a catch-all concept, causing it to lose its analytical value in security studies; meanwhile, the attempt by traditionalists to restrict the idea to military aspects misrepresents reality, and thus distorts government decision. This gap was first addressed by securitization theory in 1998.

Before continuing deliberations on securitization theory, the debate on the reconceptualization and broadening of security should be considered. As part of the review, this chapter examines two possible outcomes of this debate: human security and securitization. Human security is viewed as one solution to the debate, but has been criticized as "the dog that didn't bark,"[5] with regard to its usefulness despite its contribution to the security discourse. Securitization theory represents another answer to the debate, but is not without conceptual and methodological shortcomings. By offering an outline of the theory and the different weaknesses identified by security scholars, this chapter highlights the value of the theory although it requires further refinement. In conclusion, a possible evolution of the securitization framework is suggested.

Rethinking Security

Since the 1980s there has been an ongoing debate among the security scholars on whether to limit or expand the meaning of security. Although those in favor of expanding the meaning of security justified their position by presenting the shortcomings of the narrow definition proposed by traditionalists, the latter argued that the idea of "everything is security" poses the risk of voiding the usefulness of the security concept as an intellectual tool,[6] thus "becoming a loose synonym for 'bad.'"[7] Huysmans likewise expressed concern that security becomes a "trivial concept" when the difference between security and nonsecurity problems cannot be deliberately established.[8] Walt, for example, opposed the inclusion of nonmilitary issues such as "pollution, disease, child abuse, or economic recession" under the security umbrella,[9] because these would bring problems of intellectual incoherence[10] and political cheating.[11] Walt also asserted that although "other hazards exist, [this] does not mean that the danger of war has been eliminated,"[12] and any attempt to ignore or eliminate the role of military forces in security studies is deemed irresponsible.[13]

Walt's concern was validated by highlighting the importance of both the past and the present roles of the military. Military threat is considered as significantly less controversial than nonmilitary threat. Given that the consequences of military threat seem more apparent, opponents can simply ignore or reject the threats posed by the nonmilitary issues.[14] Nevertheless, the ambiguous nature of nonmilitary threats does not mean that these are nonexistent, or have no serious impact on the community. Indeed, Walt failed to capture the phenomenon of the contemporary world, in which disputes have shifted from military to nonmilitary forms, such as territory conflict,[15] resource scarcity,[16] and environmental degradation.[17] In this sense, the traditional framework has failed to convey the real image of reality,[18] distorting political decisions and posing a threat to the overall security of a state and the international community.[19]

Hence, current security studies require new conceptual tools and methodologies. However, the concerns of the traditionalists remain; turning the security concept into a catch-all idea is theoretically undesirable. In this catch-22 situation, the question focuses on how to broaden the scope of security to encompass nonmilitary issues, while avoiding a loss of its analytical value. One way to settle the debate is through the notion of human security.[20]

Human Security

Human security is based on the intertwined concepts of "freedom from want" and "freedom from fear." The concept of human security first appeared in the 1994 United Nations Development Program (UNDP) report titled *New Dimensions of Human Security*. In this landmark document, the idea of traditional security being synonymous with state security was applied to the individual level, or to human security. Seven components of human security were synthesized in this report: economic, food, health, environmental, personal, community, and political security.[21]

The idea of human security is plausible as humans have become the natural starting point for security discussions.[22] Yet it is subject to criticisms by various scholars, mostly on the framework's conceptual and analytical weakness in addressing the contemporary security agenda.[23] In short, developing human security into a sophisticated conceptual and analytical framework in the security discourse is still a long way off.

The Copenhagen School of Securitization Theory

The Copenhagen School offered an alternative answer to the earlier question that addresses the myriad concerns of realist, constructivist, and human security scholars. Securitization theory emanated from the Copenhagen School of security studies that is led by Barry Buzan, Ole Wæver, and Jaap de Wilde.[24] As mentioned previously, the theory stemmed from the debate on "wide" versus "narrow" concepts of security through a European Security project in the 1980s.[25] Security in the theory was regarded as an in-between concept[26] that embraces both the narrow and wide definitions of security. The Copenhagen School did not propose a universal list of definitions or delimitation of security. Instead, the school purported a meaning of security that is neither universal, nor one that is socially and intersubjectively constructed.[27] Hence, there is absolutely no "correct" or most "logical" method of defining security.[28] Regardless of history, culture, or political system, different individuals can present varied ideas on whether an issue should be cast in security terms.[29]

Security as a Speech Act

The idea of speech acts in securitization theory originated from the famous three types of acts in sentence by John Langshaw Austin. Austin refers to these as locutionary, illocutionary, and perlocutionary acts. Buzan et al. indicated the speech acts in the theory to be *illocutionary* in nature. Illocutionary denotes that the act is performed as soon as the sentence is uttered.[30] In other words, labeling something as a security issue turns it into such, although this does not necessarily mean that a real threat is present.

The meaning of security is constructed when the securitizing actor frames an issue as an existential threat to the referent object,[31] claiming the issue as having an absolute priority on the government agenda.[32] Thus, the actors invoke a right to handle such an issue with extraordinary/emergency measures to ensure the survival of the referent object.[33] In other words, if someone (the securitizer) utters that "X" is a threat, then it becomes securitized; "X" automatically becomes a high priority issue in the government agenda; thus, resources are reallocated to address "X." Based on the original securitization theory, everyone can become a securitizing actor,[34] because the success of securitization does not rely upon the political and social power or capability possessed by the securitizing actor. These conditions or authorities only influence a political interaction.[35]

Critical Condition for a Successful Securitization: Audience Acceptance

Buzan et al. justified that a complete securitization is not decided by the securitizer, but by the target audience.[36] Therefore, a speech act that presents something as an existential threat does not create securitization per se. The issue is securitized only when the audience accepts it as such.[37] When the securitizing actors fail to convince the audience via speech acts, the act is merely a *securitizing move*, or one in which the audience does not accept the discourse presented.[38] Gaining audience acceptance is a significant step toward securitization.

Based on the earlier argument that presents security as a concept framed by the securitizing actor and the audience, both traditional and nontraditional security issues can be incorporated in securitization theory. The idea likewise discourages securitizing actors from abusing the power of securitizing one issue to pursue self-interests, because the securitization success is ultimately determined by audience acceptance.[39] In addition, securitization theory delimits the definition of security by distinguishing issues in the securitization process.

Contributions of Securitization

Securitization theory has two main contributions. First it highlights a political sense of responsibility in securitizing actors;[40] second, it serves as an early warning to the referent object. Based on Wæver's argument, the securitization approach supports the explicitness behind the logic of the securitizing move.[41] Securitizing actors should clarify their reasons for securitizing one issue and not the others. Securitization does not require them to determine whether their decisions are correct or not, but simply, to be aware of the consequences of these decisions.[42] Hence, practitioners should think twice prior to deciding.

Although the threats perceived in the theory could only be existential versus real threats, securitization acts as an early warning to the referent object;[43] an issue is considered likely to yield a real threat in the foreseeable future. In the case of diseases and other threats, "prevention is always better than cure"; the most effective way to mitigate their impact is through prevention. Prevention is also vital as "it is less costly and more humane to meet these threats upstream rather than downstream, early rather than late."[44] In the notion of securitization, an existential threat usually refers to a future threat.[45] Accordingly, the state can act in advance before an existential threat evolves into a real threat.

Internal Problems of the Securitization Framework

The previous discussion has covered the core ideas embedded in securitization theory. Despite deserving much praise,[46] the theory is not without conceptual and methodological shortcomings. The major inadequacies summarized in this chapter include the lack of operationalization and differentiation, together with the presence of Eurocentrism of securitization theory in general, and the three core elements, namely "speech acts," "emergency measures," and "audience acceptance," in particular.[47] This chapter proposes an alternative framework of securitization theory that addresses the earlier concerns. Such a framework attempts to improve the theoretical restructuring and empirical usage that could "even produce anomalies for the theory in [an] interesting way."[48]

Speech Acts

Several scholars claimed that the verbal form of speech acts should include other forms of expression.[49] Other than the language form of speech acts, Hansen argued that two types of nonverbal communications are central to the context of security politics: visual and bodily communication.[50] Concerning the visual form of security, Williams, Möller, and Hansen demonstrated that security can no longer be fully assessed by focusing on the speech act alone, because contemporary political communication is increasingly embedded within televisual images,[51] photographic exhibitions,[52] and cartoons.[53]

However, in several nondemocratic countries, media is highly restricted and controlled by the government. For instance, foreign reports or websites that are suspected to have negatively represented the reputation and sovereignty of China are frequently blocked by the government. For example, despite the temporary regulations related to the Olympics that were in effect from January 1, 2007 to October 17, 2008, which granted certain freedom to foreign media, the Chinese government still prevented foreign journalists from reporting issues concerning corruption, civil unrest, and detention facilities.[54] Websites regarding pro-Tibetan independence groups and the Falun Gong were also continually blocked throughout the duration of the games.[55] Hence, the language form of speech acts remains as the significant form of expression in nondemocratic countries, such as China, whereas the media possesses a comparatively minor role in the securitization process.

In terms of the bodily aspect of speech acts, Wilkinson suggested that the centrality of speech acts in the theory excludes physical expressions of security, such as physical migration or protest actions.[56] McDonald likewise argued that an exclusive focus on speech acts excludes bureaucratic practices or physical actions of security.[57] As mentioned previously, speech acts in securitization theory are *illocutionary* in nature, which means that the utterance of words is the incident that leads to the performance of an act. Austin's explanation of this illocutionary nature of speech acts is as follows:

> It is very commonly necessary that either the speaker himself or other persons should also perform certain other actions, whether "physical" or "mental" actions or even acts of uttering further words. Thus... it is hardly a gift if I say "I give it to you" but never hand it over.[58]

Adopting Austin's idea, the utterance of the language form of speech acts should result in "physical" or "mental" actions. However, Hansen stressed that "deeds and words do not necessarily communicate the same message."[59] In other words, problems arise when securitizing actors explicitly utter a speech act, but their reactions contradict what they uttered. Ciută expounded on this phenomenon by attributing this to the securitizer's error or habit, thus reducing security utterances into mere "empty signifiers."[60] The opposite scenario is equally problematic, both theoretically and analytically: What happens when securitizing actors react to the problem to indicate emergency measures, but do not employ speech acts?

To cater for the earlier scenarios, the inclusion of "physical" reactions, that is, the emergency measures enacted by the securitizers, is thus necessary, as opposed to focusing entirely on the language or verbal form of speech acts. This suggestion resembles that of Sjöstedt, who argued that "only speaking of an issue in terms of a threat does not meet the criteria of a securitizing move, instead policy action is also required."[61] Among the ideas presented by scholars, Hansen's suggestion to consider both language and bodily practices in forming security is deemed to provide the most contribution to the advancement of speech acts, and consequently, empirical studies of securitization theory.

Emergency Mode and Measures

The conceptualization and operationalization of "emergency measures" in the securitization process remains insufficiently discussed.[62] How does the theory differentiate between "emergency" and "ordinary" politics? What measures are required in "irregular" politics? How can one determine whether to consider a certain measure an emergency or not?

Insufficient deliberation of the idea, as argued in the present study, is due to the uncertainty regarding the role of emergency measures in the securitization process. On the one hand, Buzan et al. presented emergency measures as the end product of a successful securitization: "When the speech act is supported by the relevant audience...the issue then moves out of the normal politics into the realm of emergency mode, where the issue can be dealt with through extraordinary measures."[63] On the other hand, the same authors asserted that a successful securitization can be generated without adopting emergency measures:

> We do not push the demand so high as to say that an emergency measure has to be adopted, only that the existential threat has to be argued and gain enough **resonance** for a platform to be made from which it is possible to legitimize emergency measures. [emphasis added][64]

Nonetheless, as Salter pointed out, it is hard to evaluate "resonance" in empirical studies of the securitization process.[65] Thus, he suggested that there must be policy solutions (new or emergency), whether in discourse, budget, or actual policy measures on the existential threat, and such policy solutions should be accepted by the audience.[66] In this regard, the present study suggests the inclusion of the concept of emergency modes/measures in investigating the securitization process.

Audience Acceptance

Buzan et al. justified that a complete securitization is not decided by the securitizer but by the target audience.[67] However, Wæver admitted that the idea of "audience" and "audience acceptance" remains unclear.[68] In reality, several groups comprise the audience in one operation, as opposed to a single or homogeneous group.[69] An identity securitization case involving organizations on humanitarian aid illustrates this point:[70] Vaughn identified multiple groups in the audience (e.g., the staff member of the organization that called for securitization, staff from other similar organizations, donors, and states) that the securitizer needed to convince.[71]

In terms of the relationship between the speaker and the audience, Balzacq believed that securitization should be "audience-centered."[72] He concluded that the role of the audience is significant because the "moral" and "formal" support that they provide to securitizing actors increases the probability of successful securitization.[73] This argument by Balzacq is plausible, but becomes invalid when the securitizer is a dictator, and the speaker–audience model is applied in nondemocratic settings.[74] In such an environment, the role of the audience is not necessarily as peculiar as Balzacq cited. The securitizer (usually the top-level political leader or high-ranking government officer) is not publicly elected; therefore, he has less reason to seek moral or legal support to yield audience consent and consequently, successful securitization.

Given the complex conceptualization and operationalization of audience acceptance, some scholars may evade the problems by neglecting the concepts in empirical studies of securitization. Floyd argued that the audience can be omitted in the securitization process due to an internal contradiction in the theory.[75] Furthermore, Floyd provided a rationale for removing the audience in empirical studies: "The audience is not an analytical concept, but rather a normative concept in analytical disguise, which is to say that it does not stem from actual empirical observation of how politics operates but rather from Ole Wæver's view of how politics, including security policy, should be done."[76] Floyd's formulation of securitization is given by, "securitization = securitizing move (speech acts) + security practice (emergency measures)."[77]

However, Floyd's suggestion contradicts the important notion of "intersubjectivity" embedded in securitization theory. Additionally, in the absence of audience acceptance, securitizing agents can easily manipulate or monopolize the securitization process. In Floyd's article, the intention to establish a "moral rightness of securitization"[78] turns into "immoral rightness" when the concept of "audience" is removed from the process. Rather than ignoring the role of audience acceptance, proper definition and incorporation of the concept is considered more morally, theoretically, and empirically "right." The inclusion of audience is also desirable that it benefits the democratization of the securitization process, considering that security scholars have been working on the theory.[79]

Shortcomings Regarding the Applicability of the Theory in Non-Western Contexts

One main problem of securitization theory that is addressed by various scholars is its Eurocentric nature and "democratically biased" framework.[80] Curley and Herington emphasized a criticism related to the Eurocentric securitization framework, that is, few empirical studies have been conducted on the securitization processes in non-Western, nondemocratic, or even Asian contexts.[81] Emmers et al. claimed that a problem arises when the liberal Eurocentric nature of securitization theory is grafted onto political systems in Asia, as a significant number of countries in this region are nonliberal (communist systems, monarchies, authoritarian regimes, or failed states).[82]

The present study concurs with the earlier mentioned recommendation that the framework for securitization theory requires further refinement to conduct empirical studies in the non-Western and nondemocratic contexts. The "Westphalian straitjacket" phenomenon is believed to exist in the theory,[83] with the concepts of "speech act" and "audience acceptance" assuming a Western liberal–democratic context in understanding security. The securitization process is particularly complicated in Asian countries, because the theory assumes that anyone, especially the non-state actors, can resort to "speech acts."[84] However, in authoritarian or totalitarian states, non-state actors are rather powerless as they do not possess the political resources or communication channels to utilize speech acts in prompting the government to prioritize their issues.

Another democratic assumption embedded in the theory is that the audience refers to the general population, which is similar to a democratic system in which the audience largely refers to the citizens of a nation-state.[85] Wæver acknowledged the presence of the "Westphalian straitjacket" within the theory that resulted in the problematic definition of "audience": "The present version risks being too tied to a Western democratic form of politics."[86] Wæver also suggested that the audience is not necessarily composed of the entire population.[87] Rather, the audience "actually varies according to the political system and the nature of the issue";[88] for instance, the audience broadly refers to citizens of a nation-state in a democratic system, or "the relevant audience is always case-specific," in Vaughn's words.[89]

The operationalization of audience acceptance is also problematic in nondemocratic settings. Are there political mechanisms (e.g., voting) available to the audience (or the general public, as in the original idea) to express their "acceptance" toward the securitizing move? Furthermore, is there any law or constitutional right (e.g., freedom of speech) available that guarantees audience "security" when they reject the securitizing move uttered by the securitizer?

The constructivism paradigm proposes that the understanding or meaning of a concept differs in countries with varied historical, political, economic, social, and cultural backgrounds. Hence, one should not overgeneralize, or apply the meaning of security prevailing in Western liberal countries to the non-Western world. As stated previously, biases arise when scholars and analysts adopt a Western lens in understanding the non-Western world. Moreover, non-Western countries, particularly, Asian countries, significantly differ in terms of political system, history, norms, and culture.

The analytical power of securitization theory in conducting empirical security studies weakens when the core elements of the theory do not undergo further operationalization and differentiation. Real-world situations yield mixed and partial results instead of "black and white" empirical judgments. This point is echoed by Vuori and later by McInnes and Rushton: securitization as a form of politics is not a binary division, but possesses "a continuum of success and failure."[90] Hence, the current study attempts to develop different types of securitization within the theory. The typology in this book avoids a "black and white" classification of empirical results. The revised framework and case studies in subsequent chapters respond to the concern raised by Wæver: "the current quite absolutist concept of 'securitized or not,' might be differentiated through empirical studies of mixed and partial situations."[91]

Having identified the major theoretical and empirical shortcomings of securitization theory, refining the idea of "speech act," "emergency measures," and "audience acceptance," as well as differentiating the results of the securitization process, are important. One proposed solution is to develop different types of securitization within the theory. However, the relationship between the securitization process and the overall impact of securitization on day-to-day policy making still needs to be addressed. In securitizing an issue, the development of a general and unified framework that accounts for its existence and impact on the policy-making process is important. The following section first draws insights from public policy literatures, especially from the process model developed by David Easton, and the five stages of the policy cycle suggested later by Michael Howlett, M. Ramesh, and Anthony Perl. This study proposes a synthesis of the policy process models and securitization theory.

Synthesizing the Policy Process Model and the Securitization Process

Public policy making is commonly simplified by referring to this as a process that involves a set of interrelated stages from "input" (problems) to "output" (policies).[92] David Easton first mentioned this idea in his book entitled, *A Framework for Political Analysis*, written in 1965.[93] In his book, he simplified the complex political life into a process model. As illustrated in Easton's process model, the government recognizes an issue because of the demand, support, and pressure exerted by different actors in domestic or international environment (inputs).[94] To "regulate the volume of demands or maximize the input of support" received from the environment,[95] authoritative outputs (public policies) such as "administrative decisions and actions, decrees, rules, and other enunciated policies"[96] are released. However, without a feedback mechanism, authorities are unable to determine whether such outputs can achieve their goals. Thus, the model includes a feedback loop that facilitates the flow of information back to the system, enabling the authorities to adjust, modify, or correct their previous political decisions.[97]

Easton's earliest work on public policy analysis was further developed and modified by different scholars. Howlett et al. proposed five different stages in political life, namely agenda setting, policy formulation, policy decision making, policy implementation, and policy evaluation.[98] In the stage of agenda setting, the problems come to the attention of the governments; policy formulation refers to how policy options are formulated within the government, whereas decision making means the process by which the government adopts a particular action or nonaction.[99] Placing the policy into effect is studied in the stage of policy implementation; policy evaluation relates to how policy outcomes are monitored by both state and non-state actors, and evaluation results are used to reconceptualize the policy problem and its solution.[100]

The earlier mentioned public policy process models are reminiscent of the securitization framework. A main idea in securitization is the securitizing move generated by the securitizer. In studying the speech acts and emergency measures generated by top-level leaders, one understands how policies are formulated and decided within the "black box" of a political system. Thus, a securitizing move (speech acts plus emergency measures) resembles the policy formulation and policy decision-making stage suggested by Howlett et al.

A securitizing move is successful when the audience accepts it as such. The process of acceptance is similar to the stage of policy evaluation, in which the policies or outputs are monitored and evaluated by state or non-state actors, to decide whether to continue, modify, or demolish policies within the political system. The stage of policy evaluation clarifies securitization not as a linear process, but as one that requires feedback loops that lead to reconceptualizing problems and policies; such is an alternative type of securitization. The insight provided by the process model in public policy literature significantly contributes to the dynamics of securitization.

In conclusion, the securitization framework synthesizes the policy process models, thereby maximizing the empirical capability to comprehend the securitization process in day-to-day policy making. The revised framework analyses the results of numerous case studies and of comparative studies of different stages.

A Revised Framework for Health Security Analysis

This specific study suggests a modified framework of securitization theory with different types of securitization. Three main conditions of securitization exist in constructing a typology.[101] The first is the nature of the security act uttered by the securitizing actor(s), whether positive (+SA) or negative (–SA). The second is the mode of political reaction initiated by the securitizing actor(s), classified as either emergency (+EM) or nonemergency mode (–EM). The third is the response of the audience (the civil society groups, in this case) representing either high level (+AA) or low level of acceptance (–AA) toward a particular securitizing move. The first and second dimensions constitute the securitizing move delivered by the securitizer, whereas the third dimension focuses on the acceptance of the designated audience of the securitizing move initiated by securitizing agents. Considering the three criteria, a revised securitization framework is created (Figure 2.1).

Policy Formulation and Decision-Making Stage

Speech Acts

Many aspects of this typology require further elaboration. Classifying the security act as either positive or negative signifies the perception of securitizing actors toward the issue. A speech act is coded as positive when the actors recognize the problem by uttering "security words," whereas a negative speech act indicates the absence of "security words," or represents public speeches and texts that contradict positive speech acts. Here the notion of negative speech acts attempts to resolve how securitization is identified in the absence of "security words."[102]

Buzan et al. highlighted that a successful speech act requires compliance with its internal and external conditions, which they refer to as *facilitating conditions*.[103] Internal conditions refer to correct grammar and plot structure of the speech acts uttered by the securitizing actors, whereas external conditions denote the social capital and authority possessed by securitizers in uttering.[104] These internal and external conditions are also underpinned in the revised framework, as follows:

External Conditions

The original framework suggested that everyone can become a securitizing agent.[105] However, as argued by Eriksson, "anyone may securitize an issue, but only a few put a securitized issue onto the government agenda."[106] As such, securitizing actors should be the ones to bring the securitized issue on the government agenda. Having state actors, particularly heads of government or their representatives, perform most securitization acts is not surprising,[107] because they traditionally represent

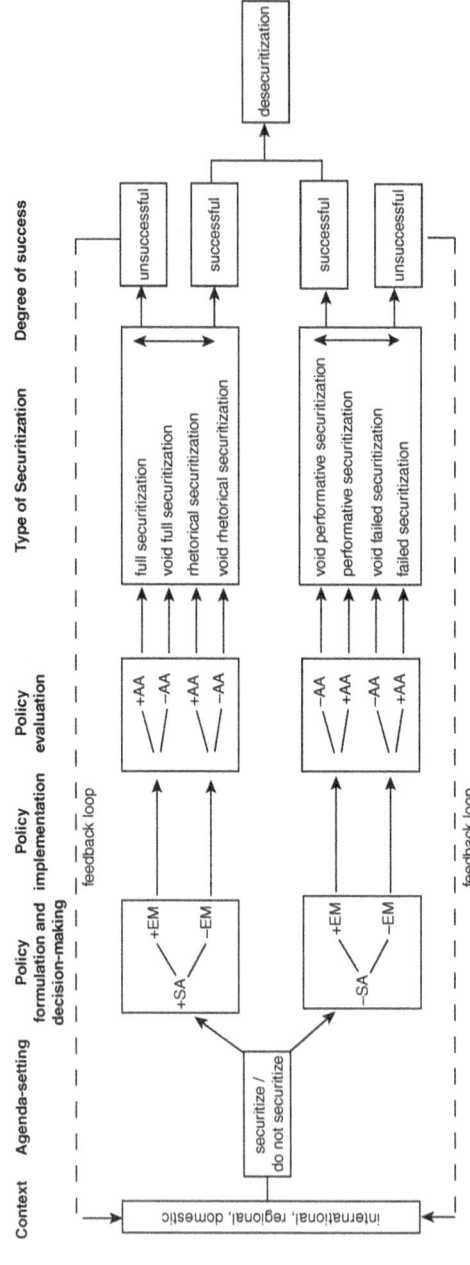

Figure 2.1 A Revised Securitization Framework for Health

the accepted voice of security that initiates effective responses to control existential threats.

In addition, national governments that define national priorities and set the security agenda often have the legitimacy and authority to mobilize various sections of the population,[108] and control most resources (legal, financial, and bureaucratic) necessary to mount a campaign against the problem.[109] These points are supported by the statement, as observed by Mechai Viravaidya, a high-ranking official in the Thai government, who remarked, in reference to Thailand's HIV/AIDS response, "Ministers are not the most powerful, they cannot demand the full cooperation of others, and they cannot order a change in the budget—but the Prime Minister can."[110] Hence, the securitizing actor in the current study particularly refers to top-level leader(s) in the national government.

Internal Conditions

Following the logic of the Austinian speech-act theory, a problem becomes a security issue when the power holders declare it to be so.[111] In this respect, an issue such as HIV/AIDS is securitized when the securitizing actor utters, "HIV/AIDS is a security threat." However, securitizing actors may not always use the exact "security words" of the securitization concept, in this case, "security" or "threat" in attempting to bring the issue into the realm of security.[112] As Huysmans pointed out, there exists a "cultural specificity" of the rhetorical structure of the speech act.[113] In other words, the usage of "security words" by securitizing agents can be influenced by political or cultural factors. In a constraining political context or traditionally repressive culture, the usage of certain phrases might be suppressed.

Likewise, linguistic factors play a crucial role in the choice of wording. The English term "security" will be absent if there are no words in other languages that exactly mean "security." Although one may find the Chinese equivalent of "security," the word may not bear the "same connotations, strength, and interpretation in that language" as the same word in English.[114] The term "security" is translated as *anquan* in Chinese. However, the meaning of *anquan* is different from "security"; *anquan* merely means "safety" instead of "security." Therefore, equivalent or related notions should be considered to determine positive and negative security acts. Using the words "great problem," "tremendous problem," or "serious problem" possibly reflects a positive security act, because the meaning of these expressions is equivalent to "security threat" in a particular culture and society.

Aside from the usage of words or phrases in a security concept, a particular logic of argument should be uttered by the securitizer to determine the presence of a positive speech act. This line of argument should constitute at least one of these elements: (1) a problem exists (existential threat); (2) the perceived problem challenges the survival of states or their people (referent objects), and (3) absolute priority and urgent handling of the problem is required. The presence of security words allows the researcher to identify the positive or negative speech acts, and the security logic in public statements or speeches of the securitizing agents.

The revised securitization framework contributes to resolve its internal problem and Hansen's concern by dividing "speech acts" into positive and negative acts, signifying securitizing actors' perception of the issue. As mentioned earlier, a speech act is coded as positive when the actors recognize the problem by uttering "security words," whereas a negative speech act indicates the absence of "security words" or the presence of public speeches and texts contradicting the positive speech acts. In the present study, the notion of negative speech acts attempts to address Hansen's concern regarding "how to identify securitization in the absence of 'security words.'"[115]

However, the speech act, whether positive or negative, does not guarantee subsequent security practices in the real-world political environment.[116] Securitizing actors can deliberately choose not to securitize an existential threat or securitize the threat via speech acts, but instead, choose not to carry out emergency measures to resolve the threat.[117] Discrepancies, in other words, exist between the securitizer's verbal and physical acts, which securitization theory has not fully addressed. Instead of solely relying on the illocutionary nature of speech acts, this book proposes to emphasize the study of the actual "physical actions" of securitizers toward the perceived threat.

Emergency Mode/Measures

The mode of political reaction is considered either as an emergency or a nonemergency. In the present study, two significant points are incorporated to distinguish between these two modes. The first one suggests that "emergency" and "nonemergency" are not absolute but relative concept.[118] What seems unusual for one political unit may be normal for another. For instance, a war can be an ordinary policy outcome in failing states, but an extraordinary measure in historically conflict-free countries. In this sense, a measure is regarded as an "emergency" when it differs from the political ideology or usual practice upheld by leadership or the government, or varies from a cultural norm that is traditionally deeply rooted in society.

The second notion is that the distinction between "emergency" and "nonemergency" is not fixed, given mixed political measures in dealing with issues in the real world. Williams held a similar idea, arguing that "not all changes in policy and practice are exceptional, even if they partake explicitly of the language of security."[119] Indeed, Wæver stated that "in the application on concrete cases, quite hopeless debates often emerge on whether something is 'ordinary' or 'extraordinary.'"[120] However, he stressed that "if the concepts of 'extraordinary measures' contains distinct subcategories, it might be easier to develop degrees of securitization without watering out the theory."[121] Considering the differentiation of subcategories proposed here, the revised framework identifies the following subcategories of emergency measures: (i) *budgetary allocation,* (ii) *policy measures and institutional arrangement,* and (iii) *legislation amendment or formulation.*

Budgetary Allocation. A dramatic increase in the national budget and resource allocation should be observed, for an issue that is previously not securitized; by means of redirecting funds from other projects or adding to existing tranches. With regard to the HIV/AIDS case, Iqbal argued that the provision of antiretroviral treatment (ART) can reflect the extent of seriousness or emergency of state response.[122] Thus, the timely provision of ARV drugs for treating HIV/AIDS is a major indicator of the spending level.

Rushton asserted that a common concern surrounding securitization is the potential effect on the spending level on the securitized issue.[123] However, if securitization is defined solely as a shift in resources to address a threat, then states with low economic power are constrained in their ability to shift an issue into emergency mode.[124] Aside from resource allocation or redistribution to new security issues, the creation of new institutions and legislation for the sake of newly defined security issues comprises other subcategories of emergency measures.

Policy Measures and Institutional Arrangement. The upsurge in budget and resources, as previously mentioned, could result in (a) the rollout of policy measures exclusively for the problem, and (b) the replacement of existing structures/systems to a novel one that particularly deals with the issue, or the establishment of new institutions alongside existing structures at the national and subnational levels. The creation of national agencies for HIV/AIDS is an example.[125] Ramiah also suggested that multi-sectoral responses within different government departments and with nongovernment sectors are usually observed within such new institutions.[126]

Legislation Amendment or Formulation. The formulation of new policy measures and institutions related to the issue is essential; however, when not implemented, these may become "dogs that can only bark." When securitizers earnestly consider the actual implementation of emergency measures, then related laws or regulations are formulated or amended to ensure the proper implementation of policies and measures.

Still with respect to the second point on emergency measures, in a real political environment, not all policy responses are extraordinary; mixed political reactions usually exist in handling the problem. However, if the securitizer considers an issue as critical, then a *full set of emergency measures* ought to be present *within* the political term of the securitizing agents. In other words, a political reaction is considered to be in "emergency mode" when *all* three subcategories exist, and in "nonemergency mode" when any or all subcategories are absent.

With both discursive and nondiscursive components, speech acts and issues in emergency mode do not create a successful securitization per se, and are only securitizing moves.[127] In theory, a securitizing move is the political reaction of the securitizers. Given the positive and negative speech acts, and the emergency or nonemergency modes, a matrix with four types of securitizing moves is generated (Table 2.1).

A full securitizing move is observed when securitizers carry out what they promised. A securitizing attempt that lacks either speech acts or emergency modes is considered a partial securitizing move. This incomplete yet valid securitizing move is crucial in classifying rhetorical and performative[128] securitizing moves, because their validity is supported by either the speech or action of the securitizer. A securitizing move that lacks both elements is termed a failed securitizing move; the issue is neither framed as a security threat nor handled in the emergency mode by top-level leaders.

In other words, a *complete* securitizing move does not exist during the speech act, but only when a relevant actor changes his or her own behavior in response to the justification of the existential threat.[129] The advantage of this revision is that examining whether "the rhetoric of the speech act is matched by subsequent security practice" becomes possible.[130] Furthermore, these four types of securitizing moves attempt to emphasize that the results of a securitizing move are not homogeneous, as offered by McInnes and Rushton in their article.[131] The construction of these securitizing moves responds to Wæver's suggestion for a deliberated study of specific securitizing moves, including "some that fail, and possibly some that succeed only partially."[132]

Table 2.1 A Matrix of Securitizing Moves

	Positive Speech Act (+SA)	Negative Speech Act (−SA)
Emergency mode (+EM)	Full securitizing move	Performative (action-laden) securitizing move
Nonemergency mode (−EM)	Rhetorical (speech-laden) securitizing move	Failed securitizing move

A valid securitizing move is the first step toward a successful securitization.[133] Buzan et al. believed that a successful securitization is not decided by the securitizer but by the audience, who determines whether to accept something as an existential threat to a shared value.[134] Simply put, a speech act that proposes an existential threat, and a securitizing agent that intends to react either in emergency or nonemergency mode, does not create a securitization in itself. The issue is securitized only when the audience accepts it as such.[135]

Following the earlier reasoning, a speech act that presents an issue as a nonexistential threat to a referent object that is handled either as an emergency or nonemergency, does not create a failed securitization per se. Failed securitization happens only when the audience rejects the issue to be so. Hence, the third dimension of the securitization process, audience acceptance, should be examined to understand the level of acceptance by designated audiences, and thus identify the extent of securitization of an issue.

Policy Evaluation

Audience Acceptance

Despite the vagueness of the concept of "audience," Wæver did specify that the "audience is those who have to be convinced in order for the securitizing move to be successful."[136] He also mentioned that in reality, several audiences are often involved in one operation.[137] Concerning Wæver's delimitation of the concept of "audience" and the revised securitization framework, at least three types of audience can be identified in different stages of a public policy cycle or securitization process: (1) audience involved in policy formulation and decision making (e.g., high-level politicians, congress, parliament, or cabinet members); (2) audience involved in policy implementation, (e.g., street-level bureaucrats, provincial, and local government officers); and (3) audience involved in policy evaluation (e.g., civil society groups, think-tank members, academic members, public policy scholars, and businessmen). Some audiences, however, are not necessarily confined to one stage; they can be engaged in multiple stages of securitization. For instance, academic scholars are involved in both policy formulation and evaluation stages, whereas civil society groups can be both implementers and evaluators.

The audience involved in policy evaluation, especially civil society groups, is singled out for this investigation. Throughout the study, "civil society groups" refer to nongovernmental organizations (NGOs) operating at the international, national, or grassroots levels, faith-based groups, businesses, international and national funding/donor agencies, media, and ad hoc groups. In this study, NGOs that particularly worked on HIV/AIDS issues are selected and examined, as illustrated in chapters 6 and 8 of this book.

The reasons for studying the acceptance of HIV/AIDS-focused NGOs are as follows: on the one hand, the state-centric nature of the original securitization theory can be addressed by including civil society groups in the securitization process. Being the only non-state "audience" (actors) in securitization, on the other hand, NGOs play a significant role in the process.[138] Rushton asserted that their role is even more prominent in developing countries where national governments have often been unable or unwilling to adequately control the pandemic.[139] Thus, Rushton argued that these participants have the power to either support or oppose the security discourse.[140] However, Rushton has not considered the fact that the political power and resources of NGOs are relatively weak compared to those in developed countries. In addition, NGOs operating in developing countries usually face some form of hardship or suppression by the national government.

HIV/AIDS-focused NGOs are an exception; they are conceived as a very interesting group compared to other NGOs operating in Asian contexts. In general, the HIV/AIDS-related NGOs are more active than other health-related NGOs. One reason is that with the help of ARV treatment, the HIV/AIDS infected individuals can look and feel well for a long time without developing late-stage AIDS. Thus, it encourages them to participate in HIV/AIDS advocacy or campaign to fight for their rights or help other HIV/AIDS infected people.

More importantly, HIV/AIDS-related NGOs in China and India have been developed with the help of the Global Fund to Fight HIV/AIDS, Tuberculosis, and Malaria mechanism. As the recipients of the Global Fund, both Chinese and Indian governments are required to include the representatives of NGOs into HIV/AIDS-related policy making and implementing processes. In addition, a designated portion of the Global Fund grants should be allocated to support the HIV/AIDS interventions of HIV/AIDS-focused NGOs. Illustrated in chapter 6 of this book, with the assistance of the Global Fund, HIV/AIDS-focused NGOs are the most outstanding health NGOs developed in China.

To reiterate, securitization is not entirely an elite-driven process, but represents an intersubjective dynamics that involves both securitizer and audience in constructing or framing the security issues.[141] In other words, how civil society groups apprehend the securitizing move created by the securitizer is ultimately the most relevant factor in determining the presence of audience acceptance toward a security act.

As defined in the revised securitization framework, "audience acceptance" denotes the *audience support of a particular securitizing move*. "Support" is composed of two dimensions: *moral* and *technical*. Moral support is indicated by the extent to which the audience holds the same perceptions on HIV/AIDS as the securitizer, whereas technical support is indicated by the extent to which the audience is involved in national policies initiated by the securitizer. The presence of both moral and technical support (high-level support) generates a valid form of securitization, whereas the absence of either or both "support" (low-level support) generates a void securitization.

In classifying acceptance (support) into moral and technical dimensions, this study attempts to address both *normative* and *pragmatic* concerns of securitization. Accordingly, without strong moral support from the audience, the securitization is considered to be in an "immoral" form. Following the same logic, the lack of strong technical support from the audience generates an "ineffective" securitization.

Outcomes of the Policy Evaluation: A Typology of Securitization

Moving beyond the three dimensions and their indicators, although not intended to be comprehensive, the eight branches of securitization are elaborated.

Full securitization is an ideal form of securitization. This occurs when top-level political leaders perform what they express in public speeches, and the audience provides strong moral and technical support.

HIV/AIDS Securitization in Thailand (1991–1995), under the Leadership of Prime Minister Anand Panyarachun

In 1991, Prime Minister Panyarachun accepted HIV/AIDS as a national security issue that was not to be regarded solely as a health problem.[142] Aside from the positive speech act, the HIV/AIDS problem was handled in an emergency mode. Chaired by Panyarachun, the National AIDS Committee (NAC) was established in July 1991.[143] A drastic change in budget distribution was observed. Under the Panyarachun administration, the Thai government's budgetary allocation for HIV/AIDS campaigns increased dramatically from US$2.6 million in 1990 to US$25.1 million, and to US$44 million in 1993.[144] In 1992, Panyarachun ordered all ministries to allocate HIV/AIDS funds and implement HIV/AIDS-related policies consistent with national funding and measures. In terms of legislation, several repressive policies against people with HIV/AIDS were repealed. The AIDS bill, which required mandatory reporting of names and addresses of HIV/AIDS individuals, was revoked by the government, and voluntary, anonymous counseling was established.[145]

Commercial enterprises such as cosmetic firms, insurance companies, and gas stations were mobilized to deliver messages on HIV/AIDS prevention to their customers and employees.[146] NGOs and Community-based Organizations (CBOs) were actively enlisted to provide support and peer education to sex workers. In 1991, only one support group existed for people infected with HIV/AIDS; a decade later, there were 400 such groups.[147] Funding from the national government for NGOs supporting HIV/AIDS in the country was shortly observed. From 1994 to 1995, funding for NGOs in Thailand surged sixfold.[148]

Strong collaboration among police, local health officials, brothel bosses, and sex workers, at both provincial and district levels, resulted in the successful implementation of the 100 percent Condom Program in 1992, although prostitution is illegal in Thailand.[149] Until 1993, action taken on the HIV/AIDS problems was primarily from the government, international agencies, and NGOs. The business sector began supporting the move in 1993, with the establishment of the Thai Business Coalition on AIDS (TBCA).[150] TBCA assists businesses in providing HIV/AIDS education to the workforce and in developing a workplace policy.[151]

Void full securitization is full securitization that is incomplete; the audience does not fully support the perception of threat, or is not involved in political reactions toward the perceived threat.

HIV/AIDS Securitization in Taiwan (2001–2008), under the Leadership of President Chen Shui-Bian

A press release by the Executive Yuan[152] on December 19, 2001 affirmed the seriousness of the HIV/AIDS problem and the government's commitment to deal with HIV/AIDS:

> We clearly know that HIV/AIDS is a **human catastrophe**. It is still an incurable disease that is **resemble to the Black Disease**...we aware that HIV/AIDS is not only a deadly disease, it also has a dramatic impact on social development, reduces the productivity, scares away the foreign investment, decreases the living standard of people, and **weakens the power of the government and society**... we attach **great importance** towards the HIV/AIDS problems... it is **not solely a medical and health problem**. [emphasis added][153]

Along with the positive speech acts, a full set of emergency measures was observed. An interdepartmental Committee for the Promotion of AIDS Prevention and Treatment was formulated by the Executive Yuan on the same day that the speech acts were made.[154] This committee, which replaced the 1985 AIDS Advisory Committee, was composed of 13 departments and agencies.[155] Members of the committee gathered nearly NT$2 billion for HIV/AIDS intervention in 2002.[156] Additionally, the Executive Yuan promised that "the budget for HIV/AIDS Prevention and Control is the priority item on the national budget," thus affirming the financial commitment of the Taiwanese government.[157]

Aside from the increase in budget and the institutional reform, several laws and regulations were formulated and amended during that period. These laws and regulations include *HIV Infection Control and Patient Rights Protection Act* (originally, the *AIDS Prevention and Control Law*) that was amended in 2007, and the *Enforcement Rules of the AIDS Prevention and Control Act* that was amended in 2006.[158] Two new regulations were enacted in 2008, namely the *Regulations Governing Reporting by Medical Personnel upon Detection of HIV Infection* (March 25, 2008) and the *Regulations Governing Payments for Costs for Laboratory Testing, Prevention and Treatment of HIV* (June 16, 2008).[159]

With regard to audience acceptance among NGOs in Taiwan, Rollet's study shows that Taiwanese HIV/AIDS-related NGOs have achieved a certain degree of maturity and sustainable financial stability over the years, and that majority of the NGOs play complementary and collaborative roles in national HIV/AIDS intervention.[160] However, out of the 11 registered HIV/AIDS-focused NGOs, only two are operating in South Taiwan—Taichung and Kaohsiung[161]—where the HIV/AIDS prevalence dramatically increased in recent years.[162] Technical support toward national HIV/AIDS programs has been confined to north Taiwan, particularly in the capital city, Taipei.

Rhetorical securitization lacks the full set of emergency measures for the securitization process, yet the security move receives strong moral and technical support from the target audience. The absence of extraordinary measures can be attributed to two reasons. First, the use of the term "security threat" is abused by top-level political leaders and officials. National authorities use the term to invoke public attention to certain issues, but the leaders do not commit to subsequent emergency actions related to their speeches. Second, top-level leaders recognize the threat, but their attention and funding are diverted to other, more pressing national problems or threats. Such concerns probably include food and water scarcity, terrorism, deadly infectious diseases, civil confrontations, and environmental degradation, especially in developing countries or failing states.

HIV/AIDS Securitization in India (1998–2003), under the Leadership of Prime Minister Atal Bihari Vajpayee

Prime Minister Atal Bihari Vajpayee delivered several HIV/AIDS-related speech acts in India in 1998, 2000, and 2002. He framed HIV/AIDS as a threat,[163] and as a global problem with a strong Indian dimension.[164] Thus, Vajpayee affirmed that controlling the spread of HIV/AIDS and caring for infected individuals were urgent national tasks.[165] Despite the presence of such positive speech acts, a full set of emergency measures was absent throughout this period. There was no top-level leadership in the HIV/AIDS-related program until 2006, and no resources and budget increment until 2004. Financial allocation for HIV/AIDS even declined from US$52.6 million for the 2002–2003 period, to US$50.7 million from 2003 to 2004. Multi-sectoral cooperation among the ministries and departments in the Indian government was equally absent.

Despite the absence of a full set of emergency measures at the national level, positive responses were noted among civil society groups, especially in business groups. Taking the Indian Business Trust for HIV/AIDS (IBT) and the Confederation of Indian Industry (CII) as an example, they co-organized a one-day meeting on *Accelerating the Business Response to HIV/AIDS: Partnerships and Action* in October 2003. During the meeting, S. B. Mookherjee, who was the Indian Minister of State for Commerce and Industry, appealed to the business community to extend its assistance to people infected with HIV/AIDS in India.[166] Indian Oil, the country's biggest company, promoted HIV/AIDS awareness among long-distance truck drivers at 4,000 of its petrol stations on national highways.

Void rhetorical securitization is an incomplete from of rhetorical securitization. This happens when the utterance of positive speech acts is not followed by a full set of emergency measures, and the audience does not provide moral or technical support to the perceived threat and to policies in response to the existential threat.

HIV/AIDS Securitization in Russia (2006–2011), under the Leadership of President Vladimir Putin

On April 21, 2006, President Vladimir Putin delivered a speech act relating to HIV/AIDS during the State Council Presidium meeting:

> This is a **serious situation** that requires us to take the appropriate action. We **need more than words; we need action**, and the whole of Russian society must get involved. [emphasis added][167]

Funding for HIV/AIDS programs increased from around US$4 million to US$150 million in 2006,[168] and to US$445 million in 2007.[169] Aside from the substantial increase in its HIV/AIDS budget, the Russian government also became the chief contributor to the nearly US$1.5 billion allocation in response to HIV/AIDS for 2006–2011.[170]

A high-level, multi-sectoral Government Commission on Prevention, Diagnostics, and Treatment of HIV Infection and AIDS was created in October 2006; representatives from 11 federal ministries and services, members of the legislature, and representatives of civil society comprised this commission.[171] However, the chairman of this HIV/AIDS Commission was not the Russian president, but the minister of Health Care and Social Development.[172]

Political reactions related to the HIV/AIDS problem were largely handled in a nonemergency mode. Financial resources for the HIV/AIDS programs were limited. Regarding ART provision, although the government planned to provide ARV treatment to 70,000 people infected with HIV/AIDS, the UN estimates that more than 75 percent of this number did not receive such treatment.[173] Furthermore, the Russian government ceased its support of the country's harm reduction program. The government likewise curtailed its funding for needle exchange, from 15 programs in 2006 to three in 2007.[174] Necessary preventive strategies are scarce in Russia.[175] Funding is especially lacking for the HIV/AIDS prevention undertaking aimed at high-risk groups, including IDUs, FSWs, MSM, and the transgender population.[176]

The harm reduction program remains extremely controversial and unacceptable at the local level. Many local bureaucrats view drug users as potential criminals. Police officers usually arrest drug users to fulfill set "targets" for drug arrests and extort money from them.[177] Thus, audience acceptance of the HIV/AIDS securitizing move is considered generally low in Russia.

Void performative securitization is observed when there is difficulty in gaining audience support due to the nature of the issue, which is either new (or newly discovered) and/or controversial.[178] Given the nature of the problem, the political leaders may choose not to frame such as a "threat" or "serious problem" via speech acts, yet react with a full set of emergency measures. This type of securitization is common in the early stages of the response to HIV/AIDS by many developing countries. The central government may avoid framing HIV/AIDS as a "threat" to national security for fear of worsening the stigma and discrimination toward HIV/AIDS-infected individuals, causing the society to perceive these individuals as "threats" instead of the disease itself.

Performative securitization implies the institutionalization of securitization. In short, pertinent measures have become intertwined with daily national policies and practices. As mentioned by Buzan et al., "If a given type of threat is persistent or recurrent, it is no surprise to find that the response and sense of urgency become institutionalized."[179] In this regard, "when we talk of this, we are by definition in the area of urgency."[180] Therefore, if HIV/AIDS was perceived as a persistent long-term problem in a country, then the utterance of "HIV/AIDS" automatically brings with it danger, vulnerability, and fear.[181] Thus, HIV/AIDS spontaneously receives specific attention and sufficient resources, although political leaders did not declare the disease as a "threat."

Buzan et al. suggested that the ultimate goal of securitization is, in fact, desecuritization. In other words, successful securitization ultimately leads to desecuritization, which means the issue no longer undergoes the process of securitization. In reality, however, the existing policies in emergency modes establish beneficiaries that pursue the continuation of securitization, whereas the emergency policies often become largely institutionalized that their cessation triggers costly legal, bureaucratic, and political battles.[182] Hence, desecuritizing an issue becomes difficult once it is securitized for a long time. Institutionalization or performative securitization is thus more often recognized in a real political environment, compared to desecuritization.

HIV/AIDS Securitization in Brazil (1995–2011), under the Leadership of President Fernando H. Cardoso (1995–2003) and Then President Luiz Inácio Lula da Silva (2003–2011)

HIV/AIDS securitization has been institutionalized in Brazil since the mid-1990s. During his term, President Cardoso reformed the national HIV/AIDS program for this to become more autonomous and centralized. Since then, the implementation of the HIV/AIDS program no longer required approval from other executive branches, and formal application for additional funding from the Congress.[183]

With the special authority granted to the national HIV/AIDS program, the budget for HIV/AIDS dramatically increased, and was largely unaffected by other urgent issues or adverse financial situations. Brazil's national spending on HIV/AIDS averaged US$56.5 million from 1993 to 2002, and exceeded US$30 million annually since 1993.[184] Budget was not even upset by the 1998 financial crisis.[185] Under the Silva administration, funding significantly augmented from US$90 million in 2003 to US$278 million in 2007.[186]

Policy and institutional change and a high level of audience acceptance have been observed since 1998, with the establishment of the interministerial National Commission to Control AIDS. The commission is responsible for reporting not only to the Ministry of Health, but also to representatives from the Ministries of Education, Labor, and Justice, the principal association of lawyers in Brazil, various universities, and four particular NGOs.[187] The inclusion of NGOs in the national policy structure for HIV/AIDS facilitated the acceptance level among civil society groups of the HIV/AIDS policy enacted by central authorities.

Void failed securitization captures the incomplete form of the failed securitization, in which the audience does not support the absent or negative rhetorical act and/or the related policy measures.

HIV/AIDS Securitization in South Africa (1999–2008), under the Leadership of President Thabo Mbeki

Negative speech acts were uttered by Thabo Mbeki throughout his presidency. He minimized the need to focus on the HIV/AIDS issue: "The government is not an NGO...focused on one particular disease. We are not a TB NGO or an AIDS NGO or a pneumonia NGO."[188] Mbeki claimed that the biggest killer in South Africa was extreme poverty, stating that "the world's biggest killer and the greatest cause of ill health and suffering across the globe, including South Africa, is extreme poverty."[189]

An interministerial committee named the South African National AIDS Council was set up in 2000 under the leadership of Deputy President Phumzile Mlambo-Ngcuka; this committee included the departments of Health, Education, Social Development, and local governments.[190] Nevertheless, this council was not widely recognized as the authoritative source of decision making on the HIV/AIDS policy due to its low-level leadership in the council.[191]

Overall, a full set of emergency measures is largely nonexistent in South Africa. The public sector did not provide any ARV treatment to infected people until November 2003 because of Mbeki's reluctance.[192] He asserted that HIV does not cause AIDS; hence, HIV/AIDS-infected individuals do not need the ARV drugs manufactured by the Western companies.[193] Health Minister Manto Tshabalala-Msimang shared the president's apprehensions regarding the so-called Western drugs, denouncing AZT and Nevirapine as "dangerous" and "poisonous" drugs.[194]

Civil society groups in South Africa staunchly disagreed with the country's failed HIV/AIDS securitizing move. Several NGOs and activists together wrote an open letter to Thabo Mbeki in 2002, urging the South African president to respond "to the global threat of HIV/AIDS by pro-actively providing ARV treatments to the infected populations, and Nevirapine to curb mother-to-child transmission."[195] On March 21, 2003, a civil campaign entitled "Dying for Treatment" was launched. In the course of this event, 200 HIV/AIDS activists marched to the Sharpeville police station to present charges of manslaughter against Health Minister Manto Tshabalala-Msimang, for not administering ARV treatment, and against Trade and Industry Minister Alec Erwin, for blocking the manufacturing of generic drugs in South Africa.[196]

Failed securitization happens when (1) an issue is of low priority on the government agenda; thus, national authorities resort to ordinary political measures in handling the issue, or (2) an issue has never existed in the country; hence, it is not included in the national agenda. In such cases, national leaders deny the existence of an existential threat and reject the launching of extraordinary measures. The audience shares the national government's value and perception that it is an unimportant issue, or handles the issue via ordinary political measures.

HIV/AIDS Securitization in China (1985–1997), under the Leadership of President Jiang Zemin and Premier Li Peng

At the onset of the HIV/AIDS outbreak, the People's Republic of China (PRC) government framed HIV/AIDS as a "foreigner disease," anticipating a confined spread of the virus in China, and that Chinese would not be infected,[197] considering that "homosexuality and promiscuity...are limited in China because they run counter to public opinion, moral standard and laws."[198] Hence, HIV/AIDS was not perceived as a threat/problem to China and its people.

The PRC government perceived HIV/AIDS as only one of the many infectious diseases that exist in the country; thus, ordinary public health measures, such as isolation and quarantine, were implemented to combat the disease. Consistent lack of attention to the seriousness of the HIV/AIDS problem was generally observed in society. A Chinese newspaper, *Liberation Daily*, commented on the initial discovery of HIV/AIDS in Yunnan in 1989: "The facts prove that AIDS has entered our country when foreigners knocked at our door and has spread in a small area [Ruili county of Yunnan]."[199] Audience acceptance remained low in China at that time.

Given the eight types of securitization, one point should be emphasized: audience acceptance does not necessarily depend on the audience being convinced about the emergency security threat posed by HIV/AIDS, or their being involved in national HIV/AIDS intervention. They may use the HIV/AIDS securitization as a means to achieve their hidden agendas. In other words, the audience may not conceive HIV/AIDS as a security/serious problem in the country, or that the national government has involved them in political reactions; however, they will espouse the securitizing move initiated by the national government.

This type of securitization is termed *false securitization*. In this type of securitization, the reason for the securitizer and audience to construct and to accept, respectively, the HIV/AIDS security frame is not due to the seriousness of HIV/AIDS and the appropriateness or effectiveness of the emergency measures. Either or both actors may treat the HIV/AIDS securitization as a means to achieve their hidden or ultimate ends.

Summary

In the last two decades, securitization theory has become one of the most successful theories developed within security studies. However, the theory is not without conceptual and methodological shortcomings. As illustrated in this chapter, most security scholars criticize in an attempt to polish the theory, suggesting its long-term benefits to scholars. In exploring existing debates on securitization theory, its major shortcomings were highlighted in this chapter: the lack of operationalization and differentiation, together with the presence of Eurocentrism in securitization theory in general, and the three core elements, namely "speech acts," "emergency measures," and "audience acceptance," in particular. This study develops a revised theoretical framework based on the identified inadequacies of the theory. A typology with eight branches of securitization is constructed, ranging from failed securitization to partial securitization (rhetorical and performative securitization), and finally, to full securitization (where the issue is presented as an existential threat, coupled with a full set of emergency measures and a high level of audience acceptance of the securitizing moves). An important point is underscored: placement varies at different periods of time. In other words, the type of securitization experienced by a certain area will not necessarily endure throughout the years.

After constructing the theoretical framework, brief case studies of HIV/AIDS securitization in different countries are offered as real-world examples to illustrate each type of securitization, as proposed by the revised framework. These case studies serve as cornerstones for revising the theory and structuring the case studies of HIV/AIDS securitization in China and India, as discussed later in the book. Through the revised framework and these two countries as examples, the study sheds light on the future development of the theory and security research. Prior to presenting in-depth studies of HIV/AIDS securitization in China and India, the relationship between security and health is discussed in the next chapter, as well as the history of the spread of HIV/AIDS in the world, and the securitization of HIV/AIDS in the international level.

Chapter 3

Health Security and HIV/AIDS

Introduction

Prior to the early nineteenth century, no one knew that diseases were caused by microbes, or so-called microscopic organisms, for they were invisible to the naked eye.[1] Lacking a plausible explanation, people at that time often viewed diseases as a form of punishment inflicted by gods.[2] Marcus Terentius Varro (116 BC–27 BC), a Roman writer, was the first to foresee the presence of tiny, invisible living organisms, in his work entitled *On Agriculture*: "Precautions must also be taken in the neighborhood of swamps, both for the reasons given, and because there are bred certain minute creatures which cannot be seen by the eyes, which float in the air and enter the body through the mouth and nose and there cause serious diseases."[3] However, this first mention of the possibility that diseases were caused by microbes took more than 1,500 years to gain full acceptance, after people eventually saw such minute creatures using a microscope or electron microscope.[4] This scientific breakthrough allowed individuals to realize the continuous "wars" fought between humans and microbes.

Microbes also played a very salient role in the numerous wars and warlike events in human history. As Smallman-Raynor and Cliff stated: "War epidemics have decimated the fighting strength of armies, caused the suspension and cancellation of military operations, and has brought havoc to the civil populations of belligerent and nonbelligerent states alike."[5] In other words, human casualties of war, from both military and civil populations, arise not only from enemies' weapons, but also from the spread of diseases. It is estimated that cholera killed at least three times more soldiers in the Crimean War than the number of soldiers being killed in the actual conflict. Furthermore, the killing power of an infectious disease is even greater than physical weapons when a society with no previous exposure to a disease (*virgin soil* infection) is struck by it.[6]

In the postwar era, the discussion of infectious diseases had moved from traditional war epidemics to contemporary security discourses—one of the seven components of human security and securitization of health. The health-security linkage implied a sense of urgency in responding to the anticipated or forecasted threat, which justified securitizing infectious diseases rather than the chronic diseases that caused 60 percent of deaths annually around the world.[7]

Among all the known viruses that cause diseases, three were singled out by Elbe owing to their tremendous impact on the global/international security agenda in the past decade: (1) the human immunodeficiency virus (HIV) that causes HIV/AIDS, which emerged in the late 1980s; (2) the corona virus that caused severe acute respiratory syndrome (SARS), which spread around the world between 2002 and 2003; and (3) the highly pathogenic H5N1 avian influenza virus that has repeatedly emerged in the past decade.[8] However, among these three epidemics, HIV/AIDS is the first infectious disease to be framed as a security threat in the international level since 2000.[9]

Some scholars cited the absence of any direct causal linkage between HIV/AIDS and security threats,[10] whereas others claimed that the collective impact of the disease on social structure and the strength of the state are obviously undeniable.[11] Although an important issue requiring many debates, such an argument is not the focus of this book. One objective fact observed in Resolution 1308 is that HIV/AIDS has been framed as a security threat in the international arena.[12] Phrased using the terminology in securitization theory, HIV/AIDS has been *securitized*,[13] whether in complete or partial, successful or failed versions.[14]

This chapter discusses the history of diseases and securitization of health. The description of the virology and route of spread of HIV/AIDS follows, with a view of understanding the disease and the threat it produces. The discussion shifts to HIV/AIDS securitization in the international level afterward.

Microbes and People

History reveals that numerous "battles" have been fought between humans and microbes from ancient times to the present, and humans usually achieved triumphs by developing natural immunity and vaccines against those diseases despite hundreds and millions of human lives lost. In 1967, Dr. William Stewart asserted that "it is time to close the book on infectious diseases, and declare the war against pestilence won."[15] Based on the list released by the National Institute of Allergy and Infectious Diseases (NIAID), however, over 80 types of pathogens were newly recognized or reemerged in the past three decades.[16] Microbes do not just surrender themselves to the human immune system and vaccines. Following Darwin's idea of evolution, microbes continuously undergo natural genetic variations and recombinations to form new strains of pathogens that adapt to adverse environments. Considering that the human immune system cannot immediately recognize these altered antigens, such as Swine Influenza A H1N1 in 2009, individuals are exposed to the pathogens and become ill.

Meanwhile, human behavior plays a significant role in the reemergence of diseases. Modern medical practice was termed as one of the disease multipliers by Caballero-Anthony;[17] the increase and sometimes improper use of antimicrobial drugs and pesticides, in particular, have led to the development of a number of resistant pathogens, such as the methicillin-resistant Staphylococcus aureus (MRSA), which is also known as the "superbug," the Tamiflu-resistant H1N1,[18] and the multidrug resistant colon bacillus found in livestock in Hong Kong. Given the success in developing penicillin, which eradicates microbes within a comparatively shorter time than the human natural immune response, antibiotics have been widely used globally for a variety of illnesses, and indiscriminately used by medical practitioners and self-medicated patients.[19] Without proper instruction on the use of antibiotics, microbes are subjected to an amount of drugs that is not enough to kill them; thus, they become powerful drug-resistant bacteria.[20] For instance, certain strains of the bacterium named *Enterococcus faecium* (*E. faecium*) have been found resistant to over 100 antibiotics produced by scientists to date.[21]

In addition to the improper usage of antibiotics, the reduced compliance with vaccination policies has led to the reemergence of several "ancient diseases," such as pertussis and measles, which were previously controllable through human immunity and specific vaccines. Low vaccination rates among the population have resulted in pertussis and measles outbreaks in Japan and the United States in 1979 and 1989, in which 13,000 and 55,000 people were infected, respectively.[22] However, a more devastating problem is that some individuals have used deadly pathogens such as smallpox or anthrax as bioweapons, because majority of the civilian population currently do not possess immunity against these "extinct" pathogens.[23] The anthrax letters sent via the US Postal Service, which infected 22 people and killed five, illustrated this point.[24] Current problems on new and reemerging diseases, along with the bioterrorism threat, have principally led to a dramatic shift in human response to these diseases, from a medical perspective to security discourse.

Health-Security Linkages

Health-security linkage is not a novel concept, being explicitly pronounced in the Constitution of the World Health Organization (WHO) backed in 1946.[25] However, this linkage did not produce an immediate shift toward an emergency mode. Such a weak linkage was maintained after the Cold War, until the human security discourse emerged with the release of the *1994 United Nations Development Program* report. Of the seven aspects of human security mentioned in chapter 2, four are directly related to human health: health security, food security, environmental security in conjunction with personal security,[26] signifying the importance of health-related security over other aspects in human security discourse.

Health is vital because it determines the survival of the human race,[27] and constitutes a key dimension of socioeconomic development.[28] Chen elaborated that human security and health are closely linked because "good health is 'intrinsic' to human security, since human survival and good health are at the core of 'security'; good health is also 'instrumental' to human security as it enables the full range of human functioning."[29] Caballero-Anthony pointed out the risk of social and political instability when health issues are sacrificed for other types of issues.[30]

In short, these arguments do not mean that the overall security of humans can be achieved by solely promoting health security at the expense of other forms of security.[31] On the contrary, good health should be attained prior to advocating other aspects of human security. Although human security discourse offers a good start for developing the health-security connection, it lacks a substantive conceptual and analytical framework for understanding health issues in security discourse. This inadequacy is countered by the analytical framework in securitization theory.

Apart from the emergence of the conceptual framework of health security within human security and the analytical framework in securitization theory, other developments have escalated the health-security linkage. Such developments include the following: the destructive impact of emerging and reemerging infectious diseases (ERIDs) and the bioterrorism threat mentioned previously; the devastating political, social, and economic implications of HIV/AIDS pandemic in the developing world;[32] and a rising awareness of the deepening vulnerabilities of populations caused by the global spread of diseases in rich and poor countries.[33] In response to these current developments, various scholars and analysts have proposed the idea of securitizing health, thereby offering an alternative means of handling problems efficiently and effectively.[34]

Despite numerous theoretical inputs, there is no coherent voice as to whether or not the logic of securitization is the best route with respect to the public health problems. As Orbinski remarked: "Is global health simply a security concern... Or is global health best conceptualized as pursing equity, justice, and fairness, and as fundamentally considering public health measures and access to health care and healthcare technologies, such as drugs, as a basic human entitlement?."[35] Protecting the fundamental values of the health provision is undoubtedly vital. However, associating health with security does not imply ignorance of these basic values. On the contrary, such a linkage retains the core value embedded in public health, while strengthening the idea through security-related strategies and tactics, which is the fundamental value of public health securitism.[36]

In particular, the idea of public health securitism can enhance the government's prioritization of public health policy. Many countries, in fact, continue to rank health relatively low on the national agenda.[37] Sadly, this phenomenon is even more palpable in many developing countries, as shown in table 3.1, for instance, Saudi Arabia spent 5.6 percent and 10.1 percent on education and military, respectively, but only 2.7 percent on health; India allocated 3.1 percent and 2.7 percent on education and military, respectively, and a mere 1.2 percent on public health issues.

Moreover, public health expenditures of developing countries are significantly lower than developed countries. Table 3.1 clearly illustrates this situation, with developed countries (United States, Netherlands, France, and Germany) allocating over 9 percent of their GDP on health, whereas the health expenditures of developing countries (India, Bangladesh, and Pakistan) are below 1.5 percent. As argued by Curly and Thomas, "The security of state resides in the security of the individual."[38] The current public health expenditure of developing countries obviously poses problems that imperil human as well as national security.

With public health securitism incorporated into public health governance, issues that are likely to jeopardize the overall health of society are securitized, resulting in an "alternative, potentially more effective, response mechanism."[39] Based on the statistics released by the WHO in 2014, chronic and infectious diseases continue to dominate as the top eight leading causes of death in the globe.[40] Nevertheless, infectious diseases have successfully gained more emphasis and discussion in both academic and political agendas.[41] Recapping the idea of securitization theory, a securitized issue is not necessarily an objective threat. In other words, the infectious disease does not necessarily have to be a leading cause of death

Table 3.1 Public Spending on Health, Education, and Military in Developed and Developing Countries

Countries	Public expenditure on health (% of GDP) in 2010	Public expenditure on education (% of GDP) from 2005–2010	Military expenditure (% of GDP) in 2010
Developed countries			
United States	9.5	5.4	4.8
Netherlands	9.4	5.9	1.4
France	9.3	5.9	2.3
Germany	9.0	4.6	1.4
United Kingdom	8.1	5.6	2.6
Norway	8.0	7.3	1.5
Canada	8.0	4.8	1.5
Japan	7.8	3.8	1.0
Australia	5.9	5.1	1.9
Korea	4.1	5.0	2.7
Developing countries			
Brazil	4.2	5.7	1.6
South Africa	3.9	6.0	1.3
Russian Federation	3.2	4.1	3.9
Thailand	2.9	3.8	1.5
China	2.7	No data	2.1
Saudi Arabia	2.7	5.6	10.1
Vietnam	2.6	5.3	2.5
Malaysia	2.4	5.8	1.6
Angola	2.4	3.4	4.2
Cambodia	2.1	2.6	1.6
Syrian Arab Republic	1.6	4.9	4.1
India	1.2	3.1	2.7
Bangladesh	1.2	2.2	1.1
Pakistan	0.8	2.4	2.8

Source: "Table 6: Command Over Resources, The Rise of the South: Human Progress in a Diverse World," *United Nations Development Program*, last modified March 14, 2013, http://www.undp.org/content/dam/undp/library/corporate/HDR/2013GlobalHDR/English/HDR2013%20Report%20English.pdf.

to justify its securitization. Conversely, the framing of the disease into a threat via speech acts by securitizing actors is essential to render everything else irrelevant when no prompt political reaction is taken.

In framing infectious diseases as threats via speech acts, using the impacts of ERIDs on domestic populations, economic growth, regional and international peace and stability as a security frame is easier.[42] Given the communicable nature of the diseases, the sense of urgency in eliminating these is noticeably stronger than in chronic diseases. In addition, when mortality rate is high, and no satisfactory treatment or vaccine is available for an infectious disease, similar to the HIV/AIDS pandemic that caused 36 million deaths and over 35 million infections since 1981,[43] securitization versus normal political responses to the disease becomes more justified.

A study of the virology, history, and spread of HIV/AIDS is important, prior to discussing its securitization. Similarly, understanding the obstacles in developing effective drugs and vaccines, as well as the ignorance and misperception of people toward the disease is vital, as all these factors help justify the seriousness of HIV/AIDS and the rationale for securitizing it.

Virology of HIV/AIDS

HIV is a lentivirus, which is one of three subfamilies of retroviruses. The other two subfamilies are oncoviruses and spumiviruses.[44] HIV was the third retrovirus detected in humans, after the discoveries of Human T cell lymphotropic virus (HTLV-I) and its close relative HTLV-II, in 1980 and 1982, respectively.[45] HIV is different from other retroviruses in terms of genetic structure and style of reproduction. Unlike the genes of most viruses, which make use of deoxyribonucleic acid (DNA) as a template to produce reverse-image molecules of ribonucleic acid (RNA), retroviruses use the viral RNA as a template to create a DNA copy with the help of a unique enzyme reverse transcriptase; next, the viral-cored DNA is incorporated into the chromosome of the infected cell and generates future generations of virus.[46] As a lentivirus, HIV is considered as a slow virus ("lenti" means slow), laying dormant for a while after getting into the hosts' cells.[47]

Once the virus enters human bloodstream, the extracellular part of HIV gp120, docking glycoprotein, binds with the membrane protein of host cells possessing the antigen CD4 receptor. This type of receptor is abundantly present on T (thymus-derived) cells, which are white blood cell that acts as "commanders" and perform a vital role in responding to infection, including identifying an invader and signaling the immune system to defend against the microbes.[48] With the tailored shape of its receptor, the CD4 antigen fits well with the spikes on the extracellular part of the virus, like a key to a locker. Once the locker is "unlocked" by the key, the virus penetrates the membrane and injects its core into the host cell. The viral core consists of two identical strands of RNA, structural enzymes and proteins that facilitate the replication of the virus.[49] Within the cytoplasm of the host cell, the viral enzyme reverse transcriptase converts the viral RNA to DNA,[50] and then copies it to make a double-stranded helix.[51] After completing the transcription, the virus-coded DNA enters the nucleus and binds into the chromosomes of the human genome with the help of another virus enzyme.[52] Next, the viral DNA alters/replaces the DNA in the T cell, forcing the host cell to produce viruses via replication, which then emerges from that infected cell to attack more cells.[53]

Given the decline in the number of T cells in the immune defense system, the host becomes vulnerable to microbes of all types, including bacterial, viral, and fungal infections that are dubbed *opportunistic infections*. Acquired Immune Deficiency Syndrome (AIDS) refers to these multiple syndromes appearing on the host that result in a total collapse of the immune system.[54] Without anti-HIV treatment, the infected individual normally dies quickly, sometimes in less than a few years, either from the virus itself or from other contracted diseases and cancers prior to entering late-stage AIDS.[55]

Such a plague was not fully apprehended or even heard of prior to the 1980s; in 1981, an occasional HIV/AIDS infection led to its discovery. This discovery only forms the tip of the iceberg; underneath, numerous investigations were conducted in the past two decades.

Tip of the Iceberg—Discovery of HIV/AIDS

The first diagnosed HIV/AIDS case in human history surfaced in mid-1981. In diagnosing a young homosexual man at the Los Angeles Medical Center in southern California, an unusual clustering of symptoms was found: an extremely pale and thin body; a mouth full of white "cottage cheese" fungal infection, and uncontrollable coughing and severe lung pain.[56] After running several tests, the medical practitioners concluded that the man suffered from *Pneumocystis carinii* pneumonia (PCP), a rare form of pneumonia caused by the protozoon *Pneumocystis carinii*.[57] PCP is only found among newborn infants, terminally ill cancer patients, and the elderly, yet rarely in young men with no prior history of illness.[58] The white yeast-like infection was caused by *Candida albicans* fungi, which could be transmitted through sexual contact.[59] Tests also revealed that the man's blood contained very few or virtually zero T cells. This young man passed away in the wake of the diagnosis, but it was not an isolated case at that time.

By the end of August 1981, 107 cases with symptoms resembling those noticed in California were found in other cities of the United States,[60] especially in New York, San Francisco, and Los Angeles.[61] Similar clinical syndromes were discovered among the homosexual community in the cities: they suffered from either PCP or Kaposi's sarcoma (KS) (the latter is a form of skin cancer characterized by purplish spots on the body,[62] limited to black Africans and Mediterranean whites),[63] or a combination of both. Toxoplasmosis (a type of brain infection) was likewise diagnosed in certain infected individuals,[64] with a marked depletion in the number of T cells.

A general impression was that the unknown disease only attacked homosexual men, which later proved to be a misleading description of the disease. The media coined the disease as "gay cancer" or "gay plague," whereas scientists named the disease Gay Related Immunodeficiency Disease (GRID).[65] However, GRID was also reported in individuals outside the homosexual community, including IDUs, hemophilia patients, blood transfusion recipients, and infants born to mothers who had GRID or were IDUs. This range confirmed that the disease did not have a homosexual bias. As a result, the name was dropped and replaced by AIDS in 1982. The new name indicated that the disease was not inborn and was characterized by a plethora of symptoms.[66]

Indeed, the collapse of the human immune system with a low number of T cells is the reason for the various infections of viruses and bacteria occurring in infected individuals. Teams of medical researchers acted on the suspicion that the disease was caused by an unknown virus attacking the human immune system, eventually uncovering the mystery virus. Dr. Robert Gallo, an American scientist who discovered the retrovirus HTLV, was convinced that he found the virus that give rise to the disease, and coined the virus as HTLV-III.[67] Unlike their American counterparts, the French scientists in the Pasteur Institute, led by Dr. Luc Montagnier, declared that the lymph-associated virus (LAV) caused the disease.[68] The mystery was ultimately resolved in 1984, when evidence revealed that HTLV-III and LAV were in fact the same virus,[69] and in 1986, the virus was renamed Human Immunodeficiency Virus (HIV).[70]

Genetic studies suggested that two types of HIV have prevailed: HIV-I is the original virus, which is responsible for 99 percent of the current pandemic, evolving in Central Africa; HIV-II is much less virulent than

HIV-I, often causing no illness, and is found primarily in West Africa.[71] In addition, both types resemble the Simian Immunodeficiency Virus (SIV)[72] found in *Pan troglodytes troglodytes*, which are black-faced chimpanzees of Central Africa.[73] This finding supported the speculation that African monkeys are the natural reservoir for SIV, and the possibility of SIV mutation and transmission from the chimpanzees to the African people through human blood contact with infected blood in times of monkey hunting.[74]

These scientific findings revealed that the disease was endemic within the African countries before the 1970s, but became a pandemic disease by 1985, and remains one of the greatest global killers to date. This trend implies that humans have been losing the battle with HIV/AIDS. Researchers were overconfident in claiming that HIV/AIDS would be under control very soon, through a cure or even a vaccine. Despite the effort of thousands of researchers, sadly speaking, we still have no cure and no vaccine for HIV/AIDS.

Combating HIV/AIDS—Controlling the Virus versus Controlling the People

HIV/AIDS Treatment

Virologists and immunologists have worked constantly to develop antiretroviral drugs that can cure the disease. Several classes of drugs are available in the market that is commonly referred to as "cocktail therapy"; these include azidothymidine, zidovudine, and retrovir (AZT); *non-nucleoside reverse transcriptase inhibitors* (NNRTIs); protease inhibitors (PIs); and *highly active antiretroviral therapy* (HAART).[75] The names of these drugs indicate their functions in preventing the virus from completing its life cycle via replication inside the nucleus of the infected cell. However, the drugs available to date can, at most, only halt or slow the infection. Once the individual stops receiving treatment, the viral infection is reactivated, or even brings about more infections than before.[76] Side effects are another problem to be resolved throughout continuous treatment.[77] Considering that the virus is a piece of genetic material that becomes part of the infected cell, the host cells are killed alongside the virus, causing additional complications.

Despite the scientific evidence, identifying newly infected individuals is challenging due to the "lenti" property of the virus, allowing it to hide in the clandestine interstices of the nucleus for years before developing symptoms.[78] In this regard, it is difficult for people to recognize the infection in the absence of symptoms, thus likely losing the "prime time" of treatment. Most importantly, vaccine development is still ongoing. Despite these scientific obstacles to the development of a drug, antiretroviral treatment (ART) is still vital at this stage, "buying time" for both researchers and HIV/AIDS infected individuals while waiting for a cure or a vaccine for the disease, averting more people from contracting the virus and losing their lives.

Vaccine Development

Since 1985, the National Institute of Health has sought to develop a vaccine to impede HIV infection.[79] However, the progress toward HIV/AIDS vaccine development is still very tough and at a relatively slow pace compared to the rate of spread of the disease.[80] Some researchers have previously been able to develop effective antibodies, but these were used against a very limited number of HIV types, and most of them failed.[81] The reason for the failure is attributed to rapid virus mutation and genetic variability.

The higher propensity for viral mutation accounts for the difference in replication methods. Unlike a DNA virus such as the smallpox virus, whose careful genetic spell-checking minimizes mistakes when it replicates, an RNA virus (HIV virus) uses RNA polymerase enzyme to copy itself. However, this enzyme is particularly liable to errors in transcription of the genetic code,[82] making every successive generation of RNA virus slightly different from its predecessor.[83] Given that the virus keeps mutating to evade the host's immune defense in every viral replication, a person may carry many variations of the virus by the time symptoms appear. Some people can be infected with both HIV-I and HIV-II, and with different groups and subtypes as well.[84]

The genetic diversity of HIV is another obstacle to vaccine development. As a matter of fact, the strain of HIV-I can be classified into three distant groups, namely major (M), outlier (O), and new (N) groups. Over 90 percent of HIV/AIDS infections belong to HIV-I group M. Within group M, nine subtypes A, B, C, D, F, G, H, J, and K, together with 15 circulating recombinant forms (CRFs) between subtypes, have been identified at the present stage.[85] Each subtype has its unique geographical distinction, mode of transmission, and type of infectivity.[86] In short, a distinct geographical area or a single person can possess either a single or a compound of several HIV subtypes. Hence, antibodies developed against one local strain may not recognize and combat varieties elsewhere.[87]

In terms of vaccine manufacture, most traditional methods (live attenuated, whole-killed/whole-inactivated, and subunit vaccines) are made from the pathogen itself, employing weakened or inactivated organisms to stimulate antibodies, thereby protecting people from disease infection.[88] However, none of these approaches can be applied to vaccine development for human HIV/AIDS infection, because there is no "proof of concept" that the infected individual recovers spontaneously and that the virus is altogether eradicated inside the body. In this sense, vaccinologists fear that some viral particles may survive during the sterilizing process and infect subjects in times of clinical testing.[89]

The "lenti" characteristic of the virus, the capability of hiding in the host cell, high viral mutation tendency, and genetic diversity of the HIV, thwart researchers' efforts in combating and controlling the epidemic. Regardless of obstacles, researchers continue to hope for successful therapies and vaccines in the near future. Dr. Anthony Fanci, an HIV/AIDS researcher and head of the National Institute of Allergy and Infectious Diseases, commented on the ongoing challenge: "The obstacles to success are scientific obstacles, and I am cautiously optimistic that we will overcome these obstacles with scientific solutions."[90] His statement seems plausible; however, scientific advancement merely represents half of the resolution to the problem. Although scientists are working in the background in the drug and vaccine industry, what other people do in the front end is unclear.

Social and Human Attitudes and Behaviors Regarding HIV/AIDS Spread

To date, the development of HIV/AIDS vaccine purportedly remains unsuccessful, implying the vulnerability of the human immune system to the virus. Ironically, HIV/AIDS is a highly preventable disease. It is neither an airborne nor a waterborne disease, and is transmitted in limited ways: bodily fluid, blood, and mother-to-child. Prevention is thus the best and effective "vaccine" currently available for HIV/AIDS. As Montaginer asserted, "The rush for a cure, while important, should never overshadow the push for prevention."[91]

A range of HIV/AIDS preventive methods is undoubtedly promising and effective, including "HIV/AIDS testing, counseling, education, behavior change programs, condom distribution, drug and alcohol abuse prevention, needle-exchange programs, prevention of mother-to-child HIV transmission, and male circumcision."[92] Some scientists denote these prevention methods as the "AIDS vaccine" available at present.[93] However, why does HIV/AIDS continue to spread and threaten humans worldwide? As Karlen stated: "Ignorance, however, is a destructive luxury when infections again threaten to take more lives than war and famine."[94]

The ignorance of people to the HIV/AIDS problem has partly caused the dysfunction of this "AIDS vaccine." Individuals and governments remain in denial about the seriousness or even existence of the disease.[95] Ignorance of the disease in the early 1980s by the American government resulted in HIV/AIDS infection in both local and overseas hemophiliacs, especially in some Asian countries, via the transfusion of contaminated and unscreened blood products. The same ignorance has led to unprotected sex behaviors and needle sharing among the risk groups. Finally, the misperception, stigmatization, and discrimination of people living under this epidemic can be attributed to the same lack of knowledge by the general public. Overall, history shows that ignorant attitudes helped spread the disease from the United States to the rest of the world in the form of different risk behaviors such as receiving HIV/AIDS-contaminated blood transfusion, engaging in unprotected homogeneous and/or heterogeneous intercourse, using shared needles to inject drugs, and an HIV-positive mother conceiving or breastfeeding an infant.

The securitization of HIV/AIDS is deemed to be one of the many political reactions toward the HIV/AIDS problems. As argued in the following section, HIV/AIDS securitization is a desirable political option that addresses HIV/AIDS problems, especially in developing countries such as China and India, where stigma and discrimination are strongly attached to the disease and, at the same time, health budget is unsustainable as the economy has yet to reach full-fledged development.

Securitization of HIV/AIDS in China and India

According to Buzan et al., "[securitizing] actors can choose to handle a major challenge in other ways and thus not securitize it. The use of a specific conceptualization is always a choice—it is not possible to decide by investigating the threat scientifically."[96] Simply put, the epidemiological seriousness of HIV/AIDS in China and India does not guarantee that securitization occurs: it is a political choice for securitizers to decide whether securitization is the best or most desirable option to address the HIV/AIDS in their respective countries.

The reason for not securitizing HIV/AIDS may be due to negative outcomes and the dilemma of HIV/AIDS securitization. Undoubtedly, the history of HIV/AIDS reveals flawed approaches that have violated human rights and worsened the spread of the epidemic. For instance, in China and India, those infected with HIV/AIDS are quarantined, and barred from serving in state institutions or even receiving school education, orphan care, and health care.[97] Other countries refuse to issue visas to HIV/AIDS-infected visitors or even people coming from countries with high HIV/AIDS infection rates. Having said that some countries have experienced negative outcomes from securitizing HIV/AIDS, securitization itself is not necessarily the root of the problem. Rather, the negative outcomes are largely due to an inappropriate implementation of HIV/AIDS-related emergency measures by the authorities at the national or local levels.

Elbe elaborated the normative dangers of securitizing HIV/AIDS: (1) violation of human rights and civil liberties due to the control, and power shifts away from the civil society to the state institutions; (2) manipulation of the "threat-defense" logic to restrict national interests and fund the armed forces and elites; and (3) opposition to the grassroots HIV/AIDS activities that aim to normalize social perceptions of HIV/AIDS-infected individuals.[98]

Having admitted these normative dangers, Elbe concluded that securitization theory cannot resolve this complex dilemma; however, "raising awareness of its presence did allow policy makers, activists, and scholars to begin drawing the links between security and HIV/AIDS in ways that at least minimize some of these dangers."[99] In other words, pursuing the securitization of HIV/AIDS despite some unavoidable negative outcomes is still worthwhile. Additionally, the securitization of HIV/AIDS is more beneficial to the developing countries that possess a higher prevalence rate of HIV/AIDS, but at the same time, underestimate or neglect the devastating effects of the pandemic. The benefits are twofold: (1) reducing HIV/AIDS-related stigma and discrimination in society, and (2) maintaining a sustainable budget for HIV/AIDS-related programs.

Reduce HIV/AIDS-Related Stigma and Discrimination

Stigmatization and discrimination of people living with HIV/AIDS are obvious in many Asian countries where health workers and the general population have an inaccurate comprehension and misperception of how HIV/AIDS is transmitted.[100] They perceive that causal contacts such as sharing toilets and utensils, or shaking hands with an infected individual results in contacting the disease. HIV/AIDS stigma is often layered on top of many other stigmas associated with high risk groups such as MSM, FSWs, and IDUs, as well as their related behaviors such as promiscuous sex, sex outside of marriage, and illegal drugs injection.[101] In this sense,

HIV/AIDS stigma among infected individuals is inevitably deepened in society, posing a threat to preventive and treatment measures such as condom use, HIV/AIDS voluntary testing, the quality of health care received, and social support from the government and communities.

Rai argued that "stigma and discrimination about HIV/AIDS in society could only be removed when prominent figures including politicians and sport stars start discussing about HIV/AIDS in public."[102] In other words, the adverse attitude toward HIV/AIDS-infected individuals can be alleviated when government officials and top-level leaders take the lead in talking about HIV/AIDS openly in public.[103] Securitization as a top-down political reaction can mitigate stigma and discrimination of the general public against individuals with HIV/AIDS, eventually raising the awareness and preventing the spread of HIV/AIDS especially in less developed countries. In the securitization process, top-level political leaders typically declare HIV/AIDS as a security threat, implying changes in the attitudes and strategies of the government. With altered attitudes toward HIV/AIDS, political leaders can act as role models in changing people's perception on the disease. Concurrently, HIV/AIDS-related knowledge can widely prevail in society via media, discussion groups, and forums. Thus, HIV/AIDS stigma and discrimination is reduced when people are properly educated about HIV/AIDS.

Maintain a Sustainable HIV/AIDS-Related Budget

The securitization of HIV/AIDS helps support the sufficiency and sustainability of the budget related to HIV/AIDS treatment and prevention in developing countries, especially in an economic downturn. The crucial reason for the need for budget sufficiency is that HIV/AIDS treatment is very heavy, in terms of the cost and duration of treatment. The cost of ARV drugs is much higher in developing countries than in developed countries due to the former's limited medical resources. Once an individual is infected with HIV/AIDS, he or she has to receive ARV treatment endlessly for the rest of his or her life. Moreover, the government is burdened if the infected people are young.[104] Budget sustainability is as crucial as sufficiency from the medical perspective. The virus frequently mutates to avoid the attack of the host's immune system; hence, novel ARV drugs should be continuously developed.

Nevertheless, the dearth of budgets and instability of funds are the major obstacles in less developed countries in Asia, where all the political, economic, and social systems are in the developing stage. Thus, public health policy is usually not prioritized by the government. In the case of a chronic disease such as HIV/AIDS that requires long-term strategies and commitment, the government may not have sufficient resources to support the policy, resulting in incomplete treatments, preventive measures, and educational programs. The budget fluctuates in these countries since their funding usually comes from foreign aid, which is subject to the prevailing economic situation. The securitization of HIV/AIDS denotes that the government gives a higher priority to the prevention and spread of the disease than other sociopolitical issues, and the government commits to allocate or reallocate resources to yield a sufficient and sustainable budget to address the epidemic.

Furthermore, health is not a prioritized issue in developing countries, thus public expenditure on health is relatively low in developing countries such as China and India. Despite the fact that HIV/AIDS has been declared as a security threat by national leaders, resource scarcity can still resist the shift of political reactions to emergency modes, posing a daunting challenge in fully securitizing HIV/AIDS in developing countries.[105]

This gap creates opportunities for international institutions and funding agencies to alter the norm and facilitate the political responses of the national governments toward HIV/AIDS in their respective countries. In other words, HIV/AIDS securitizing moves can be fully implemented with the help of international agencies. Resolution 1308 of the United Nations Security Council (UNSC) and the Global Fund to Fight HIV/AIDS, Tuberculosis, and Malaria (GFATM) are believed to have exerted a prominent influence on HIV/AIDS securitization in normative and technical manners at the state level.

Securitization of HIV/AIDS in China and India: Normative and Technical Influences of International Institutions and Other Countries

Normative Influences

In the UNSC meeting in January 2000, then US vice president Al Gore claimed that HIV/AIDS was a security issue as "it threatens not just individual citizens, but the very institutions that define and defend the character of a society. The disease weakens workforces and saps economic strength. HIV/AIDS strikes at teachers, and denies education to their students. It strikes at the military, and subverts the forces of order and peacekeeping."[106] In July 2000, the UNSC passed Resolution 1308, acknowledging the urgent need to address HIV/AIDS that threatens the stability and security if left unchecked. The adoption of Resolution 1308 in 2000 appears to represent a powerful speech act, framing HIV/AIDS as a threat to national and international security rather than as a "mere" development or public health problem.[107] The priority of HIV/AIDS issues at the international level was reconfirmed in the UN's documents: the *2001 Declaration of Commitment on HIV/AIDS*,[108] the *2006 Political Declaration on HIV/AIDS*,[109] and the *2011 Political Declaration on HIV/AIDS*.[110]

Along with the rhetorical security frame, global spending to address HIV/AIDS has risen exponentially since 2000. In 1999, global expenditure on the HIV/AIDS response was just under US$900 million; it had risen to approximately US$16 billion by 2009.[111] Several funding agencies and programs related to HIV/AIDS treatment and prevention have been formulated after 2000. The G8 set up the GFATM (also refers to Global Fund) in 2002. One year later, the Bush administration launched the President's Emergency Plan for AIDS Relief (PEPFAR). Launched between 2003 and 2008, PEPFAR aims to spend US$15 billion "to turn the tide against AIDS in the most afflicted nations of Africa and the Caribbean."[112] WHO launched the "3×5" campaign that aims to get three million people on ARV treatment by 2005,[113] whereas the Multi-Country HIV/AIDS Program of the World Bank has provided more than US$1.3 billion for grants and concessional loans to help governments respond to HIV/AIDS issues.[114]

Technical Influences

Among the international funding agencies, the Global Fund is the most renowned and major contributor to the HIV/AIDS interventions in both China and India. The engagement with the Global Fund's funding policy is deemed to transform the primary HIV/AIDS governance mechanism and the way HIV/AIDS-related policy is formulated and funded in national governments.[115]

Countries receiving the Global Fund are required to have a designated system and structure to manage the use of the grants. These include Principal Recipients (PR), a local fund agent (LFA), together with a multi-sectoral Country Coordinating Mechanism (CCM).[116] PR is a country organization, either governmental or nongovernmental, that receives funds and implements and monitors programs, and is accountable for the use of the grants; LFA, on the other hand, is an independent professional organization that helps the Global Fund ensure the proper use of the funds and verify the progress of the programs in recipient countries. The CCM is a country-level partnership, overseeing the implementation of successful applications.[117] The Global Fund requires CCMs to include a broad representation from the government, nongovernment organizations, civil society, multilateral and bilateral agencies, and private sectors.[118]

It is believed that the Global Fund in general and the structures of PR and CCM in particular facilitate and guarantee the political and financial capability of civil society groups in participating in national HIV/AIDS policy-making and implementation processes in recipient countries.[119] For instance, in the existing government structure in China, civil society has only limited channels to participate in policy-making and implementation processes. Thus, the multi-sectoral structure of CCM contributes to enhance the government's commitment to involve civil society groups in national HIV/AIDS prevention and control measures.[120] Michel Sidibe, executive director for the Joint United Nations Program on HIV/AIDS, also noted that "the Global Fund to Fight AIDS, Tuberculosis, and Malaria was helping to bring innovation and make a difference in [the] most-affected countries by establishing a new link among the government and civil society and NGOs to work together."[121]

Aside from the increase in participation, financial supports for NGOs working on HIV/AIDS-related programs were augmented via the Global Fund. As the PR in the country, the Chinese government is required to disburse a designated portion of the grants to HIV/AIDS-related civil society groups operating in the country.[122] Overall, the Chinese authorities committed over US$43 million to support HIV/AIDS-focused civil society groups in round 3, 4, and 5 of the Global Fund.[123] In India, among the 10 PRs for the different rounds of the Global Fund, five of them come from civil society groups. They include Emmanuel Hospital Association, India HIV/AIDS Alliance, Tata Institute of Social Sciences, Indian Nursing Council, and IL and FS Education and Technology Services Ltd,[124] who receive financial endowments from the Global Fund.

Twilight of HIV/AIDS Securitization at the International Level

Recently, both China and India have faced the same problem regarding the abatement of the normative and financial support at the international level. The reason for the reduction of support is twofold. The first reason is that the international HIV/AIDS securitizing move generated by the UNSC in 2000 has been gradually faded out in recent years. The world's priority has shifted from HIV/AIDS to general public health issues, such as maternal and child health and primary health care system. As stated by a respondent [R2] working in an international NGO in China: "There is a shift in the funding pattern globally. The focus of my organization, national government, and international funding agencies have shifted from HIV/AIDS to more general health issues such as reproductive health care. This shift is because a more visible impact can be seen in dealing with more general health issues."[125] Another respondent [R7] also stressed, "It is a global phenomenon that the level of funding on HIV/AIDS interventions is decreasing. The reason is that the leaders and donors believe that lots of efforts have been exerted on HIV/AIDS interventions, but the sign of improvement is not obvious."[126] Hence, the amount of international funding that is specific for HIV/AIDS has been curtailed or redirected to other public health issues.

On the other hand, after the 2008 Olympic Games and the 2009 Commonwealth Games held in China and India, respectively, international organizations and funding agencies perceived that these two countries are financially capable of supporting their own HIV/AIDS programs. Thus, international funding agencies such as Ford Foundation, MSF, and Clinton Foundation have reduced their support for the HIV/AIDS prevention and treatments in some countries, or even withdrawn from these countries. The Clinton Health Access Initiative (original name was Clinton Foundation) and Bill and Melinda Gates Foundation in India, on the other hand, have announced that they will no longer continue to support the HIV/AIDS programs in both countries.

Despite the expression of international concerns and the cutback in funding for HIV/AIDS issues, China and India have reacted differently to the international health-threat priority in recent years. The Chinese government decided to maintain the 2004-full HIV/AIDS securitizing move, whereas it failed in India. Further elaboration regarding the political reaction toward HIV/AIDS in China and India is seen in chapters 5 and 7, respectively.

Summary

The first diagnosed HIV/AIDS case in human history surfaced in mid-1981 in the United States. Given its "lenti" property, high viral mutation tendency, and genetic diversity of the virus, HIV/AIDS has become a powerful infectious disease that remains incurable. HIV/AIDS was officially pronounced to be a security issue by the UNSC Resolution 1308 in 2000, claiming that the pandemic may pose stability and security risks if left unchecked.[127] Concerns have been raised regarding the full acceptance of

HIV/AIDS securitizing moves by the nation-state members. Nevertheless, HIV/AIDS securitizing moves are deemed to have been generated at the international level since 2000.

At the national level, although HIV/AIDS securitization is viewed as a desirable political reaction toward the problem, HIV/AIDS cannot easily become a priority issue particularly in developing countries such as China and India. In addition, resource scarcity is able to thwart the emergency measures enacted by the national government even if HIV/AIDS is framed as a security threat. Arguably, HIV/AIDS-focused international institutions and related programs play a very significant role in providing normative and technical support to the states in securitizing HIV/AIDS.

Securitization theory, as an analytical tool in security studies, sheds some light on the political response to HIV/AIDS within Asian countries. China and India have become testing sites for government responses toward the HIV/AIDS issues using the refined securitization framework that was discussed in chapter 2. Before proceeding to the China and India case studies, chapter 4 examines the evolution of the health care system and its implication on the HIV/AIDS-related problems in both countries.

Chapter 4

The Changing Face of Public Health Care Systems in China and India

Introduction

The previous chapter illustrated some of the biological and epidemiological characteristics of HIV/AIDS, the development of the linkage of health and security, and also how HIV/AIDS has been securitized at the international level since 2000. Chapters 5–8 explain how HIV/AIDS is being securitized in China and India at the national and subnational levels. While it is necessary to understand how HIV/AIDS has become a health security problem in China and India, it is also imperative to understand the HIV/AIDS threat within the context of the public health care systems in the two countries. The organization and financing of a health system has crucial implications on the system's ability to detect, treat, and control an epidemic.

This chapter offers an overview of health governance in China and India, with a particular focus on the evolution of the public health care systems and the implications of the changes toward HIV/AIDS problems. Illustrating the public health care system in China and India in a comparative perspective, it is argued that the shift in economic focus from the 1980s onward have created wide repercussions for the two public health care systems, especially in rural areas. This chapter highlights the implications of economic reforms and post-reform public health care system on the spread of HIV/AIDS in China and India.

Pre-Reform Systems of Public Health Care in China and India

In 1949, Mao Zedong established the People's Republic of China (PRC) to build a new China that could transcend the United Kingdom and catch up with the United States (*chaoying ganmei*).[1] To achieve this goal, Mao drew upon lessons from the Soviet Union and outlined them in his 1956 speech, titled "On Ten Major Relationships."[2] The concept of equality was emphasized in economic development: equality in industrial development between coastal and interior regions of China as well as equality between heavy and light industries and agriculture.[3] A balanced regional economic development was achieved through interregional transfers of investment resources;[4] such transfers entailed the flow of fiscal resources from rich to poor regions to reduce the variations of their development process.

Mao's objective of equality was also embedded in the provision of health care. The first National Health Conference in August 1950 laid down the major themes of health care policies, namely access to health care and prevention before cure.[5] Given the aforementioned objectives, health care services were indiscriminately provided by a three-tiered network composed of brigade (village) stations, commune (township) health centers, and county hospitals in the rural areas of China.[6] This network used an integrated system with a formal bottom–up referral process for patients.[7] Prior to the 1978 economic reform, preventive health campaigns played a prominent role in the provision of public health care. Preventive health care measures, such as mosquito control and clean water projects, infectious disease vaccination, and other public health services, were largely subsidized by the central government and provided by anti-epidemic stations at county levels, together with the commune and village clinics.[8]

Mao further strengthened health measures in rural China in 1965. At that time, universities and medical schools were closed for five years so medical students and faculty members were sent to the countryside to render three- to six-months medical training to thousands of peasants and urban youth. These individuals later became the "barefoot doctors" that provided preventive and basic health services to rural residents in almost all brigades[9] and therefore enabled basic health services to reach rural areas or remote counties.[10] In addition, a commune-based cooperative medical scheme (CMS) was established; under CMS, the village collective ran and financed health clinics and paid the barefoot doctors to offer primary medical services to the villagers.[11]

Although domestic economic planning was conducted only after independence in 1947, the blueprint of India's modern public health system was defined during the colonial era.[12] In October 1943, the Government of British India appointed a committee, chaired by Sir Joseph Bhore, to survey the state of public health in India and submit recommendations for future development.[13] The *Report of the Health Survey and Development Committee*,[14] also referred to as the *Bhore Committee Report*, was published in 1946. The report recognized the vast rural–urban disparities in existing health service provisions and focused on health care for the rural population.[15] The main ideas in the report included (1) free health service regardless of one's ability to pay; (2) preventive health care as a vital part of the health program; (3) health at people's doorsteps; (4) people's participation in health care; and (5) integrated structure for preventive and curative services.[16] On the basis of the Bhore Committee Report, latter reports—including those of the 1961 Mudaliar Committee, 1966 Jain Committee, 1974 Kartar Singh Committee, 1975 Srivastava Committee, and 1980 Indian Council of Medical Research and Indian Council of Social Science Research (ICMR-ICSSR) Joint Panel[17]—sought to articulate the foundations of comprehensive rural health service provision in India.[18]

India embarked on economic and social development in 1947 after earning its independence. Economic policies were inspired by the Soviet-style central planning and driven by five-year plans that had been designed by the National Planning Commission since 1950.[19] The general objective of development planning in India was the eradication of mass poverty.[20] Acknowledging the extent of poverty in rural India, in contrast with China, Indian policymakers rejected the idea of simple redistribution of financial resources among the Indian states[21] because both the rapid growth of income and national product and the equitable distribution of resources are equally important in poverty eradication.[22]

As far as the health care system was concerned, policymakers also developed a three-tier health care delivery system in rural India.[23] This structure includes subcenters (SCs), primary health centers (PHCs), and community health centers (CHCs), in which a formal bottom–up referral system is also available.[24] At the lowest level, SCs served as the first contact point between the community and the primary health care system. Manned solely by paramedical staff—one male health worker and one auxiliary nurse–midwife or female health worker[25]—each SC was responsible for providing basic health care services, such as maternal and child health, family welfare, nutrition, immunization, and control of infectious diseases.[26] PHCs were managed by at least one medical officer and

14 paramedical staff[27] whose core activities included curative, preventive, and family welfare services.[28] CHCs provided specialized health services that were run by four medical specialists and 21 paramedical and other staff.[29]

"Health for All" is believed to be achieved via the three-tier system of health care in both China and India. Government-owned and -operated health care centers facilitated the physical access of health services using an effective referral system among the tiers. In China, expenses related to the health care delivery system were largely granted by the central government prior to the economic reform. By contrast, India assigned state governments as main contributors; the central government played only a residual role in funding the health care services. In essence, all health centers in India were established and financed by the state governments; the central government provided assistance to all SCs in India after April 2002. Expenditures in this sphere were directed ultimately toward the construction of a user-free oriented public health system.[30]

Universal access to public health care and improvement in people's health condition during the pre-reform era were successful in rural sectors of China and India. One of the greatest achievements of the Mao administration was the dramatic improvement in health care provision in rural China where majority of the population lived at that time. By the end of the 1970s, the CMS had covered more than 90 percent of the entire rural Chinese population and accounted for 20 percent of national health care spending at its peak in 1978.[31] Infant mortality rate dropped from 200 per 1,000 live births to 34, and life expectancy increased from 35 years in 1952 to 68 in 1982.[32] In India, strong leadership and commitment also led to far-reaching developments in health services during the first two decades of independence (1947–1967). This period was called the Golden Two Decades of Public Health in India.[33] Among the accomplishments was the increment in life expectancy from 33 years in 1947 to 49 years in 1970, and subsequently to 63 years in 1998.[34] Another was the drop in infant mortality rate in rural areas from 146/1,000 live births in 1961 to 72/1,000 in 1999, and subsequently to 61/1,000 in 2007.[35]

Notwithstanding these accomplishments, the early success of comprehensive public health care provision was unsustainable in both countries because of insufficient financial resources. It is ironic that the cutback of health care services in both countries was attributed to the economic policies or reforms that were implemented either by national governments or international organizations from the 1980s onward.

Economic Reforms in China and India

Economic reform in China and India consisted of two distinct phases. In China, the first phase started when Deng Xiaoping came into power in 1976, and the second phase commenced in 1992 in Deng's "southern tour" (*nan xun*), during which he advocated the deepening process of market liberalization and reform.[36] In other words, both phases of the economic reform were entirely driven by the Chinese government as it aimed to restore an economy that had been upset by internal political struggles, especially the Great Leap Forward (1958–1961) and the Cultural Revolution (1966–1976). Economic growth generated by subsequent reforms could likely reinforce the performative legitimacy of the communist regime.

In India, the first economic phase began with the inception of partial liberalization during the mid-1980s under the leadership of Rajiv Gandhi, and the second phase was ushered in by comprehensive economic liberalization after 1991.[37] Slightly different from its Chinese counterpart, the reform in the mid-1980s was largely initiated by the Indian government partly because of the internal disturbance during the national Emergency from June 1975 to March 1977. In contrast, international institutions and organizations played a key role in enforcing the latter reform in 1991, which was the result of a liquidity crisis in India's balance of payments.[38]

The 1991 liquidity crisis was concurrently triggered by several global events at that particular historical period, including the collapse of India's chief trading partner, the Soviet Union;[39] the ongoing Gulf War in 1991 that led to an upsurge in the price of imported oil,[40] as well as the suspension of remittances from Indian workers in the Gulf.[41] At the time the country nearly defaulted on its loans. It had less than US$2 billion in its foreign exchange reserves, which was barely sufficient for two to three weeks of imports.[42] As a result, economic reform was one of the preconditions for the Indian government to accept the bailout deal offered by the International Monetary Fund (IMF). Accordingly, the latter economic reform in India was deemed to enforce by the international institution and organizations.

Economic policies were implemented regardless of who initiated the reforms and aimed to alter the traditional centrally planned economy into a market economy. Liberalization measures, such as the creation of a free market where farmers could sell their extra agricultural products at unregulated prices after meeting the quota given by the state,[43] as well as the opening up of several coastal provinces with the provision of preferential investment policies and treatment for embracing foreign direct investment, were conducted by the Chinese government in rural and urban areas, respectively.[44] The 1991 economic liberalization in India was imposed in the name of structural adjustment programs (SAPs) by the IMF and the World Bank as part of its loan obligation. Similar to its Chinese counterpart, the adjustment measures mostly consisted of liberalization efforts in the area of foreign and domestic trade and in the financial system, such as delicensing, deregulation, flexible exchange rates, and tariff cuts.[45] Unlike in the Chinese economic reform, additional stabilization measures were simultaneously carried out in India on top of the structural adjustment measures. The former measures aimed to restore the balance of payments and combat the fiscal crisis in the short run, whereas the latter mainly emphasized economic growth in the medium- and long-terms.[46]

Undoubtedly, these reforms have produced desirable economic outcomes, as indicated by the annual gross domestic product (GDP) growth rate. The average GDP growth in China was 9.6 percent per year[47] and that for India was 5.7 percent annually during the first two decades of economic reforms.[48] Despite these impressive economic performances, two of the adverse consequences became the factors associated with the mounting incidence of HIV/AIDS in China and India: the enlarged economic disparity between the urban and rural regions and the collapse of the health care system in the post-reform era.

Urban–Rural Economic Inequalities and Disparities in China and India

Coastal provinces or states received economic support from the national government at the start of the reform because conditions in the coastal areas were relatively more suitable for economic growth than the conditions in other areas. Coastal areas were characterized by a large number of skilled workers, a high level of technology and managerial sophistication, and relatively well-developed infrastructure.[49] They were also more geographically suited to trade with international markets.[50] To this end, there were more preferential investment policies and treatment granted to these areas.[51] These policies indeed resulted in a large influx of investment and allowed these provinces or states growth at faster rates than the periphery did. Yet, it also worsened the regional socioeconomic disparities between the coastal and interior parts of both countries. The core–periphery disparity was further amplified by China and India's pursuit of policies designed to maximize their countries benefits from economic globalization; where each country pursued integration into the global market by concentrating efforts on developing the urban areas owing to the preexisting and more favorable environment to conduct businesses than the rural areas possessed.

Implications for HIV/AIDS in China and India

Persistent poor socioeconomic development in rural areas led to a relatively high unemployment rate in the peripheral areas. In such conditions, young and educated people from rural areas migrated to urban areas seeking better employment opportunities.[52] Given the high standard of living in the cities, migrant workers usually left their families behind and stayed in the cities for a long time without returning home. Having left their social environment and the usual normative constraints they were more likely to engage in certain nontraditional activities, such as engaging in unsafe sex with one or more partners or becoming sex workers.[53] In peripheral areas characterized by economic backwardness and high unemployment rate, some individuals remained in the rural part of the country and risked engaging in illegal activities, such as sex work or drug trafficking, to make a living.[54] These behaviors are several of the main causes of HIV/AIDS spread in China and India, which is further illustrated with the six case studies in the latter chapters of this book.

It can be concluded that the disparities between urban and rural residents resulted from the economic reforms, leading to some behaviors that were conducive to the spread of HIV/AIDS. Yet, the basic and significant reason for the failure to respond to this epidemic is the collapse in the rural health care system under the economic reforms in the respective countries.

Collapse of Post-Reform Systems of Public Health Care in China and India

Health Priority Setting and Level of Spending

Drèze and Sen argued that policy priorities and political preoccupations tend to change during periods of market-oriented economic reform, thereby marginalizing certain social sectors.[55] The major effect on health care provision in China and India is the declining priority for public health. Discarding the ideology of egalitarianism to embrace pragmatism, Deng Xiaoping openly declared that economic growth was the paramount policy goal of the party-state and the source of its legitimacy in China.[56] In other words, economic development received the highest priority in China during the 1980s. In India, the economic crisis in the early 1990s also led Indian policymakers to place a high priority on economic growth, just as China did.[57]

One symptom of the focus on economic-led development is the reduction of government spending on health care. Between the late 1980s and 2002–2003, the central government spending on health as a proportion of total health spending decreased from nearly 30 percent to just over 15 percent in both countries.[58] Both countries deliberately curtailed the level of public health expenditures in pursuing economic development and performative legitimacy of the regimes. In doing so, the Indian government could meet the requirements of the SAPs in relation to the cutback on public expenditure. Notwithstanding India's commitment to the idea of "adjustment with a human face," interest payments to the IMF drastically constrained the government's financial capacity to fund health care programs.[59] In China, as argued by Yip and Mahal, health was simply "viewed as a consumption activity rather than a productive good and therefore was given lower priority in government funding."[60] Thus, health priority in China and India declined in the wake of economic reforms.

Having said that economic reforms in India caused the decline of health priority on the government agenda; health care, however, has never been a priority per se.[61] As noted in the previous chapters, public expenditure on health care as a proportion of GDP is lower in India than in most other countries. In addition, most of the public health programs in India heavily rely on international or foreign monetary support. For example, over 85 percent of the budget in the first and second phases, and 75 percent in the third phase of the HIV/AIDS intervention program in India, were granted by international funding agencies and bilateral governments,[62] whereas at least 80 percent of China's expenditure on HIV/AIDS interventions came from the Chinese government.[63]

Public health services in rural India were extensively displaced by family planning programs,[64] thereby causing a devastating effect on overall health care services.[65] Instead of health care, population control became an overriding priority at the national level. Budget for family planning surged from Rs 6.5 million under the First Plan (1950–1955) to Rs 65,000 million under the Eighth Plan (1991–1995).[66] With the Family Planning Program (FPP) and the general health services integrated under the Ministry of

Health and Family Welfare, most of the so-called health funding was allocated to the FPP.[67]

Decentralization and Privatization

In times of economic reforms, China and India both trimmed the public expenditure on health through decentralization and increased privatization of services. One of the measures implemented during the Chinese economic reform was the decentralization of health at the subnational level.[68] Simply put, health care provision became a responsibility of the local authorities. In the course of the Chinese economic reform in the 1980s, rural communes were dismantled; the implication was that no further resources would be given by the central government to communes in financing cooperative medical insurance, paying barefoot doctors, and funding health centers and subsidized preventive programs.[69] As a result of the central government disinvestment in health and the collapse of the communes, the proportion of the rural population covered by the medical insurance drastically dropped from 90 percent to less than 10 percent in the 1970s–1980s.[70] Medical coverage dwindled in poor provinces as local governments did not have the financial resources to maintain adequate health care. For instance, 22.2 percent of the population in urban areas were covered by cooperative medical insurance, but merely one percent to three percent in poor provinces was covered in 1998.[71]

In India, the constitution holds Indian states responsible for more than 80 percent of the overall developmental expenditure in public services and health care services,[72] although the central government may provide pertinent direction and support.[73] In sharp contrast to China, decentralization of health care occurred in India prior to the economic reform that commenced in the 1980s. However, the financial capability of states in providing health care services was constrained by lack of funding. One of the imperative liberalization measures taken by the national government was a cut in tax rates. States with a major share in revenue from taxes experienced drastic curtailment from 22.15 percent in 1992–1993 to 8.96 percent in 1993–1994, and a further cut to 7.26 percent in 1994–1995.[74]

Reduced fiscal assistance from the central government to the states severely affected low-income states that were more dependent on resources from the central government than others. In response to the shrinking fiscal resources from the central government, states had to curtail local health care expenditure. States with high growth rates were able to respond better to the reform and largely reallocated the necessary resources to health.

However, the poorer states, particularly the special-category ones, "have reacted to lower central devolution by reducing their human development expenditure."[75] Medical and public health expenditure per capita disproportionately declined in poorer states such as Bihar, Madhya Pradesh, Rajasthan, Uttar Pradesh, and Orissa.[76] A sharp decline in health budget (from 13.23 percent to 8.13 percent and from 9.63 percent to 6.17 percent, respectively, during 1990–1991 and 1993–1994) was especially observed in Bihar and Orissa.[77]

Given the decentralized investment and spending decisions, political commitment of local governments serves as a critical factor in the level of health care provision in India. Public health was rarely an important topic in election campaigns in most of the Indian states except Tamil Nadu and Kerala.[78] Surviving an election was a concern for local authorities in India, but the main incentive for the local governments in times of economic reforms (even in the present time) is to pursue economic performance at the expense of long-term development planning, let alone health care provision.[79]

Cutbacks on public spending for health at both the central and local government levels are viewed as a precursor to the expansion of privatized and user-paid health care services in both China and India.[80] The collapse of the communes brought about the rapid emergence of private village health stations in rural China.[81] In addition, the dissolution of CMS also meant the elimination of barefoot doctors in China. Without financial support from the communes, many barefoot doctors opted to work full time as farmers because of the introduction of open markets for agricultural crops. Doctors who decided to remain in medicine sought profits to support their salaries and delivery of health care services.[82]

Government spending on rural health care declined but the cost of care was disproportionately surging in China and India.[83] Following the privatization of health care facilities, public sector health providers are expected to generate revenues to cover their operational costs through a 15 percent to 20 percent hike on the wholesale price of drugs.[84] Given such financial incentive, several health professionals prescribe excessive medicine or sell expensive drugs to the patients.[85] Most of the patients in rural China have to foot their own medical bills because of the collapse of the CMS. The absence of medical insurance compensation and the unreasonable increment in health care cost resulted in individual out-of-pocket spending as a share of total health spending augmented from 21 percent to 58 percent between 1900 and 2002.[86]

Unlike in the Chinese health care system, no specific health insurance schemes were available before 2003 for the rural population of India. The state government was supposed to offer low cost or free health services to individuals who could not afford private health care services.[87] However, the health service provided by the public sectors was notorious for poor-quality services, such as substandard sanitation of health centers, shortage of drugs, untrained medical staff, and frequent absenteeism of medical practitioners.[88] In addition, patients were routinely charged for services that were supposed to be free in many states.[89] These problems pushed several well-off individuals toward expensive private doctors, whereas impoverished patients either opted for self-medication or received poor-quality health care services. Poor-quality health services and the effect of the economic reform resulted in a further boom of private hospitals and practices. Considering the limited regulation of the private sector, out-of-pocket payment in India increased from 70 percent in 1987–1988 to over 80 percent in 2002–2003.[90]

Implications for HIV/AIDS in China and India

HIV/AIDS cases were first discovered in the two countries during the mid-1980s, the same period when economic reforms were beginning in China and India. Considering the limited amount of resources at the start of the reforms and the government ambition to "grow fast," Chinese and Indian political leaders viewed economic development as a far more tempting choice over the provision of health care, let alone HIV/AIDS-related treatment and prevention. Perceiving HIV/AIDS simply as one of the traditionally low-priority "medical" or "health" problems in the early years, both governments failed to allocate required resources to tackle the HIV/AIDS problems, thereby resulting in the continuous spread of the epidemic in their respective countries.

As illustrated in chapters 5 and 7 of this book, the prevailing low priority for the HIV/AIDS problems in China and India improved when top-level political leaders declared HIV/AIDS as not only a public health issue but also a problem "linked to economic development…and national security and prosperity."[91] Moreover, the issue "has [also] become one of the most serious socioeconomic and developmental concerns."[92] In other words, the Chinese and Indian leaderships having reframed HIV/AIDS as directly related to economic growth have therefore placed a higher priority on the health care sector. This implies that the public health priority agenda and the budget allocation can be bolstered when the health–economy linkage is established, especially in developing countries where economic policies are always a paramount priority on the government agenda.[93]

Following the introduction of market reforms and privatization of health care, village health clinics in China were comprehensively privatized, and prolonged underfunding was observed in many subcenters in India. Serving as the first contact point between the rural community and the primary health care system, these clinics were expected to promote HIV/AIDS-related campaigns, education, as well as disease monitoring and surveillance. However, health systems paid less attention to the aforementioned non-revenue-generating undertakings in an effort to maintain their operational profits. Thus, infected individuals may unintentionally spread HIV/AIDS to others because they know nothing about the transmission modes nor methods for its prevention. Overlooking the disease surveillance, numbers on people infected with HIV/AIDS were consistently underreported or even unreported by the subnational governments in both countries, thereby causing the loss of the "prime time" to control the HIV/AIDS spread in the early period in China and India.

Most rural people are unwilling to go to clinics because of the upsurge out-of-pocket medical expenses. They would rather take whatever drugs are available on the market to relieve their symptoms. However, these inappropriate practices usually lead to the condition worsening and/or spreading. This scenario is also observed in individuals with HIV/AIDS in rural China and India. However, many infected individuals are possibly not tested and do not know their status.[94] Rather than identifying the disease as HIV/AIDS, they simply name it based on the symptoms, such as "strange illness," "nameless fever," "high fever," or "pneumonia."[95] Individuals infected with HIV/AIDS hence simply take according drugs to relieve these symptoms. Once the disease develops into late-stage AIDS, the affected individuals and their respective families experience further poverty. If the infected person is the breadwinner, then the family bears the very expensive treatment and drugs for the breadwinner's survival.[96] Despite the free HIV/AIDS medication through the HIV/AIDS-specific programs, the medical cost of treating opportunistic infections caused by the weakened immune system is not covered by the programs or government-sponsored insurance schemes.[97] The collapse of the rural public health care system after the economic reforms, to a certain extent, led to the HIV/AIDS spread in China and India.

Summary

This chapter illustrated and compared the evolution of the public health care system in China and India, within a policy environment that prioritized economic performance over social welfare. In particular, it analyzed the impacts of the economic reforms on the health care system and service delivery, and the implications of the HIV/AIDS spread in the two countries. Both the Chinese and Indian governments started with the good intention of providing affordable or free basic health care for rural populations. However, the ideology of "grow-first" redirected policymakers toward more profit-driven objectives. A major reason for this decline was that the Chinese and Indian leaderships have not seen health care as directly related to economic growth and health care, therefore, received a low priority for investment. As a result of this shared priority, health budgets were drastically curtailed in both China and India via the twinned processes of decentralization and privatization. The resulting urban–rural social and economic disparities coupled with the downturn in China's and India's health systems provided a fertile environment for the far greater spread of HIV/AIDS than could have been the case.

Chapter 5

Securitizing HIV/AIDS in China

Introduction

This chapter looks into the development of the HIV/AIDS securitizing moves in China using the securitization process model constructed in chapter 2. With the absence of positive speech acts and a full set of emergency measures, this chapter argues that the HIV/AIDS securitizing move largely failed in the early years in China. Given the seriousness of the HIV/AIDS problem and the increase in the awareness and commitment of the Chinese government to the disease, the HIV/AIDS securitizing move has been dramatically transformed in recent years. This chapter contends that a full securitizing move has been generated since 2004, with the presence of explicit positive speech acts plus all three subcategories of emergency measures in its political reaction. This chapter also shows that such a level of securitizing move has been maintained and even strengthened in China to date.

An illustration of the historical and current overview of the HIV/AIDS epidemic in China is presented first to offer a general background of the HIV/AIDS problem in the country. The development of HIV/AIDS in China has been simplified into three phases, namely introduction phase (1985–1988), spreading phase (1989–1994), and expansion phase (1995–present). Using the framework structured in chapter 2, HIV/AIDS-related political responses are analyzed chronologically; thus, the shift from failed to full securitizing move is demonstrated. The HIV/AIDS policy analysis offered in this chapter attempts to generate a comprehensive picture of the policy-making process within the Chinese government.

Overview of the HIV/AIDS Epidemic in China

Introduction Phase (1985–1988)

The first HIV/AIDS case was identified in an American tourist in Beijing in 1985.[1] Subsequently, four Chinese hemophiliac patients in Zhejiang, who received treatment with Factor VIII supplied by the United States Armour Pharmaceutical Company, were infected with HIV/AIDS.[2] Between 1985 and 1988, 11 HIV-positive individuals and three late-stage AIDS patients were reported in China,[3] and they were either foreigners or overseas-Chinese who had returned.[4] In 1989, the first local Chinese HIV-positive individual was then recorded. Based on newspaper reports, the infected person was a shop assistant in Beijing who had homosexual relations with foreigners.[5] Given that the early HIV/AIDS infections in China were viewed as foreign or imported cases, Zeng Yi, vice president of the Chinese Academy of Preventive Medical Sciences, assured that China had no sources for HIV/AIDS.[6] However, his claim was then disproved when the outbreak of HIV/AIDS was reported among 146 Chinese heroin users in Dehong in Yunnan Province in late 1989.[7]

Spreading Phase (1989–1994)

The first indigenous cases of HIV/AIDS infection were identified and concentrated among 146 IDUs near Ruili, Yunnan in 1989.[8] With increased drug availability along the Chinese borders and its penetration into the province, drug abuse and HIV/AIDS problems rose concurrently and dramatically across Yunnan and other Chinese provinces. Between 1989 and 1990, HIV/AIDS spread to IDUs beyond Yunnan's borders to the neighboring cities, and along the major heroin trafficking routes to Guangxi, Xinjiang, Sichuan, Guangdong, and other Chinese provinces.[9] Despite the widespread prevalence of the disease in other provinces and cities, more than 80 percent of China's HIV/AIDS infection was concentrated in Yunnan due to the higher proportion of IDU population in this province.[10] The total HIV/AIDS infected population in China rose to 194, including 153 Chinese citizens and 41 foreign residents, by the end of 1989.[11]

IDUs accounted for 100 percent of reported HIV/AIDS cases in China in 1989.[12] However, the HIV/AIDS outbreak was observed in former blood plasma donors in the east-central provinces of China in the mid-1990s.[13] Five provinces, including Henan, Hebei, Hubei, Anhui, and Shaanxi, accounted for 80.4 percent of HIV/AIDS infections among

69,000 commercial blood sellers and recipients of blood and blood products in 2005.[14] Understanding this particular mode of transmission in China is critically important because HIV/AIDS started spreading rampantly through blood selling with unhygienic re-transfusion of red blood cells in China.[15] However, only in mid-2000 did the problem receive wide international and a certain level of central government's attention to the "AIDS villages" (*aizibing cun*) in central China after Journalist Elizabeth Rosenthal wrote several articles about the malpractice of blood and plasma collection in Henan.[16]

The first local HIV/AIDS infections among plasma donors were reported in 1995.[17] It was suggested that the plasma donors were infected by HIV/AIDS between 1994 and 1996; however, the number of infected individuals peaked in 1995.[18] By the end of 2006, the number of confirmed HIV-positive individuals was 35,232, with 75.3 percent of the infections attributed to commercial plasma donations.[19] An unofficial survey estimated that as many as one million people in Henan were infected with HIV/AIDS through unhygienic and unregulated blood collection in the 1990s.[20]

Expansion Phase (1995–Present)

In the past decades, the HIV/AIDS infection in China has been associated with the high risk groups such as IDUs and former plasma donors in geographically peripheral disparate regions. In recent years, these two modes of HIV/AIDS transmission have been under control. Despite the improvement, HIV/AIDS infections via IDU are still prevalent in peripheral provinces due to the proximity of the Golden Triangle.

Sexual transmission (both heterosexual and homosexual), surpassing IDU, and blood selling have become the main routes of HIV/AIDS transmission in China. In 2011, approximately 48,000 new HIV/AIDS infections were reported in the country.[21] Among these new cases, nearly 82 percent of those were transmitted via sexual contact, including over 29 percent via homosexual transmission.[22] The HIV/AIDS infections via homosexual transmission were particularly more serious in some urban areas. Based on the 2011 figures, the HIV/AIDS prevalence among MSM population is almost 10 percent in the urban cities such as Chengdu and 20 percent in some southwestern cities.[23]

Aside from the HIV/AIDS infection among the homosexual population, an upsurge in the number of infections via unprotected sexual contact was also found among senior men (aged 50 years and above)[24] and male college students (aged between 20 and 24 years) in recent years.[25]

The number of HIV-positive senior Chinese men surged from 483 in 2005 to 3,031 in 2010;[26] meanwhile, 1,252 students (21 percent of the total number of students being tested) were found to be HIV-positive between January and October 2011.[27]

The estimated number of HIV-positive individuals is 780,000 by the year 2012.[28] Based on the definition of the WHO, China is a low prevalence state, with an HIV/AIDS prevalence of 0.1 percent.[29] Despite the low prevalence rate, the HIV/AIDS problems are concentrated in some geographical areas, including Yunnan, Guangxi, Henan, Sichuan, Henan, Xinjiang, Guangdong, Chongqing, Hunan, and Guizhou.[30] These provinces account for 79 percent of the total HIV/AIDS cases in the country.[31]

Development of the HIV/AIDS Securitizing Move in China

Having discussed the historical and current HIV/AIDS situations in China, the development of HIV-related political reactions enacted by the national government are illustrated. Using the lens of the securitization framework, the HIV/AIDS policy development can be divided into four stages: (1) failed securitizing move between 1985 and 1994; (2) performative securitizing move from 1995 to 2000; (3) rhetorical securitizing move between 2001 and mid-2003; and (4) full securitizing move from 2004 onward. In each stage, the perceptions of the government toward HIV/AIDS and their political responses are explained at length.

Failed Securitizing Move (1985–1994)

As previously mentioned, early HIV/AIDS reported cases were primarily contracted overseas or by imported blood products.[32] Hence, the PRC government held a relatively hostile view of the disease, as HIV/AIDS was regarded as the consequence of favoring Western liberalism and capitalism over socialism.[33] In addition, the Chinese authorities also believed that there could only be a very limited spread of the virus in the country, and thus the Chinese would not be infected,[34] arguing that "homosexuality and promiscuity... are limited in China because they run counter to public opinion, moral standards and laws."[35] In this regard, the Chinese government perceived HIV/AIDS as a foreigner disease with a prejudiced view and without considering it as a security threat to the nation. Hence, speech acts uttered by the political leaders were largely negative in the early years.

Rather than containing the virus, the Chinese government reacted to the problem by cracking down on prostitution, drug smuggling and drug addiction, and banning imported blood products.[36] In particular, the government barely had an emergency measure related to the prevention of and treatment for HIV/AIDS-infected IDUs. Drug trafficking and drug abuse are illegal in China. Chinese law stipulates that offenders may be sentenced to prison if they smuggle ten grams or more of heroin, and could receive the death penalty for smuggling more than 50 grams of heroin.[37]

Aside from the legal aspect against drugs, drug abuse has long been considered as a "social evil" in the eyes of Chinese officials.[38] Before the foundation of PRC in 1949, there were over 20 million opium abusers—five percent of the total population at that time—in China due to the abundant availability of Indian opium after the first and second Opium Wars. In this regard, strict measures were implemented by the 1949 PRC government to eradicate illegal drug abuse through national antidrug campaigns (1950–1952).[39]

The Chinese government was slow in implementing HIV/AIDS prevention and control measures for HIV/AIDS-infected IDUs because of the illicit nature and officials' hostile perception of drug problems.[40] Accordingly, the Methadone Maintenance Treatment (MMT) and Needle Syringe Program (NSP) were nearly nonexistent after the first outbreak of HIV/AIDS among IDUs in 1989. The government eventually grappled with the drug problems by launching the harm reduction program from 2004 onward.

With regard to the mode of political reaction, HIV/AIDS was largely managed in a nonemergency mode with the absence of budget allocation for HIV/AIDS interventions. In terms of emergency measures related to policy and institutional arrangement, the Ministry of Public Health and Customs officials swiftly banned the importation of blood products and strengthened the Customs inspection of people entering China after the initial HIV/AIDS cases were announced in 1985.[41] HIV/AIDS was then listed as one of the country's major infectious diseases in 1986.[42] In the same year, the *Frontier Health and Quarantine Law of the People's Republic of China* was issued, aiming to prohibit individuals carrying infectious diseases such as HIV/AIDS from entering China.[43] The National AIDS Committee was also set up, and the National Program for HIV/AIDS Prevention and Control was launched by the Committee in 1987.[44]

The formulation of HIV/AIDS-related legislation was then observed. The first national set of regulations particularly on the prevention and control of HIV/AIDS—*Regulations Concerning the Monitoring and Control of AIDS*—was promulgated in January 1988.[45] The regulation states that individuals entering China must fill out a health form; individuals who intend to stay in China for more than one year must submit an HIV/AIDS negative certificate; and HIV/AIDS-contaminated blood and blood products are prohibited from being imported to China.[46]

The *Law of Infectious Diseases Prevention and Control* of 1989 that declared HIV/AIDS to be a notifiable disease was then issued in October 1991.[47] Under this law, diagnosed HIV/AIDS cases should be reported to the local health authority within six hours in cities and 12 hours in the countryside. The law also requires HIV/AIDS-infected individuals to be quarantined, and their name and address should be reported.[48] However, the aforementioned laws regarding isolation and quarantine of HIV/AIDS infected people were ineffective in halting the spread of the disease in China.[49] The early measures were only intended to cease the entry of HIV-positive people or blood products, but not the virus itself.

Instead of addressing HIV/AIDS, government officials largely responded to the problem by criminalizing drug use and drug trafficking as stated in the *Decision of the Standing Committee of the National People's Congress on the Prohibition of Narcotic Drugs* in 1990.[50] This government actuation palpably affirmed the absence of positive speech acts and a full set of emergency measures. Hence, political reactions toward HIV/AIDS failed to advance securitizing moves.

A significant shift with regard to HIV/AIDS securitizing moves has been identified since December 1994, as the Chinese authorities were among the 42 state-representatives who signed the Paris Declaration at the International AIDS Summit.[51] The 1994 declaration called for political commitment and obligation of the national governments to address HIV/AIDS problems by formulating national HIV/AIDS-related policies in the respective countries.[52] Since then, significant progress has been made in China in terms of budget allocation, policy and institutional arrangement, and legislative formation, albeit the absence of a positive rhetorical act. Thus, HIV/AIDS securitizing move has shifted from failed to performative version since 1995.

Performative Securitizing Move (1995–1999)

Performative securitizing moves toward HIV/AIDS issues were observed in China from 1995 to 1999. Unlike in the previous period, this period saw the implementation of a full set of emergency measures as evidenced by budget reprioritization, new institutional arrangement, and legislation formulation. Regarding the emergency responses in the financial aspect, the Ministry of Finance set up a special fund for HIV/AIDS prevention and control in 1996, with the initial contribution of five million yuan[53] (approximately US$0.8 million).[54] This special funding was augmented to 15 million yuan (US$2 million) in 1998, and the amount remained stable between 1998 and 2000.[55]

The Chinese government also formulated several laws and regulations related to HIV/AIDS prevention and control. To decide the focus of the HIV/AIDS policy, the *Recommendations on Strengthening AIDS Prevention and Control* was issued by the State Council and the Ministry of Health in 1995.[56] In the following year, the *Regulations on the Management of Blood Production* based on the *Law of the People's Republic of China on the Prevention and Control of Infectious Diseases* was then released by the Ministry of Health,[57] due to the sharp increase in HIV/AIDS cases among commercial plasma donors in central China in the early 1990s. This regulation stipulates the rules for plasma collection and the importance of blood testing at the collection sites and processing factories.[58] Blood-related legislation was strengthened in the *Law on Blood Donation* issued in 1998, which states that all blood collected for transfusion should be from voluntary donors.[59]

Aside from these laws and regulations on HIV/AIDS interventions, the national government also stipulated the regulation of the *Responsibilities of Ministries and Departments of State in AIDS Control and Prevention* in 1997 to mobilize all government departments and sectors to participate in HIV/AIDS prevention and control programs.[60] On top of the formulation of new laws and regulations, new institutional arrangements regarding HIV/AIDS interventions were made as well. The State Council AIDS Coordinating Committee was set up in 1998.[61] This interministerial body, chaired by the vice premier Li Lanqing, aimed at coordinating 34 ministry and department officials to put forth a national campaign against HIV/AIDS in China.[62] This committee thereafter outlined an HIV/AIDS-related legal framework called the *National Long and Medium Term Plan for Preventing and Controlling the Spread of HIV/AIDS (1998–2010)* in 1998. Under the 1998 framework, a new institution—National Center for AIDS/STD Control and Prevention (NCAIDS)—was thus established in July 2001.[63]

Despite the fact that the national government laid down its emergency measures and mandated the financial, institutional, and legal departments to implement them, the Chinese government took 13 years (from 1985 to 1998) to formulate the blueprint for the HIV/AIDS prevention and control strategy; meanwhile, 37 percent of all governments around the world had a pertinent plan in place within 18 months after the first case was discovered.[64] In addition, the committee had difficulties coordinating with separate ministries due to the lack of political commitment. The committee members have met only four times since its establishment in 1998.[65]

Aside from the relative lack of political will in responding to the health threat, legislative inconsistency and bureaucratic resistance have also undermined the performative securitizing moves. That the criminalization of drug use was further reinforced with the enactment of antidrug laws—*Procedures for Compulsory Drug Addiction Rehabilitation*—in 1995, illuminated the former problem.[66] The latter issue was seen in 1999. The State Family Planning Commission broadcasted new television advertisements promoting condom use to prevent HIV/AIDS infections. However, the State Administration for Industry and Commerce stopped the broadcast the next day.[67] The commission was accused of violating the law by advertising sex-related products.

Overall, performative securitizing moves toward HIV/AIDS issues were observed in China during this period. Arguably, however, emergency measures for HIV/AIDS interventions were largely ineffective due to the lack of budget, weak political commitment, and poor policy coordination within different government departments. Furthermore, similar to the previous period, positive speech acts were largely absent in China in times of this period. Ramiah asserted that the Chinese leadership was extremely reluctant to speak or acknowledge HIV/AIDS as a national problem before 2004.[68] However, the latter section shows that the Chinese authorities have started to rhetorically acknowledge the HIV/AIDS problem in the international meeting since 2000. However, considering that a full set of emergency measures did not follow the rhetorical speech acts, the HIV/AIDS securitizing move remained rhetorical.

Rhetorical Securitizing Move (2000–2003)

The HIV/AIDS problem in China was brought to the brink of full securitizing move in 2000. Participating in an international meeting, President Jiang Zemin broke the Chinese government's silence on HIV/AIDS, and admitted that the disease was not solely a health problem, urging for more prevention and control of the epidemic at both domestic and international levels:

> I fully agree with you that HIV/AIDS is **much more than a health problem**. We shall **never underestimate the impact of the disease on families, communities, and even the whole society**. The Chinese government **attaches great importance** to the prevention and control of HIV/AIDS and has been **waging a nationwide campaign against the epidemic**. [emphasis added][69]

After the president's positive speech act in 2001, several "first time" events related to HIV/AIDS in China took place: HIV/AIDS patients' testimonials and stories, a TV drama about an HIV-positive businessman, and a radio announcement related to safe sex were broadcasted. The Chinese government and international drug companies entered into a negotiation for the price reduction of HIV/AIDS drugs.[70] Most importantly, the Chinese government publicly admitted that the widespread prevalence of HIV/AIDS in Henan was mainly due to plasma selling. For HIV/AIDS infection via unsafe blood selling in Henan has been a sensitive issue in the eye of the Chinese government, the acknowledgment was viewed as the most outstanding breakthrough in this period of time. Following the acknowledgment, a total of 950 million yuan (US$115 million) was allocated to rebuild more than 250 blood banks in 20 central and western provinces and autonomous regions.[71]

However, the HIV/AIDS securitizing move was considerably rhetorical because of the absence of a full set of emergency measures that was in line with Jiang's positive speech act. New policy and institutional arrangements were largely absent after Jiang's rhetorical claim, with the exception of a dramatic augmentation of HIV/AIDS-related budget and the formulation of a legal framework for HIV/AIDS interventions. The central government funding for HIV/AIDS interventions was increased from 100 million yuan[72] (US$17 million) in 2001 to 390 million yuan[73] (US$73 million) in 2003. Regarding the legislation formulation, *China's Action Plan for Reducing and Preventing the Spread of HIV/AIDS (2001–2005)* was enacted by the State Council AIDS Coordinating Committee in 2001.[74] This national-level legal framework specifically required the subnational governments to provide HIV/AIDS-related prevention and treatment services in their respective jurisdictions.[75]

The HIV/AIDS securitizing move was further developed due to the devastating SARS epidemic and the formation of the new government chaired by President Hu Jintao and Premier Wen Jiabao in March 2003. Positive speech acts related to HIV/AIDS reflected the recognition of the seriousness of the HIV/AIDS situation:

> Hu: HIV/AIDS prevention, care and treatment is a **major issue pertinent to the quality and prosperity of the Chinese nation.** [emphasis added][76]
>
> Wen: Dealing with HIV/AIDS as an **urgent and major issue** is related to the fundamental interests of the whole Chinese nation. [emphasis added][77]

Gao Qiang, the executive vice minister of Health, further expressed the official proposition on the HIV/AIDS issue:

> HIV/AIDS is a **common enemy of the whole mankind** as it **seriously threatens public health and safety.** The Chinese government has attached

great importance to HIV/AIDS prevention and treatment and has treated it as a **strategic issue** for social stability, economic development, **national prosperity and security**, making it a **first priority** of the government work. [emphasis added][78]

The Chinese top-level political leaders also physically demonstrated their commitment toward HIV/AIDS interventions on World AIDS Day in 2003. Premier Wen Jiabao and Vice Premier Wu Yi visited HIV/AIDS-infected individuals at Ditan Hospital in Beijing. Vice Premier Wu also visited infected people in Wenlou, Shangcai village in Henan.[79]

Having recognized the health threat posed by HIV/AIDS, political leaders likewise translated their positive speech acts into pragmatic actions. With the financial assistance of the Global Fund and other international funding agencies, the government launched a five-year (from 2003 to 2008) China Comprehensive AIDS Response Program (China CARES) in early 2003 to contain the spread of HIV/AIDS and mitigate its impact on the country.[80] Based on the HIV/AIDS prevalence, 127 sites in 28 provinces were selected to implement local-specific HIV/AIDS intervention activities in the target project sites that covered 83.3 million people.[81] Positive outcomes were achieved in this five-year national HIV/AIDS program. Between 2003 and 2008, there was a 67 percent increment in the number of people who underwent tests for HIV/AIDS; 23,000 individuals enrolled in ARV treatment and 93 percent of HIV-infected pregnant women received preventing mother to child transmission (PMTCT) through the China CARES program.[82]

The aforementioned positive speech acts were reinforced by other positive outcomes such as the upsurge in the budget allocation for the HIV/AIDS programs. Aside from the government's original commitment of 120 million yuan (US$19 million) to the HIV/AIDS programs, an extra 270 million yuan (US$42 million) was allocated to China CARES to provide free ART, care, and support in HIV/AIDS hard-hit areas.[83] Prior to the China CARES program, around 100 people had access to ART,[84] and HIV/AIDS drugs were limited to a few coastal cities of the country.[85] The additional financial allocation resulted in the increase in the number of people receiving free ART, from 100 in 2001 to 5,000 in 2003.[86] However, a full securitizing move was presumed to have been generated only after 2004 because of the explicit speech acts given by the government, increase in budget allocation, and the institutional and legal formulation in relation to the HIV/AIDS threat.

Full Securitizing Move (from 2004 Onward)

In 2004, China's HIV/AIDS prevention and control policies were restated in the *State Council Notice on Strengthening HIV/AIDS Prevention and*

Control, which is also known as State Council Document Number 7. This document explicitly frames the HIV/AIDS problem in China as a security issue:

> HIV/AIDS prevention and control is linked to economic development, social stability, and **national security and prosperity**. **Long-term commitment to respond to HIV/AIDS is hence necessary**. [emphasis added][87]

In late 2010, China's HIV/AIDS prevention and control policies were further strengthened in the *State Council Notice on Further Strengthening HIV/AIDS Prevention and Control* (State Council Document No. 48). Resembling the previous Document No. 7 enacted in 2004, positive speech acts were identified in this latter document:

> HIV/AIDS prevention and control is linked to health condition of the people, economic development, **national security** and **prosperity**. The Chinese Communist Party and the State Council **have attached great importance** to HIV/AIDS prevention and treatment. [emphasis added][88]

In addition to positive speech acts, a full set of emergency measures has been formulated from 2004 onward, which is illuminated as follows:

Budgetary Allocation

There has been a substantial increase in financial allocation to the national responses to HIV/AIDS in China. The national budget for HIV/AIDS interventions was raised from US$2 million in 2000 to US$126 million in 2004. In 2011, the budget has reached to US$293 million.[89] Continuous budgetary allocation for HIV/AIDS interventions is also promising, as the national government has included HIV/AIDS testing, education, and drug coverage measures in the country's Twelfth Five-Year Plan (2011–2015).[90] The provision of ARV drugs has been further enhanced since 2004. The number of HIV/AIDS-infected adults receiving free ARV drugs increased from 5,000 in 2003 to around 15,000 in 2004 and over 130,000 in 2011.[91]

Policy and Institutional Arrangement

National and local leaders started to formulate HIV/AIDS-related institutional arrangements. In early 2004, the State Council AIDS Working Committee (SCAWC) was set up to replace the previous committee that was established in 1998.[92] SCAWC is the primary body in charge of national HIV/AIDS policymaking in China.[93] Headed by Vice Premier and Minister of Health Wu Yi, the committee consists of vice-ministers from 29 key ministries and organizations, as well as the vice-governors of the seven provinces mostly affected by HIV/AIDS, including Guangdong, Guangxi, Henan, Hubei, Sichuan, Xinjiang, and Yunnan. In addition, two of the major national policies were formulated in 2004, namely the Four Free and One Care Policy,[94] and also harm reduction program.[95]

In the harm reduction program, drug addiction treatment and needle and syringe exchange are provided freely through the MMT program and the NSP respectively. Launching the needle exchange program was sanctioned by the Ministry of Public Security because such strategies give the appearance of encouraging drug abuse. However, the Chinese government overcame this implementation obstacle by changing the name of the program to "needle social marketing." This program aims to advance the commercial availability and accessibility of needles, and provides free needles and information regarding safe injecting practices.[96]

HIV/AIDS-Related Legislation

The Standing Committee of the National People's Congress (NPC) passed the revised version of the *Law on Communicable Diseases Prevention and Control* in August 2004,[97] stipulating that the government should strengthen HIV/AIDS prevention and control measures.[98] In addition, the clause, "individual blood collection is banned," was added to the infectious disease prevention and control law, showing the government's acknowledgement of the rampant HIV/AIDS spread in the central province of Henan.[99] Another clause stating that the "state offers free medical treatment for impoverished infectious disease patients" was also included in the revised law, highlighting the importance of protecting the legal rights of infected individuals to receive free HIV/AIDS-related medical treatment and care.[100]

Most importantly, the revised law marked the first time that China targeted HIV/AIDS issues in national legislation.[101] These effects also added an independent clause on HIV/AIDS prevention in infectious disease and control law.[102] The clause states that "governments at all levels must strengthen HIV/AIDS prevention and control work in a bid to curb further spread of the disease. Detailed measures could be stipulated by the State Council."[103] In other words, the law entrusts a higher body—the State Council—to stipulate regulations on HIV/AIDS prevention and control measures. This sea change implies that HIV/AIDS has been prioritized in the national agenda, and the disease is no longer framed as a public health problem that solely requires the response from the Ministry of Health. Rather, the epidemic has been framed as a national security problem that has impacted on economic development, social stability, national security, and prosperity, calling for collaboration and cooperation at all government levels. The Chinese government has revised the 1988 *Certain Regulations on the Monitoring and Control of AIDS* to remove the ban on foreigners entering the country with HIV/AIDS since April 2010.[104] The removal of the travel ban implies the government attitude to abate stigma and discrimination toward HIV/AIDS-infected individuals. Furthermore, the government showed its anti-HIV/AIDS discrimination stance when Premier Wen Jiabao announced in December 2011 that existing laws and regulations that naturally discriminate against HIV/AIDS individuals should be amended.[105]

In 2011, the Ministry of Civil Affairs started revising the law regarding the registration of civil society groups in China. The ministry pledges that the revised law will help civil society groups register more easily in China, as they will be able to register at the local department of civil affairs without the prior approval of a "supervisory body."[106] The revision of the law on social organization registration also shows the political commitment of the national government by supporting the civil society organizations' participation in national HIV/AIDS intervention programs. Based on these laws and amendments on the regulations, the national government is deemed to have put considerable efforts to alleviate HIV/AIDS stigma and discrimination, as well as support HIV/AIDS-related civil society organizations in participating in national HIV/AIDS control and prevention undertakings.

The previous sections of this chapter showed that full HIV/AIDS securitizing moves have by and large prevailed within the Chinese government since 2004. In the full securitizing move, the Chinese government has established a link between the HIV/AIDS problem and health condition of the people, economic development, national security, and prosperity.[107] Such linkage changed the face of HIV/AIDS; now it is treated differently from other infectious diseases and health issues. For instance, since 2003, top-level Chinese leaders have made high-profile visits to HIV/AIDS patients every year; since 2004, free ARV drugs have been administered to HIV/AIDS-infected individuals, as well as free education to "HIV/AIDS orphans" through the Four Free and One Care Policy; and the State-Council level institution and HIV/AIDS-specific legislation were formulated in 2004 and 2006, respectively. Such political commitment toward HIV/AIDS problems was further confirmed by a government official in the Ministry of Health [R37]: "The Chinese government allocates financial, political, and human resources...Societal mobilization [civil society participation] is the most extensive one amongst other diseases."[108] Despite the national government's support, resistance is still felt at the subnational level. The following section highlights the fact that bureaucratic resistance at the local level compromises the positive effect of the full HIV/AIDS securitizing moves in China.

Emerging Issue: Bureaucratic Resistance to Full HIV/AIDS Securitizing Moves in China

Despite these proactive political measures in the course of full securitizing moves, local bureaucratic resistance to the implementation of national policies arguably exists side by side with the positive scenarios. Bernhard Schwartlander, UNAIDS country coordinator, commented that China needs to take the response to HIV/AIDS to the provincial, county, and community levels and "translate policies into action."[109] Subinay Nandy, UNDP China Country Director, cited some "inconsistencies" in China between regulations, and "divergences" between national and provincial laws, and between laws and their application, especially at the local level.[110] Taken together, the implementation of national policy measures and regulations, to a certain extent, is problematic at the subnational levels in China.

The implementation of the Four Free and One Care Policy enacted by the national government has encountered problems at the provincial and local levels. A respondent working in an INGO [R8] noted that "the policy is very good and effective; however, since every province and city is different in terms of their economic and epidemiological situation, implementation level is varied in different parts of China."[111] Another respondent [R7] commented on the variation in the policy implementation level: "Local governments in Beijing and Shanghai may have better policy implementation, but the level of implementation is problematic in remote areas."[112]

Taking Henan as an example, the implementation of the Four Free and One Care Policy in the province showed that the national policy had not been properly carried out and had been distorted by local government officials. The Henan government promised to deliver monthly coupons worth between US$12 and US$36 to cover the medical cost of the peasants living in Shangcai.[113] In addition, families experiencing economic hardship were exempted from paying agricultural tax.[114] However, local officials took away aid money and resources from the people in need.[115] More seriously, the farmers living in Xiongqiao were compelled by the local authorities to pay the tax, and were charged about US$ 3 per month for the "free" drugs delivered under the Four Free and One Care program.[116]

The chairperson of a local NGO [R31] put forward a reason for the discrepancy in policy implementation at the local level: "Policy is abstract, so the local government can easily ignore its duties."[117] Dr. Gao Qi of the Chinese University of Hong Kong further explained this point, stating the following: "The definition of 'One Care' is too vague. The original idea of the central government is to request the local government to provide care and support to HIV/AIDS infected individuals. However, there is no standard to measure whether the level of 'Care' is sufficient. Thus, different outcomes turn out in different places. For some local officials, they do not care about the patients as the officials will not get a promotion or an increase in GDP in their jurisdictions for caring for HIV/AIDS-infected people."[118]

Instead of receiving care from the local governments, HIV/AIDS-infected individuals and their family members were badly treated by the local officials. In Henan, due to the myriad cases of HIV/AIDS infection, the courts in this province refused to take the cases relating to HIV/AIDS.[119] Having no medical care and given the courts' refusal to their cases, HIV/AIDS infected people and their families usually attempted to make a petition—a system that was granted to seek justice from high-level authorities—requesting treatment.[120] Aside from seeking treatment, the villagers also petitioned to seek compensation for acquiring the disease from the local government-run hospitals, clinics, or blood collection stations.

The petitioning system is related to the official civic service evaluation system, in which subnational governments are subject to bureaucratic penalties if large numbers of petitioners from particular areas gather in Beijing.[121] In this regard, the local officials, with the help of public security authorities, imposed house arrest on potential petitioners to prevent them from leaving the village and leveling their charges to the NPC.[122]

Even if the petitioners escaped arrest and arrived in Beijing, they were likely to be locked up in "black jails" or "black houses" for days or months. These black jails were used to detain petitioners who come to Beijing, and were located inside state-owned hotels, nursing homes, and psychiatric hospitals.[123] Additionally, these secret jails in Beijing were purportedly run by the officials of Henan.[124]

Aside from Henan, bureaucratic resistance to HIV/AIDS-related measures had also been recognized in other peripheral areas of the country. For instance, reports revealed that both current and former drug users were humiliated by public security officials in Kunming. The police detained drug users, denied them access to such services as MMT and NSP, and put them in drug rehabilitation centers where they were neither provided drug-dependency treatment nor HIV/AIDS prevention or treatment service.[125]

Acts of humiliation were also observed among HIV/AIDS-focused NGOs helping drug users in Kunming. It was reported that an IDU activist was detained by the police in Kunming who compelled him to undergo a urine test in 2009.[126]

Bureaucratic resistance to HIV/AIDS-specific activities is observed not only in the peripheral areas, but also in economically developed cities such as Shanghai. Shanghai is deemed to be the leading city in China to positively address HIV/AIDS problems among the MSM community. In 2009, the city hosted the country's first gay pride festival—Shanghai Pride 2009. The state media *China Daily* described the event as having "profound significance" to and "a showcase" of the social progress in China.[127] However, the organizers of the festival were told by the municipal public security bureau to cancel two film screenings at a local bar because the venue lacked licenses to stage films.[128] Similar stories of homosexual events that were ceased by the local authorities did repeat in the subsequent year. The nation's first public homosexual beauty pageant—Mr. Gay China Pageant—originally held in January 2010, was then cancelled at the last minute due to inadequate documents.[129] Furthermore, in April 2011, the municipal public security bureau detained 60 patrons and employees at a gay bar in Shanghai without explanation for the arrest.[130]

After all, the national government has reacted positively and staunchly toward the HIV/AIDS infection via blood selling in Henan, and apparently exhibited more tolerance to homosexuality and injecting drug use due to the fear over the spread of HIV/AIDS among MSM and IDUs. Nonetheless, the local authorities have their own ways to execute the policies that compromise the constructive effects of national measures on HIV/AIDS control and prevention.

In China, the fully operated HIV/AIDS securitizing move at the national level, as previously illustrated, can be compromised by bureaucratic practices at the local level. Curley argued that bureaucrats have the power to "railroad, slow down, and thwart the securitizing policies and directives of elites,"[131] and their capacity and compliance to a large extent can affect the outcome of such extraordinary policies. Bureaucratic incapacity can be accounted for scarce human and financial resources as well as poor administrative and management skills, which "impede the bureaucracies' ability to 'follow through' with the securitizing decision of political elites."[132] Having the capacity does not guarantee the emergency measure implementation; genuine compliance is another vital factor to look into. Indeed, a popular Chinese proverb captures the idea of this notion: *Shang you zheng ce, xia you dui ce* (The local governments have their own ways to implement the policy made by the central government). Local officials may have the capacity to work out the policy, but when the central policy conflicts with the interests of the local government, the latter may instead execute the program in its own ways to safeguard its interests, thereby altering the main tenets of the emergency policy from the national government.[133] This condition implies that although the securitizers, especially in a nondemocratic political system, possess "important resources and sources of authority"[134] that give them considerable political power to initiate a securitizing move, the securitizing agents are likely to encounter difficulties and obstructions to deliver the securitizing move at the local level without winning the active cooperation of bureaucrats.

Summary

The first HIV/AIDS case in China was reported in Beijing in 1985. Since then the epidemic has spread throughout the country. The development of HIV/AIDS epidemic over the decades has been divided into three phases: introduction phase (1985–1988), spreading phase (1989–1994), and expansion phase (1995–present). In the introduction phase, HIV/AIDS infections were mostly found among the foreign nationals and later Chinese haemophiliac patients. The spreading phase was marked by a large number of localized HIV/AIDS infections in the southwest and central part of China, among IDUs and former plasma donors. HIV/AIDS epidemic has been spreading in China since the mid-1990s. Unlike the mode of infections in previous phases, unprotected sexual contact has now become the main route of HIV/AIDS transmission in China.

Over the past decades, the Chinese government has made tremendous efforts to contain the spread of the epidemic after years of denying the problem of HIV/AIDS in the country. Political commitment is evident in the utterance of the seriousness of HIV/AIDS, as well as the implementation of HIV/AIDS national policies in different periods of time. Using the revised securitization framework constructed in chapter 2, this chapter aims to analyze the evolution of the national HIV/AIDS policies in China. National responses toward the epidemic have been divided into four stages: failed securitizing move (1985–1994), performative securitizing move (1995–1999), rhetorical securitizing move (2000–2003), and full securitizing move (from 2004 onward).

In the early period, the Chinese government held a negative perception on the epidemic, and believed that HIV/AIDS was only a foreign disease. Thus, the speech acts uttered by the political leaders at that time were largely negative. Regarding the policy response to the epidemic, financial commitment to support HIV/AIDS programs was not fully recognized; thus, there was no full set of emergency measures. Without positive speech acts and a full set of emergency responses, the securitizing move undoubtedly failed in the early period. Early national policies were also deemed to be ineffective to halt the spread of the epidemic, because HIV/AIDS-related policies were primarily about restricting the entry of HIV/AIDS individuals into China and criminalizing drug use and narcotics trafficking.

This chapter demonstrated that a full securitizing move toward HIV/AIDS has developed since 2004. Positive speech acts were identified, and the top-level leaders linked HIV/AIDS problems to economic wellbeing, social stability, and national security and prosperity.[135] Rhetorical security acts have been expeditiously translated into performative acts as well. In other words, the political reaction is now operated within an emergency mode. A full set of emergency measures, including a significant increase in the financial support for the HIV/AIDS-related policies, formulation of HIV/AIDS-related policies and institutions, and establishment of its related legislation, have been implemented since 2004.

Having illuminated the presence of positive speech acts and emergency measures post-2004, this chapter showed that the 2004 full securitizing move has been continued within the Chinese government, that is, the HIV/AIDS issue is still perceived as a top-priority issue in the national government agenda, with scale-up efforts in terms of budgetary allocation, policy and institutional arrangement, and legislation. However, the bureaucratic resistance prevailing at the local level may inevitably compromise the constructive influence of full HIV/AIDS securitizing moves in China.

Chapter 6

Audience Acceptance in China: Case Studies in Beijing, Shanghai, and Kunming

Introduction

Based on the revised securitization framework, a securitizing move was generated by the utterance of positive or negative speech acts and the performance of political measures within emergency or nonemergency modes. The development of HIV/AIDS securitizing moves in China could be divided into four phases: failed securitizing move (1985–1994); performative securitizing move (1995–1999); rhetorical securitizing move (2000–2003); and full securitizing move (from 2004 onward). With the presence of positive speech acts (+SA) and a full set of emergency measures (+EM), the previous chapter also revealed that the 2004 securitizing move had been sustained in the national government to date.

With regard to positive speech acts in recent years, the national government announced in 2010 that "HIV/AIDS prevention and control is linked to health condition of the people, economic development, national security, and prosperity. The Chinese Communist Party and the State Council have attached great importance to HIV/AIDS prevention and treatment."[1] Hence, HIV/AIDS was framed as a top-priority issue via speech acts uttered by top-level Chinese leaders.

The national government had reacted and was reacting to the HIV/AIDS problem within an emergency mode (+EM), with scale-up efforts in terms of budgetary allocation, policy and institutional arrangement (e.g., Four Free and One Care Policy and State Council-level HIV/AIDS Committee), and legislation (e.g., *Regulation on AIDS Prevention and Control*). The form of HIV/AIDS securitizing move that prevailed from 2004 onward was simplified as follows:[2]

(+SA) + (+EM) → Full securitizing move

Identifying the type of securitizing move, however, was only the halfway stage of studying securitization. As stated in securitization theory, the securitizing move produced by the policy makers would ultimately turn to securitization once it was accepted by the designated audience. Defined in the revised framework in chapter 2, "audience acceptance" referred to the *support of the audience toward a securitizing move*. The idea of "support" was composed of two dimensions: *moral* support and *technical* support. Moral support indicated the extent to which the audience held the same perceptions on HIV/AIDS as the securitizer; meanwhile, technical support indicated the extent to which the audience had been involved in the national policies by the securitizer. In China's case, the presence of high-level moral and technical support (+AA) denoted the generation of a *full securitization*, whereas the absence of either or both dimensions of high-level support (-AA) denoted a *void full securitization*, illustrated as follows:

Full securitizing move + (+AA) → Full securitization

Or

Full securitizing move + (-AA) → Void full securitization

This chapter attempts to uncover the level of audience acceptance (support) in three locales—Beijing, Shanghai, and Kunming—toward the full HIV/AIDS securitizing move. Individuals working in NGOs located in these three cities were the target audience in this study.

To contextualize the case studies, a section on the overview of HIV/AIDS situations in the cities is first illustrated. To capture "what the audience already knows" about the prevailing HIV/AIDS securitizing move in their local contexts,[3] an elaboration of the local understanding of the security aspect of HIV/AIDS in each city is provided prior to the section on audience acceptance. To determine the local understanding toward the full HIV/AIDS securitizing move, respondents were asked whether: (1) HIV/AIDS was the most serious public health problem in the eyes of the Chinese government; and (2) HIV/AIDS was the top-priority issue in the national government agenda; the justifications for their answers are also described.

Acceptance levels in each city are demonstrated and analyzed in the subsequent section through the interview materials obtained in the fieldwork and the existing secondary data. More precisely, the level of moral and technical support of the interviewees in the selected cities are compared and contrasted. The issue of the type of HIV/AIDS securitization in China is identified afterward.

Overview of HIV/AIDS Situations and Local Understanding of Full Securitizing Moves in Selected Cities

Beijing: Overview of the HIV/AIDS Situations

Beijing reported its first HIV/AIDS infection in 1985 in an American tourist.[4] By the end of May 2010, the city had registered 7,672 HIV/AIDS cases since the first identified infection.[5] Among the HIV/AIDS infected individuals, 74.3 percent of them were migrants,[6] a group that accounts for about a quarter of the city's population.[7] Sexual transmission and IDU were the two major transmission modes in the capital city. Among the new cases found in Beijing in 2009, 68 percent were infected via sexual contact and 12 percent were caused by IDU.[8]

HIV/AIDS prevalence remained low in Beijing compared to the rest of China. However, HIV/AIDS was still an important issue to be dealt with in the capital city due to the high population mobility, posing a great challenge for the HIV/AIDS prevention and treatment in the city.[9] Aside from the HIV/AIDS interventions among migrants, several respondents also observed the rapid growth in HIV/AIDS infections among MSM in China in general and Beijing in particular.[10]

Local Understanding of Full HIV/AIDS Securitizing Moves

The findings obtained from the interview sessions show that a majority of the respondents in Beijing believed that the national government perceived HIV/AIDS as the most serious public health problem to be dealt with.[11] Several respondents in Beijing justified their views by citing the *institutional arrangements* the government had taken to respond to HIV/AIDS problems in the past years. A country program manager of an INGO

[R5] highlighted the interdepartmental cooperation of the national HIV/AIDS institution: "The government set up the AIDS Control Committee to grapple with HIV/AIDS. The members in this committee include officials not only from the Ministry of Health, but also from the Public Secretary Bureau, Ministry of Commerce, and Ministry of Finance."[12] Moreover, a respondent [R3] working in an NGO in Beijing claimed that "the most serious public health problem in the eyes of the national government should be HIV/AIDS. It is because a State Council-level institution for HIV/AIDS is present, yet similar institutions do not exist for other diseases."[13] A project development director of an INGO [R9] added that "the Vice Premier is the leader of the AIDS Committee, showing that the government is highly concerned about the HIV/AIDS problem in China."[14]

Regarding the prioritization of HIV/AIDS in the national government agenda, over half of the respondents said that HIV/AIDS had become a top priority issue in the national government agenda.[15] For instance, a project manager working in an INGO [R8] contended that "HIV/AIDS is a relatively high priority issue in the national government agenda. In the government's report, I can see the political leaders relatively pay more attention to HIV/AIDS problems."[16] Another respondent [R9] highlighted the precedence of HIV/AIDS over other contagious diseases: "Compared to other infectious diseases such as SARS, HIV/AIDS is the first or second priority issue in the national government agenda."[17] Taken together, the findings reveal that a high-level understanding of full securitizing moves was observed among respondents in Beijing.

Shanghai: Overview of the HIV/AIDS Situations

The first HIV/AIDS case in Shanghai was detected in a foreigner in 1987.[18] The city recorded the first local cases in a Chinese woman and her partner in 1991.[19] Since then, there had been a substantial increase in the number of HIV/AIDS reported cases in the city, from 18 in 1994 to 191 in 1998. As of October 2010, the city had reported 5,992 HIV and 1,213 late-stage AIDS cases, since the first case was discovered in the city.[20] Sexual intercourse was the prominent route of HIV/AIDS transmission in Shanghai. In 2010, nearly 80 percent of the registered HIV/AIDS people in the city were infected via unprotected sex.[21]

HIV/AIDS infections via homosexual route had particularly increased in Shanghai. The Shanghai Center for Disease Control and Prevention had conducted surveys among MSM population in the city since 2005.[22] One of the surveys indicated that the infection rate among MSM in Shanghai mounted from 1.5 percent in 2005 to 4.1 percent in 2006 and 7.5 percent in 2007.[23] Figures released in 2009 showed that homosexual transmission made up 26.5 percent of the new HIV-positive cases, whereas drug use accounted for 18.4 percent.[24]

Unlike commercial sex and narcotic use, homosexuality was legalized in China in 1997,[25] but it had been listed as a psychiatric disorder under the *China Psychiatrics Classification and Diagnostic Criteria* until 2001.[26] In general, homosexuality was largely unaccepted in Chinese society. The media condemned homosexuals (*tongzhi*), labelling them "depraved, debilitated, or ill."[27] In the past, MSM were often arrested and charged with hooliganism or disturbing public order when they met in public areas.[28] Although such incidents are less frequent nowadays, stigma and discrimination still indelibly remained in China. In addition, due to the sociocultural pressure that emphasized the continuity of paternal lineage, some Chinese MSM had concurrent relationships with male sex partners and with women (wives or girlfriends).[29] More importantly, HIV/AIDS-related stigma and social pressure had contributed to the decrease in the use of HIV/AIDS prevention devices, leading to the upsurge of HIV/AIDS-infected cases among the MSM population as well as their female partners.[30] Regarding the future trend of HIV/AIDS in the city, all the respondents observed that the HIV/AIDS prevalence among MSM would steadily surge in Shanghai.[31]

Local Understanding of Full HIV/AIDS Securitizing Moves

In the course of the interview sessions, half of the respondents in Shanghai claimed that HIV/AIDS was the most serious problem in the eyes of Chinese authorities.[32] Although the respondents did not confirm the Chinese authorities' perceptions on the seriousness of HIV/AIDS, they asserted that "the government is highly concerned about the problem"[33] or "the government feels it is a serious problem."[34]

Regarding the prioritization of HIV/AIDS issues, none of the respondents in Shanghai believed that HIV/AIDS was the top-priority issue in the government agenda. For instance, a leader of a local NGO [R31] noted that "the first priority is food safety and some other social issues. Although CDC officials come out and say something on December 1 [World AIDS Day] every year, they cannot represent the stance of the Ministry of Health."[35] In this sense, local understanding toward full HIV/AIDS securitizing moves was relatively lower among respondents in Shanghai compared to those in Beijing.

Kunming: Overview of the HIV/AIDS Situations

The first case of HIV/AIDS infection was reported in 1989 in Yunnan.[36] In the early stage of the epidemic, people referred to the epidemic pattern as "Ruili Epidemic Pattern," because the first outbreak was identified and concentrated among 146 IDUs near Ruili.[37] A survey conducted between 1989 and 1990 revealed that over 50 percent of IDUs in Ruili were HIV-positive.[38] Subsequently, the epidemic expanded geographically to Dehong and the rest of Yunnan.[39] By 1999, all 16 prefectures of Yunnan had reported the HIV/AIDS cases.[40] The high HIV/AIDS prevalence in Yunnan was attributed to its geographical proximity to the "Golden Triangle"—Myanmar and Thailand in the west and southwest and Laos in the south—which was one of the biggest sources of opiates and the leading heroin-producing region in the world.[41]

Based on the 2011 figures, 93,567 people in the province had been infected with HIV/AIDS since the first case was discovered.[42] A recent study revealed that the cumulative reported cases in Yunnan were concentrated in the prefectures of Dehong, Honghe, Lincang, Dail, Wenshan, and Kunming.[43] Kunming, the capital and largest city in Yunnan, was selected to exemplify the emerging problem of drug use and HIV/AIDS in this area.

Given its favorable geographical location in the province, Kunming has become the leading international transportation hub in southwestern China, with a rail connection to Vietnam and road links to Myanmar and Laos. Its advance development in transportation system, however, has also facilitated narco-trafficking activities from Myanmar to China.

Beyrer et al. identified two major trafficking routes for Myanmar heroin to China and then to other countries. The principal route is from the Myanmar Wa and ethnic Shan areas, across into Yunnan, by road to Kunming, and then by air or land to Baise, Nanning, Guangzhou or Hong Kong, and to the west.[44] The second route also begins in eastern Myanmar, leads to Kunming, and then goes north and west, through Chengdu, Sichuan Province via China National Highway 213, across western China to Urumqi in Xinjiang Province, and then across the Chinese border to Kazakhstan.[45] As a result, Kunming has become the main hub for heroin trafficking from Myanmar to Yunnan, and then to Hong Kong and Macau. Myanmar-exported heroin then flows overseas to Australia, Taiwan, Europe, and North America via sea and air.[46]

Increased drug flow had resulted in the rise in HIV/AIDS cases, especially among IDUs in Kunming. According to the study conducted by Bacaër, the number of HIV/AIDS cases via IDU infection in Kunming surged from 4 in 1990 to 1,433 in 2002.[47] Currently, the cumulative number of HIV/AIDS cases in Kunming was over 15,000.[48] Regarding the mode of HIV/AIDS transmission, the official report released in October 2010 revealed that IDU remains the major HIV/AIDS transmission route in the city (44.37 percent), followed by sexual transmission (26.73 percent), and mother-to-child infection (0.48 percent). The remaining 28.42 percent falls under the unknown category.[49]

Considering the future trend of the HIV/AIDS situation in Yunnan in general and Kunming in particular, an HIV/AIDS consultant [R26] predicted that "due to its culture and history, IDU remains the main HIV/AIDS transmission mode in Yunnan."[50] Holding a similar idea, a program officer of an INGO [R28] contended that "the number of infections will surge among IDUs in Yunnan."[51] Aside from the spread of HIV/AIDS via IDU, an officer of an INGO [R20] further pointed out the seriousness of HIV/AIDS infections among MSM in Kunming: "In some cities such as Kunming, the HIV/AIDS prevalence is over 10 percent among MSM population."[52]

Local Understanding of Full HIV/AIDS Securitizing Moves

Regarding the local understanding of the full HIV/AIDS securitizing move, based on the data collected during the interviews, the majority of the respondents in Kunming apprehended that "HIV/AIDS has been treated as the most serious health problem by the national government."[53] Some respondents in Kunming justified their views, stating that the *financial commitment* of the government toward HIV/AIDS had outweighed that toward other infectious diseases such as TB. A respondent working in an INGO [R24] asserted that "in terms of financial resources, HIV/AIDS has received larger resources than other diseases."[54] Similarly, R20 noted that "in terms of resource allocation, HIV/AIDS receives the largest amount of resources from the central government."[55]

Aside from the financial pledge toward HIV/AIDS, Dr. Zhang Kaining, director of Yunnan Health and Development Research Association, unequivocally acknowledged the *institutional arrangement* for its response to HIV/AIDS, stating that:

> The central government recognizes HIV/AIDS as the most serious problem in China. In the State Council, there is an HIV/AIDS leading group composed of 14 departments. In the Chinese context, "group" is understood as "committee." The **power of this leading group is greater than a department**... if you request budgets from the Ministry of Finance for

TB measures, the Ministry will tell you to go to the Ministry of Health. However, if you request money for HIV/AIDS interventions, the Ministry of Finance will give money to you right away as the **political power of the HIV/AIDS leading group is greater than the Ministry of Finance.** [emphasis added][56]

Concerning the prioritization of HIV/AIDS, again a majority of respondents in Kunming claimed that HIV/AIDS was a priority in the national government agenda.[57] Dr. Zhang Kai-ning explained the reason for the priority: "Only HIV/AIDS measures have inter-departmental cooperation. Thus, only HIV/AIDS is a high concern in the State Council."[58] A vice director of a drug treatment center [R22] likewise mentioned the precedence of HIV/AIDS over other health problems: "More attention and better policies are present for HIV/AIDS issues. You cannot see the same amount of resources allocated in other diseases such as diabetes. Only HIV/AIDS patients can receive free ARV treatments offered by the government."[59]

Semi-Summary

Overall, the previous sections reveal that existing literature regarding the HIV/AIDS transmission mode in the core and peripheral parts of the country was consistent with the realities in China—the major HIV/AIDS mode in Beijing as well as in Shanghai (core) was unprotected sexual contact, whereas HIV/AIDS infections via IDU was prevalent in Kunming (peripheral).[60] However, the upsurge in the prevalence of HIV/AIDS among MSM was a worrisome trend in all three selected cities, requiring further favorable political reactions.

In terms of the local understanding of full HIV/AIDS securitizing moves, majority of the respondents in Beijing and Kunming perceived that the Chinese authorities treated HIV/AIDS as the most serious health problem in China and the top-priority issue in the national government agenda. The respondents also believed that the rhetorical acts of the political leaders were staunchly reinforced through the existence of the institutional arrangement in Beijing, and both the institutional arrangement and financial commitment in Kunming. Unlike the perceptions of the respondents in Beijing and Kunming, not a single respondent in Shanghai perceived that HIV/AIDS took the precedence over other health problems in the national government agenda. In this sense, the level of understanding toward full securitizing moves was higher among respondents in Beijing and Kunming than those in Shanghai.

Having illustrated the comprehension of the HIV/AIDS securitizing moves in local contexts, the following sections demonstrate the level of moral and technical support toward the HIV/AIDS securitizing moves in Beijing, Shanghai, and Kunming. Following an analysis regarding the moral and technical supports observed in the cases, the level of overall audience acceptance and the type of HIV/AIDS securitization in China is presented.

Audience Acceptance Toward the Full HIV/AIDS Securitizing Moves

Level of Moral Support

During face-to-face interviews, participants were inquired whether they perceived HIV/AIDS as the most serious public health problem in China in comparison to other public health problems or diseases. The subsequent sections show the similarities and differences of the interviewees' responses and justifications for their views.

Similarities

Most of the respondents in both Beijing and Shanghai believed that HIV/AIDS was the *single most serious* public health problem in China.[61] Several respondents in Beijing justified their views by citing the devastating impacts of HIV/AIDS problems on the national stability and prosperity and the survival of the population. Consider the following responses:

> If we do not deal with this problem [HIV/AIDS], it will affect the **national prosperity** and **life of the general public**. [emphasis added][62]
>
> HIV/AIDS is an infectious disease that will **increase the mortality rate of the population**, which has a great impact on the **economic development and stability** of the **Chinese government**. [emphasis added][63]

With the exception of two respondents in total in Beijing and Shanghai,[64] the majority of the respondents in Beijing and Shanghai, respectively, perceived HIV/AIDS as *one of the most serious* problems in China.[65] Consider the following views:

> In terms of the number of infections, TB and malaria are more serious than HIV/AIDS. With regard to the HIV/AIDS prevalence, the prevalence is higher only in some provinces. In general, HIV/AIDS prevalence is low in

China. Therefore, HIV/AIDS is only one of the most serious public health problems.[66]

HIV/AIDS is not the most serious public health problem in China. HIV/AIDS problems exist because of historical incident—blood business—in China. SARS is as serious as HIV/AIDS. Fake drugs and TB are also serious public health problems facing China.[67]

Differences

In Kunming, an HIV/AIDS consultant [R26] thoroughly explained the severity of the disease: "HIV/AIDS is a serious problem as the incubation period is long and thus people may not know their positive status and infect other people unintentionally; stigma problem is serious in China. Hence, many people are reluctant to conduct VCT [Voluntary Counselling and Testing]; also, HIV/AIDS problem is closely linked to poverty. Those migrants have a relatively poor situation and their knowledge on HIV/AIDS prevention is limited. In addition, they do not have enough money to support HIV/AIDS-related treatments once they are infected with the disease."[68] Despite what has just been said, findings indicated that only a small portion of the respondents in Kunming believed that HIV/AIDS was the most serious public health problem in China.[69]

The majority of the respondents admitted that *HIV/AIDS was not the most serious or HIV/AIDS was not a serious public health problem in China at all*. A vice director of a drug treatment center [R22] expressed that "the mortality rate of some diseases is higher than that of HIV/AIDS. Thus, HIV/AIDS is not the most powerful infectious disease."[70] R24 likewise noted that "other diseases such as hepatitis, cancer, high blood pressure, and HPV [Human Papillomavirus] are more serious than HIV/AIDS."[71]

Notwithstanding the burgeoning development of HIV/AIDS intervention programs, several respondents still believed that HIV/AIDS was not the most serious problem in the country. For instance, a project officer of a national NGO [R25] stressed that "HIV/AIDS is not a serious problem in China at present. The government has increased its effort in dealing with the problem. International organizations have also played a role in it."[72] R24 also stated that "based on the current situation, HIV/AIDS is not the most serious disease in China... The government has allocated lots of resources and paid great attention to the disease... the budget for HIV/AIDS increased continuously every year."[73]

Level of Technical Support

The level of technical support can be reflected by the extent to which the audience has been involved in HIV/AIDS-related political measures that are operated in an emergency mode. In the course of the interview sessions, the respondents were invited to comment on NGO involvement in the national HIV/AIDS control and prevention undertaking. The following sections depict the similarities and differences of the responses of the NGO respondents.

Similarities

Based on the empirical data, over half of the respondents in Beijing,[74] Shanghai,[75] and Kunming[76] recognized that NGOs had been engaged in the national HIV/AIDS control and prevention programs. However, the justifications for the government commitment to NGO involvement were similar among respondents in Shanghai and Kunming, and different among those in Beijing.

One of the most striking trends in the comments of respondents from Shanghai and Kunming was their indication that NGO activities were largely controlled by the government albeit the increase in NGO engagement in national HIV/AIDS policies. For instance, the founder of an HIV/AIDS-related self-help group in Shanghai [R29] explained that "to some extent, the government supports the NGOs' work. However, the government also manages to control NGOs' activities."[77] R24 expounded the reason for resisting NGOs' involvement: "While the authorities recognized the work done by NGOs, they feared that grassroots NGOs may link HIV/AIDS to [sensitive political issues such as] human rights. Thus, the government suppresses the work of NGOs, but at the same time helps NGOs participate in HIV/AIDS interventions."[78] Holding a similar viewpoint, R26 stated, "The Health Department recognizes the work of grassroots NGOs. In the policy of SCAWC, it encourages more NGOs to work in this area. For other departments, however, they are unfamiliar with NGOs' work and thus are reluctant to support NGOs. Officials are afraid that the NGOs talk about sensitive political issues such as human rights."[79]

In particular, some respondents in Kunming said that the Chinese government was "forced" to involve NGOs in national HIV/AIDS policies due to the international pressure. Consider the following quotations regarding their experiences working with the government:

> The central government does not want civil society groups to participate due to the political sensitivity of NGOs after the 1989-incident. However, due to the **pressure from the international governments and bilateral partners** of the Chinese government, the government is **forced to involve** civil society groups. [emphasis added][80]
>
> We have a cooperative relationship with the government, but this relationship is only on the surface. NGOs are the "chesses" of the government; the

Chinese authorities fully control the activities of NGOs. If we behave well, they will give us more money. In fact, the government does not want to cooperate, but due to the problems coming to the surface, the government has to be **accountable to the international governments**, and thus needs to cooperate with NGOs. [emphasis added][81]

These statements palpably demonstrated the respondents' overwhelming sense of distrust and suspicion toward the central government's intention to fully involve civil society groups in the national HIV/AIDS policies.

Differences

Unlike the respondents in Shanghai and Kunming, respondents in Beijing believed that the national government was willing to cooperate with NGOs, because the Chinese government held a more pragmatic view of NGOs in recent years. A program officer working in an NGO [R3] commented, "There has been a dramatic improvement in the perception of government toward NGOs and civil society groups, although some worries still exist within the government. However, the central government's concern is whether the NGOs can bring better changes to the country and the people."[82] More quotations in relation to NGO involvement in the national HIV/AIDS interventions are as follows:

> Cooperation has been increased between the Chinese government and HIV/AIDS-related NGOs in the areas of treatment, care, and prevention. The government can make use of the advantage of NGOs in reaching out to those target populations that cannot be reached by government officials otherwise.[83]
>
> In the past, our relationship with the government was not good, but now it is much better. The government sent officials to visit our center to learn the management strategy of our organization... They are more willing to cooperate with the grassroots NGOs because they can see the effectiveness of the NGOs' work.[84]
>
> Dialogue and communication have been increased between the government and NGOs. The government also involves NGOs in the policy-making process... Grassroots representatives are present in the CCM [Country Coordination Mechanism of the Global Fund].[85]

Another respondent [R6] undoubtedly believed that "the government will involve more grassroots NGOs in HIV/AIDS interventions in the coming two or three years, because the Chinese authorities have realized that some work cannot be accomplished by the government alone."[86] The aforementioned comments suggested that a relatively harmonious relationship had been established with the government and NGOs operating in Beijing.

In sum, majority of the respondents in all selected cities agreed that HIV/AIDS-related NGOs had been involved in national HIV/AIDS programs. However, an overwhelming sense of distrust and suspicion toward the central government's intention prevailed among the respondents working in Shanghai and Kunming, whereas a more harmonized relationship was observed with the government and NGOs in Beijing.

Using the language in the revised securitization framework, the level of moral support toward the full HIV/AIDS securitizing move was relatively *stronger* in Beijing and Shanghai than in Kunming. With regard to the level of technical support toward the full securitizing move, the empirical data showed that technical support was strong in all selected cities.

Analysis of the Audience Acceptance of Full HIV/AIDS Securitizing Moves

Moral Support

The previous section illustrated the moral support of the individuals working in NGOs toward the full HIV/AIDS securitizing move generated by the Chinese top-level leaders. Compared to the respondents in the selected Chinese cities, majority of the respondents in Beijing and Shanghai perceived HIV/AIDS as the *most serious public health problem* in China, whereas respondents in Kunming asserted that other epidemics were more threatening in the country than HIV/AIDS.

Considering the graveness of the disease in an epidemiological perspective, more people in China were infected with TB than HIV/AIDS, although the mortality rate of TB was lower than that of HIV/AIDS.[87] The figures in 2011 revealed that 154,000 were estimated to be in the late-stage of AIDS, whereas the number of HIV-positive individuals had reached 780,000.[88] Nevertheless, recent figures released by the Ministry of Health in March 2011 reported that the number of infectious TB individuals in China had exceeded five million, and the number of suspected TB-infected individuals had reached 500 million, accounting for 45 percent of the entire population in China.[89] Considering the epidemiological situation, TB is a far more serious and threatening problem than HIV/AIDS in China.

Despite the severity of TB over HIV/AIDS problems in China, only a small portion of the respondents in Beijing and Kunming declared that

"TB is more serious than HIV/AIDS in China."[90] For example, a country program manager of an INGO [R5] stated that "TB is the most serious public health problem as it has a higher infection rate and more people are living with TB than HIV/AIDS."[91] Another respondent [R20] believed that "TB is more serious than HIV/AIDS...yet the government's effort in dealing with TB is not enough. Basic TB treatments are insufficient because lots of TB patients are infected with MDR-TB [multidrug resistant tuberculosis]."[92]

Instead of TB, a couple of respondents in Beijing and Shanghai in particular considered HIV/AIDS as the *single* most serious public health problem among other diseases.[93] A project manager of an INGO [R8] asserted that "in terms of the epidemiological and medical aspect, TB is the most serious public health problem in China... However, in terms of the devastating impact on economy, lifestyle, and moral value of people, HIV/AIDS is the most serious one among the three."[94] Another respondent [R26] claimed that "TB and malaria are solely public health problems. HIV/AIDS is related to social behaviors such as injecting drug use or unprotected sex. Hence, HIV/AIDS is a more complicated problem in comparison to other diseases."[95]

Moreover, the respondents justified that HIV/AIDS was not only a public health problem, but also a social problem because of the stigma and discrimination attached to the disease and the infected individuals. The stigmatized condition of HIV/AIDS made the respondents believe that HIV/AIDS was more serious than TB and other infectious diseases. This perspective was demonstrated in the following quotations:

> HIV/AIDS is not only a medical problem; it is also an ethical problem, because **stigma** is usually attached to the HIV/AIDS patients. [emphasis added][96]

> In terms of the number of infections, more people are infected with TB than HIV/AIDS. However, HIV/AIDS killed more people than TB...the difference of HIV/AIDS from other diseases is that HIV/AIDS has **a stigmatized condition**. [emphasis added][97]

> For TB and malaria, the resource for treating the diseases is open [easily accessed]. The patients are easily recognized, the treatment is more affordable, and these two diseases are relatively easier to be treated. However, HIV/AIDS is a hidden disease, which is attached with **social stigma**. [emphasis added][98]

> Epidemiologically speaking, HIV/AIDS is a serious public health problem...the economic and social problem that HIV/AIDS can generate is more than what we can imagine. For example, if a person gets cancer, he will tell his family members and friends and thus he will receive support and care from them. However, if the individual infects with HIV/AIDS, he

will not tell others as **misunderstanding and stigma** prevail in our society. [emphasis added][99]

HIV/AIDS is not **only a public health problem**; it is also **a social problem**. If it is solely a health problem, then we should deal with the OIs treatment and control the transmission rate. However, we can see nowadays companies reject to hire HIV-positive individuals. Medical doctors refuse to conduct operations on HIV/AIDS patients... People are **afraid of HIV/ AIDS more than TB**. In fact, people are afraid of the TB disease itself, not the people who are infected... Overall, **stigma** is seriously prevalent in society and families of those HIV/AIDS infected individuals. [emphasis added][100]

The general public has different perceptions on individuals living with these two diseases. If you are infected with HIV/AIDS, people will stay away from you. After all, **TB is more serious due to its high infection rate** in China. **HIV/AIDS is more serious because of the discrimination** of the general public towards the disease and the people living with HIV/AIDS. [emphasis added][101]

Intriguingly, a number of Beijing respondents were undecided on whether HIV/AIDS or TB was the *single* most serious public health problem in China. Instead of viewing HIV/AIDS and TB as separate issues, they perceived TB as *one of the problems of HIV/AIDS*.[102] Similar to the issue raised by Beijing respondents, Lin Oi-chu, chief executive of Hong Kong AIDS Foundation, claimed that "HIV/AIDS and TB have become twins: HIV/AIDS-TB co-infection is getting more serious in China."[103] TB is one of the common opportunistic infections (OIs) found in HIV/AIDS-infected individuals.[104] As such, the number of HIV/AIDS and TB infections would mount simultaneously if no appropriate and effective HIV/AIDS control and treatment measures were carried out in China.

Empirical data on audience perception toward HIV/AIDS shows that the positive speech acts uttered by securitizers have been diffused and shared among audiences in selected cities with various intensities. In short, the level of moral support was comparatively *stronger* in Beijing and Shanghai, and *weaker* among Kunming audiences.

The intersubjectivity of HIV/AIDS threat-framing was deemed to be constructed between the securitizers and the audience. However, divergences appeared between their security justifications. Only two respondents in the selected cities justified their views by stating the devastating impacts of HIV/AIDS on national stability and prosperity and the survival of the population.[105] Majority of the respondents justified their views by citing the *stigma and discrimination attached to HIV/AIDS*, thereby making the epidemic the most serious public health problem in China.

Technical Support

Based on the empirical data collected during the interviews, majority of the respondents in the selected cities believed that HIV/AIDS-focused NGOs had been involved in national HIV/AIDS programs.[106] In fact, due to the SARS and HIV/AIDS crises and the persisting deficiencies in health care provisions in China since the economic reforms of the 1980s and 1990s, the Chinese government had encouraged the development of health NGOs to respond to the health challenges and address the gaps in the health care provision of the government.[107] HIV/AIDS-focused NGOs were perceived as the most outstanding grassroots health NGOs developed in China.[108] The political recognition of the HIV/AIDS-focused NGOs had been highlighted by multiple statements delivered by various top-level government officials since 2004. In 2004, Vice Premier Wu Yi stated, "We should mobilize all the partners in society to participate in the fight against HIV/AIDS. We need to improve our policies and strategies to build a better environment for the society to participate in the response, and try our best to facilitate the involvement of all sectors."[109]

In 2005, Vice Health Minster Wang Longde asserted that the Chinese government would give more support to HIV/AIDS-focused NGOs as they played a significant role in HIV/AIDS interventions.[110] In 2006, he again stressed the importance of NGOs engagement: "Government efforts alone were not enough to fight HIV/AIDS given a population of 1.3 billion people and more NGOs needed to join the fight."[111] In 2008, deputy director of the SCAWC and vice minister of health Gao Qiang urged "all sectors to take their responsibilities and obligations in response to HIV/AIDS, so as to achieve sustainable development of its operational mechanism.[112] He also emphasized multi-sectoral cooperation and NGO involvement in the containment of the HIV/AIDS epidemic."[113] In 2011, vice-health minister Yin Li publicly claimed that "civil societies play an indispensable role in effective HIV/AIDS interventions led by the government and the [Red Ribbon] forum helps form a long-term partnership between the two."[114]

The participation of the Global Fund in the national HIV/AIDS programs strengthened the involvement of HIV/AIDS-focused NGOs in China. The Global Fund accepted China's application in 2003.[115] Between 2003 and 2011, the Chinese government received US$548 million in grants from the Global Fund.[116] Half of these grants (approximately US$260 million) were solely dispensed to HIV/AIDS.[117]

The Global Fund enhanced the commitment of the Chinese government to involve civil society groups in national HIV/AIDS prevention and control measures. The Global Fund requires its recipients to have a full range of stakeholders, embracing the government, bilateral and multilateral donors, the private sector, and civil society (includes government- and individual-organized NGOs, affected communities, and faith-based organizations) took part in the CCM.[118] With a view to meeting the criteria of the Global Fund, the Chinese government opened a seat for HIV/AIDS-related NGOs' representatives to participate in the CCM.[119] The existing government structure did not allow for the full involvement of civil society in China; the CCM thus provided valuable opportunities for civil society groups to engage in policy making related to HIV/AIDS.[120]

The Global Fund also required the PRs (China CDC or the National Center for AIDS/STD Control and Prevention) to disburse a designated portion of the grants to HIV/AIDS-related civil society groups operating in the country.[121] Following the instruction, the Chinese government pledged 25 percent of the US$24 million budget from Round 4 of the Global Fund to NGOs in 2005.[122] The Chinese authorities likewise allocated 70 percent of the US$10 million budget from the Round 6 project to both government-organized and individual-organized NGOs in 2008.[123] Overall, the government contributed over US$43 million to support HIV/AIDS-focused civil society groups in Rounds 3, 4, and 5 of the Global Fund.[124]

The financial commitment of the Chinese government to civil society groups was likewise observed in its Social Mobilization Program, in which the government allocated 2.66 million yuan (US$0.42 million) to support Round 6 of the Global Fund in 2007.[125] In 2008, the Chinese government allocated three million yuan (US$0.48 million) to support Round 6 of the Global Fund, whereas 0.43 million yuan (US$0.07 million) financed the pertinent programs in Round 5.[126] Table 6.1 shows the numbers of government- and individual-organized HIV/AIDS-focused NGOs established in China since 2004 because of the constructive political atmosphere and promising financial resources in the country.

The importance of NGO involvement in national HIV/AIDS programs was notably highlighted in Round 6 of the Global Fund. Implemented between 2008 and 2012,[127] Round 6 specifically aims to "mobilize and support civil society and NGOs' participation in scaling up China's HIV/AIDS prevention and control activities."[128] In Round 6, the Chinese government promised to: (1) support NGO participation in implementing activities; (2) strengthen the capacity of civil society and NGOs; and (3) provide sustained support and create a supportive environment during the program implementation.[129]

Several respondents mentioned in times of interview the profound influence of the Global Fund in general and Round 6 in particular. For example, Lin Oi-chu commented, "Round 6 of the Global Fund acts as a pushing force for the government to involve more grassroots NGOs in HIV/AIDS interventions."[130] An officer of Home AIDS [R25] similarly believed that "due to the requirement of the Global Fund, many grassroots [HIV/AIDS-focused] NGOs have been developed in China."[131] Moreover, Round 6 of

Table 6.1 Proliferation of HIV/AIDS-Focused NGOs in China

	Before 2003	2003	2004	2005	2006	2007	2008	2009	Unknown Date
PLWHA Support groups	7	4	10	13	11	16	12	3	3
MSM	17	4	11	11	29	26	9	5	0
Sex workers	4	1	1	3	1	6	8	1	1
IDUs	2	0	3	2	2	3	6	3	0
Research institutions	4	0	1	3	0	0	0	1	0
Mass organizations	4	0	0	0	0	0	0	0	0
Others	14	6	3	7	8	8	12	5	2
Total	52	15	29	39	51	59	47	18	6
Total (cumulative)	52	67	96	135	186	245	292	310	316
Increase (%)	N/A	28.8	43.3	40.6	37.8	31.7	19.2	6.2	N/A

Source: *2009/2010 China HIV/AIDS NGO Directory* (People's Republic of China: National Centre for AIDS/STD Control and Prevention, China CDC and China HIV/AIDS Information Network, 2009).

the Global Fund is linked to the establishment of civil society groups, which resulted in the proliferation of HIV/AIDS-related NGOs in China.[132]

The 300 million yuan (US$46 million) worth of financial support specifically for HIV/AIDS offered by the Global Fund in 2011 assures the continued augmentation of HIV/AIDS-related funding in the country in the coming years.[133] Minister of health Chen Zhu stated that "in the coming five years, the Chinese government will constantly increase its financial support of social organizations, particularly those that work to control and prevent HIV/AIDS."[134]

Types of HIV/AIDS Securitization in China: Full HIV/AIDS Securitization

A comprehensive picture regarding the type of HIV/AIDS securitization in China could be generated by identifying the level of moral and technical support among the NGO respondents in three selected cities. Half of the 30 NGO respondents in three selected cities viewed HIV/AIDS as the single most serious problem in China. Regarding the level of NGO involvement in national HIV/AIDS programs, likewise over half of the respondents in the selected three cities believed that NGOs had been engaged in national HIV/AIDS interventions. The empirical data suggested that a *full HIV/AIDS securitization tended to develop in China*, with high-level moral and technical support toward full HIV/AIDS securitization generated at the national level. Despite the high-level technical support observed in this study, the HIV/AIDS-related grassroots NGOs in selected cities, constituting the majority (by number) of the audience,[135] had faced considerable predicament in involving themselves in the HIV/AIDS interventions.

Factors Hindering Technical Support: Restrictive Legal Status of Grassroots NGOs

During the face-to-face interviews, a number of Chinese respondents stated that grassroots NGOs had less access to financial resources. Consider the following responses:

> The national government did allocate resources in HIV/AIDS interventions. However, the funding remains inside the government and never goes down to the grassroots level.[136]

> The government has put a lot of money on HIV/AIDS interventions. However, I doubt that not many grassroots NGOs have benefited from this money... The local officials did not let grassroots NGOs do the work. Budgets from the central government and international organizations have fallen into the hands of GONGOs [government-organized nongovernmental organizations]... we do not know whether the money has been used on PLWHA [people living with HIV/AIDS], or has been used to pay the management fees.[137]
>
> Although the government has set this percentage, most of the budget is taken by the GONGOs instead of the grassroots NGOs. GONGOs are also counted as civil society groups, but the difference is that they have heavy support from the government. The person in charge of these GONGOs is a government official or someone who has a close relationship with the government. What the grassroots NGOs can finally get is not much.[138]

A program officer working in an international NGO [R2] in Beijing explained that the unregistered nature of grassroots NGOs in China was a major problem that hindered the flow of money into grassroots organizations, stating that:

> The amount of money is already sufficient to enact a substantial response. However, the problem is how those unregistered grassroots NGOs can get this money from the government. In fact, it is difficult for them to register in China, so it is hard for them to get the money. It is also difficult for an individual NGO to receive funding.[139]

As a matter of fact, grassroots NGOs in China were often unregistered or registered with the Ministry of Industry and Commerce (MOIC).[140] However, only NGOs registered with the Ministry of Civil Affairs (MOCA) or one of its local bureaus were legally recognized by the Chinese government.[141] Several grassroots NGOs were not formally registered in the MOCA because of strict registration criteria. For instance, an organization must possess minimum assets of 100,000 yuan and have a "professional management unit"—usually a government department—that acts as a supervisory body to the organization.[142]

However, fulfilling the two requirements was not easy for grassroots NGOs. The financial situation was problematic in many grassroots NGOs due to the limited source of funding. On the one hand, most grassroots NGOs received little financial support from the government as they usually did not possess political ties with the government. Moreover, grassroots NGOs seldom obtained donations from local communities because (1) newly developed NGOs did not have good track records that enabled them to win the trust of the locals;[143] and (2) donors could not receive tax breaks for their donation to unregistered NGOs.[144] Such aforementioned financial predicament was forthrightly described by a program coordinator working in a grassroots NGO in Beijing [R6]:

> We do not have stable sources of funding; we do not even have a stable office. We have received some grants from the China–Bill Gates Project. However, the level of funding we can receive is based on the number of patients using our service. In addition, this funding does not include the transportation fee and other expenses such as wages. We do not receive any money from social donation. The future development of our organization is problematic. We cannot hire full-time staff as they cannot get the social insurance [as the organization is not legally registered].[145]

On the other hand, it was also difficult for grassroots NGOs to find a "management unit" in order to register in the MOCA. Most government departments simply rejected their applications as they feared the consequences of taking responsibilities for grassroots organizations.[146] Even though NGOs managed to find a management unit to support their registration, R6 further explained that the financial situation was in fact constrained by the respective management unit:

> What makes our financial situation worse is that based on the government regulation, every grassroots NGO should find a management unit to manage the funding they have been granted from the government. [In other words], funding is not directly given to the individual grassroots NGO. The unit will even charge us 5 percent of the budget granted for the management fee.[147]

Grassroots NGOs registered under the MOIC likewise encountered problems with regard to the amount and source of funding. As registered commercial entities, grassroots NGOs were required to pay a five percent tax on any revenue, even for funding received for nonprofit purposes.[148] As such, stated by R22, "International donors are dissatisfied with their money being used to pay taxes; thus, they are reluctant to support grassroots NGOs registered under the MOIC."[149]

Aside from these criteria, the *Interim Procedures on the Registration and Administration of Private Non-enterprise Organizations* (1998) set the non-competition principle of NGO establishment, that is, similar organizations with the same scope of business could not operate in the same administrative region.[150] Hence, this regulation further limited the registration of grassroots NGOs in China. Numbers of grassroots NGOs working on HIV/AIDS have remained unregistered in China because of these legislations. This situation impeded the ability of grassroots NGOs to obtain funding and carry out their activities.[151]

The unregistered status of many grassroots NGOs also resulted in the difficulty in receiving financial support from the central government. Without direct and sustainable financial assistance from the government, grassroots NGOs were often financially dependent on relatively small grants and subcontracts provided by the China CDC, or small-term endownments granted by international funding agencies.[152] However, Thompson and Lu pointed out that NGOs reliance on foreign funding in the absence of domestic support fueled government suspicion, prompting fears that NGOs were subversives, attempting to undermine the government through western-supported "peaceful evolution."[153]

Instead of unregistered NGOs, the central government intended to support and partner with registered grassroots NGOs or organizations that were closely affiliated with the government, specifically the GONGOs. Chinese officials believed that majority of the civil society groups could not be trusted on the proper spending of the Global Fund money, whereas government agencies such as GONGOs were more trustworthy.[154] For instance, the central government had invested money on registered grassroots NGOs and GONGOs through the Social Mobilization Program since 2002.[155] The budget and the number of organizations being funded in this program have steadily expanded throughout the years. Initially, 21 organizations received a combined funding of US$0.25 million, which augmented to 60 organizations receiving a total of US$1.46 million in 2010.[156]

Curley mentioned that "subordinate" or "co-opted" organizations such as GONGOs often benefit from their institutional arrangements with the state.[157] To illustrate this point, R6 described the disparity in the amount of grants obtained by GONGOs and grassroots NGOs:

> Ditan hospital, which is a GONGO, can receive 180,000 to 260,000 yuan from the government; grassroots NGOs can only get 20,000 to 30,000 yuan. The amount of money is definitely insufficient to support grassroots NGOs' work (such as holding activities, interventions, transportation, communication, and other expenses). The chairperson of the Ditan hospital gets the salaries from the government hospital plus allowances from the HIV/AIDS budget.[158]

The way in which the Chinese government performed in relation to funding allocation, as previously described, violated the regulation of the Global Fund. Having failed to allot 35 percent of the US$283 million HIV/AIDS grant to community-based organizations as pledged, consequently, the Global Fund stopped its 2011 funding to Chinese HIV/AIDS programs in early 2011.[159] According to a report released by an NGO called Global

Fund Watch, China only managed to dispense less than 11 percent to NGOs working on HIV/AIDS.[160] A program officer of an INGO [R2] further pinpointed the failure of CCM to distribute the right portion of the Global Fund grant to grassroots NGOs: "The CCM is dominated by government officials and representatives from GONGOs. Only a few representatives are from grassroots NGOs and civil society. Meng Lin is one of the very few NGO representatives on the board of CCM."[161]

In an interview with a high-ranking government official in Shanghai [R33], he clearly expounded the reasons for the Global Fund grant withdrawal in early 2011:

> First, the Global Fund required at least 25 percent to 30 percent of the grant should be given to grassroots NGOs. However, the government has failed to achieve this requirement. Second, the management fee in some provinces is too high. Third, one of the elements in the RCC program [Rolling Continuation Channel Program] is related to budget aggregation (monetary contribution by both the national government and the Global Fund). However, the Chinese government has not allocated enough money for the aggregated budget. Lastly, the Global Fund debated countries such as those in Africa are more in need than China. The Global Fund representatives believed that China is rich enough to support its own programs, as China has successfully held the Olympic Games as well as the World Expo.[162]

After the negotiation between the Chinese authorities and the representatives of the Global Fund, the Chinese government pledged to dispense at least 25 percent of the Global Fund grant to NGO work.[163] However, that Chinese authorities are delivering the correct proportion of funding to grassroots NGOs as promised required further scrutiny.

Repression of HIV/AIDS-Focused NGOs and Activists

Aside from the restrictive legal status of NGOs, coercion and suppression of NGO activities were likewise observed in China. Although there had been formidable effort by NGOs at the grassroots level to help HIV/AIDS-infected individuals, government response to the rise of vigorous NGOs, to a certain extent, had been suspicious and even hostile.[164]

The quality of being too outspoken could trigger harassment from the government, which risked the very survival of organizations whose primary mission was to serve those suffering from HIV/AIDS.[165] Financial dependence on foreign funds was also problematic, because authorities could use those NGOs as tools of foreign powers to influence their own affairs. For example, local authorities in Xinjiang shut down the Snow

Lotus HIV/AIDS Education Institute in October 2006, a proactive HIV/AIDS advocacy group sponsored by the Global Fund.[166] Aside from repression, a 2007 report revealed that Chinese authorities banned HIV/AIDS activists (50 Chinese and foreign experts and activists) from launching a conference in Guangzhou for fear of foreign intervention in the politically sensitive subject, HIV/AIDS.[167]

In this sense, the power of the NGOs to constrain securitizer decision was relatively weak in China. Additionally, the audience that challenged the security/nonsecurity frame put forth by the securitizers could be viewed as threats to national security at best, and could face imprisonment at worst.[168] Hence, authorities have stifled numbers of HIV/AIDS activists through imprisonment, house arrest, or assault. Dr. Wang Yanhai and Dr. Gao Yaojie were two of the prominent Chinese HIV/AIDS activists that fled to the United States due to the recurrent pressure and disturbance exerted by Chinese authorities.[169]

False Securitization

As explained in the previous section regarding the restriction and suppression of civil societies and HIV/AIDS activists, it was argued that the full HIV/AIDS securitization generated in China was suspected to be *false securitization*. Based on the discussion in chapter 2, positive speech acts, a full set of emergency measures, and high-level audience acceptance could be identified in false securitization, which were characteristics of full securitization. However, audience acceptance of a particular security frame was not necessarily due to the seriousness of the issue.

The relatively restrictive media and internet access in China could restrict the chance of an audience to expose the contrary arguments or evidence of a particular issue. Thus, morally supporting a securitizing move was easier for an audience. In addition, the level of moral support was more stable for a longer period of time, because the bottom-up initiative in securitizing a new issue or challenging the existing securitization was rather limited in an authoritarian regime such as China.

On the other hand, due to the legal and political repression of grassroots NGOs in China, the audience could and/or would not challenge established ways of thinking regarding securitization.[170] For the sake of reaching a *modus vivendi*, some HIV/AIDS-focused grassroots NGOs had largely avoided direct confrontation with the government and simply focused on their core missions,[171]

This setup could even prompt some audiences to join the state elites in calling for "more security."[172] Civil society groups relied heavily on their connections with government agencies, because no legal and democratic mechanisms existed to guarantee the influence of the audience in the securitization process.[173] Having good relationships with state agencies was the *sine qua non* for securing organizational resources and survival.[174] Accordingly, government constraints could be loosened or waived for organizations that had strong connections with government agencies.[175] For example, grassroots NGOs in China that were closely affiliated with the government could receive more financial and human resources, and had a higher chance of being selected in the bidding process of national HIV/AIDS programs. Therefore, some NGOs would obey any government stance to receive financial and political support at the expense of their opinions and judgments toward HIV/AIDS securitization.

Summary

Using the primary data collected from Beijing, Shanghai, and Kunming, as well as the existing secondary resources, this chapter illuminated the level of moral and technical support of individuals working in HIV/AIDS-related NGOs in the respective cities toward full HIV/AIDS securitization. A comprehensive picture of the overall level of audience acceptance and the types of HIV/AIDS securitization was identified in China after uncovering the level of moral and technical support in the selected cities.

Empirical data revealed that full HIV/AIDS securitization was observed in China, with an overall high-level moral and technical support among the respondents in selected cities. Respondents justified their moral support by pointing out that HIV/AIDS was the most serious problem because of the stigma and discrimination attached to the disease, which complicated the according prevention, control, and treatment of the disease. Technical support for HIV/AIDS securitization enhanced as seen in the growing involvement of HIV/AIDS-focused NGOs in national HIV/AIDS programs, which were recognized by the individuals working in HIV/AIDS-specific NGOs. The Global Fund played a significant role in facilitating NGO participation in national HIV/AIDS programs.

Albeit the augmentation in financial and technical assistance for HIV/AIDS-related NGOs, respondents pinpointed that grassroots NGOs did not benefit from this development because of their unregistered status, suspicion, and suppression by Chinese authorities. The restrictive legal status and suppression of HIV/AIDS-related NGOs and activists cast doubt on the authenticity of full HIV/AIDS securitization in China. Instead of viewing HIV/AIDS as the most serious problem, the audience agreed with the perception of the securitizers to gain more financial or political support, or avert coercion and suppression from the government.

Chapter 7

Securitizing HIV/AIDS in India

Introduction

Similar to its Chinese counterpart, HIV/AIDS securitization failed in early years in India. The seriousness of the HIV/AIDS problem and the increased awareness and commitment of the Indian government toward the disease had dramatically changed the securitization of HIV/AIDS. This chapter argues that a full HIV/AIDS securitizing move with explicit positive speech acts and a full set of emergency measures was generated in 2004. However, it also shows the weakening of full HIV/AIDS securitization in current years as a result of the withdrawal push.

In this chapter, a brief illustration of the historical (1986–2005) and current (2007–present) overview of the HIV/AIDS epidemic in India is given. The overview was divided because a revised estimated HIV/AIDS figure was released in 2006 using the new estimation method.[1] The revised 2006 figures are deemed to have altered the whole picture of the HIV/AIDS epidemiological situation in India. The HIV/AIDS-related policy response is analyzed chronologically using the revised securitization framework. As such, the change from a failed to a full securitizing move and the fade-out of the 2004 security move to post-2010 is demonstrated. A post-facto analysis of the HIV/AIDS-related policies offered in this chapter attempts to generate a comprehensive picture of the development of HIV/AIDS securitizing move within the Indian government.

Overview of the HIV/AIDS Epidemic in India

Historical Epidemiological Situation (1986–2005)

The first cases of HIV/AIDS in India were reported in 1986, when two medical practitioners identified six HIV-positive samples among a group of 102 FSWs in Chennai, Tamil Nadu.[2] In the same year, Mumbai also reported its first HIV/AIDS case in a FSW.[3] Initially, the epidemic was concentrated among high risk groups (HRGs), primarily FSWs and IDUs in several areas, such as Mumbai and Pune in Maharashtra, Chennai, and Pondicherry in Tamil Nadu in southern India, and Manipur in the northeastern part of the country.[4] These areas would be home to three-quarters of the infected people in India.[5]

However, the spread of HIV/AIDS was not geographically restricted. By 1995, 24 of the states and union territories in India had already reported HIV/AIDS-infected cases.[6] The disease finally reached all states and union territories of the country by the late 1990s.[7] The number of HIV/AIDS infections rose from 3.7 million in 1999 to 5.1 million in 2005,[8] which was nearly a 40 percent increment over a six-year period.

In 1999, the National AIDS Control Organization (NACO) divided all states and union territories in the country into three groups in accordance with the HIV/AIDS prevalence in respective areas. Group 1 included Maharashtra, Tamil Nadu, Karnataka, Andhra Pradesh, Manipur, and Nagaland. HIV/AIDS prevalence among antenatal women was more than 1 percent in this group. Among these six states, Maharashtra and Manipur were the top two states with the highest HIV/AIDS prevalence.[9] Gujarat, Goa, and Pondicherry belonged to Group 2 where HIV/AIDS infection rates were less than 1 percent among antenatal women, but more than 5 percent among high-risk populations. The remaining states and union territories were placed in Group 3 where HIV/AIDS prevalence was less than 1 percent among antenatal women, and below 5 percent among HRGs.[10]

A reversed figure of the estimated number of HIV/AIDS infected people—2.5 million—was released in 2006.[11] The number of sentinel sites not only increased from 703 to 1,122 in 2006, but this new estimation also encompassed the HIV/AIDS testing results of the general population (102,000) during the third National Family Health Survey (NFHS-III).[12] In addition, data from the second round of national Behavioral Surveillance Survey (BSS-2) and the first round of the Integrated Biological Behavioral Assessments (IBBA) survey were used for the revised estimate.[13] This new method was also applied to "back calculate" HIV/AIDS prevalence in the previous years since 2002.[14] Results of the back calculation revealed that HIV/AIDS prevalence was stable from 2002 to 2005, and then declined in 2006.[15] Despite the reduced number of HIV/AIDS cases, a 2006 report alarmingly estimated that 11 million people would die from late-stage AIDS in the next 20 years if no effective measures to combat the disease were implemented.[16]

Current Epidemiological Situation (2007–Present)

Based on the latest figure, approximately 2.1 million people were living with HIV/AIDS in India, with an adult HIV/AIDS prevalence of 0.3 percent in 2012.[17] Regarding the modes of transmission among HIV/AIDS reported cases, heterosexual contact remained the most prominent mode of transmission (87.4 percent), followed by parent-to-child (5.4 percent), IDUs (1.6 percent), homosexual (1.3 percent), blood and blood products (1.0 percent), and the remaining 3.3 percent fell under the unspecified category.[18]

In terms of the geographical distribution of HIV/AIDS cases in India, four southern and western industrialized states (Maharashtra, Karnataka, Tamil Nadu, and Andhra Pradesh) and two northeastern states (Manipur and Nagaland) were identified as the six states with the highest HIV/AIDS prevalence in the country, which accounted for over two-thirds of the total HIV/AIDS burden of the country.[19] HIV/AIDS spread primarily through heterosexual contact in the southern states, whereas IDU is the predominant mode of transmission in the northeastern states.[20]

The existing data indicated that relatively fewer HIV/AIDS cases have been reported in northern and northwestern India. However, this result may not be equivalent to low HIV/AIDS prevalence, as this may be simply a result of poor surveillance system and low reporting of the epidemic in these regions. S. Samraj, executive director of Christian AIDS National Alliance, commented on the reporting problem in India: "HIV/AIDS prevalence for those labeled as 'low prevalence state' is not low since there are many risk factors in these areas: migration and women trafficking. Also, the surveillance systems are relatively poor; thus, many cases are not found or reported."[21] Gopal Mukherjee, program manager of Family Health International, likewise stated that "some states that have been categorized as Category D does not mean the HIV/AIDS prevalence is the lowest among Indian states, rather it means 'unknown prevalence' as these states do not release reports regarding HIV/AIDS situations in their respective states."[22]

Development of the HIV/AIDS Securitizing Move in India

Having discussed the historical and current HIV/AIDS problems in India, the development of HIV/AIDS-related political responses enacted by the national government is analyzed using the revised securitization framework. HIV/AIDS-related policy development within the Indian government is divided into five stages: (1) failed securitizing move (1986–1991); (2) performative securitizing move (1992–1997); (3) rhetorical securitizing move (1998–2003); and (4) full securitizing move (2004–2009). The perception of the government toward HIV/AIDS and its political responses are explained in each stage. Unlike its Chinese counterpart, the full securitizing move in the latest development of HIV/AIDS political responses (2010 onward) in India is no longer present within the Indian government. In other words, the security frame of the HIV/AIDS threat has debilitated at the national level. Hence, the latest/fifth stage of the HIV/AIDS securitizing move (2010 onward) in India is referred to in this chapter as the "fading-out of the full securitizing move."

Failed Securitizing Move (1986–1991)

Resembling the Chinese responses, a strong sense of denial of the actual threat posed by HIV/AIDS in the Indian government in the early years was evident.[23] Government officials viewed HIV/AIDS as a "western disease,"[24] and "a disease of the poor, the illiterate, the prostitutes and the deviants."[25] Government officials attributed the rise of HIV/AIDS infection figures to "the increasing influx of foreigners."[26] Positive speech acts were absent at that time because officials by and large denied the existence of HIV/AIDS in the country.

Shortly in the wake of the first cases were detected in 1986, measures related to legislative formulation and policy and institutional arrangement were enacted in response to HIV/AIDS problems. As a legislative political response, the government issued a quarantine law for HIV/AIDS cases in 1987.[27] Under this law, all foreign students and foreigners staying in India for more than a year should undergo a mandatory HIV/AIDS test;[28] infected individuals are repatriated to their place of origin.[29]

In addition to the quarantine law, the Indian officials proposed AIDS Prevention Bill forbidding Indian commercial sex workers from having sex with foreign clients in 1988.[30] One year later, the Indian government further suggested that the Bill should include the clause requiring HIV/AIDS infected individuals to disclose their identity. The bill was also proposed to empower medical practitioners to test and isolate suspected individuals, and introduce criminal penalties for the transmission of HIV/AIDS by professional blood donors.[31]

Aside from the enforcement of the legislation, the Indian government reacted to the disease in terms of policy and institutional establishment. An AIDS task force and the National AIDS Committee were established in 1986.[32] One year later the committee launched a three-year NACP under the Ministry of Health and Family Welfare (MoHFW) with the financial assistance of the World Bank.[33] Accordingly, measures such as surveillance, blood screening, and health education, were thereby carried out via the NACP.[34]

Aside from the 1987-NACP a Medium-Term Plan (1990–1992) was ushered in particularly in Tamil Nadu, Maharashtra, West Bengal, and Manipur and in the four metropolitan cities of Delhi, Mumbai, Chennai, and Calcutta.[35] HIV/AIDS interventions including information, education, and communication (IEC) campaign, surveillance system establishment, and safe blood supply were launched under the plan.[36]

Despite the rollout of the 1987 program and the 1990 plan, a full set of emergency measures was yet to be developed because of limited budgetary allocation for HIV/AIDS prevention and control. S. Samraj commented that "the Ministry of Health and Family Welfare did not focus on HIV/AIDS interventions from 1986 to 1992."[37] Instead of HIV/AIDS, the priority of the Indian government at that time was malaria, which was allocated with half of the health budget.[38] As such, the HIV/AIDS securitizing move in India failed during this period.

Performative Securitizing Move (1992–1997)

HIV/AIDS securitizing moves were transformed from a failed to performative attempt in 1992. With the financial assistance from the World Bank, NACO was set up in 1992 to formulate national HIV/AIDS policies.[39] NACO implemented the programs set forth by NACPs in different phases. State AIDS Control Societies (SACS) and Municipal AIDS Control Societies were thereafter established in all states union territories, and large cities to implement the central policies in their respective jurisdictions.[40] According to a NACO official [R47], the programs in each state were reviewed every three months, and annual reports were submitted to NACO every year.[41]

The total expenditure in the first phase of NACP (1992–1999) for the national program reached Rs. 4,541.8 million (US$99.6 million).[42]

The program was funded by the Indian government (Rs. 643 million or US$14.1 million), plus a loan of Rs. 3,830.4 million (US$84 million) offered by the World Bank, and a co-funding of Rs. 68.4 million (US$1.5 million) granted by the World Health Organization Global Program on AIDS.[43] During the NACP-I, an annual sentinel surveillance system was set up to monitor HIV/AIDS prevalence trend in the country.[44] To raise the public knowledge and awareness of HIV/AIDS, the national government launched an IEC program and "social marketing" for promoting condom use.[45] With respect to HIV/AIDS-related legislation change, the previously proposed AIDS Prevention Bill violated human rights was eventually withdrawn by the Indian government in late 1992.[46]

The previously mentioned early measures were yet inadequate in curbing the spread of the disease. The estimated number of HIV/AIDS-infected cases in India rocketed from 1.75 million in 1994 to 3.7 million in 1999.[47] Furthermore, the uniform national strategy for addressing the heterosexual mode of HIV/AIDS transmission was ineffective in north-eastern states such as Manipur,[48] where over 90 percent of HIV/AIDS infections were found among IDUs.[49] Positive speech acts were nonexistent during this period albeit extra budget allocation, policy, and institutional reformation. Hence HIV/AIDS securitizing moves were argued to be merely in their performative stage.

Rhetorical Securitizing Move (1998–2003)

Positive speech acts regarding HIV/AIDS have been identified in India since 1998. Prime Minister Vajpayee framed HIV/AIDS as a "scourge" and "threat" in his public speech in 1998,[50] in which he explicitly stated that:

> The experience of countries that have been successful in containing this **scourge** [HIV/AIDS] tells us government, business and society have to fight this **threat** collectively... There is no reason why we cannot forge such a partnership against HIV/AIDS in order to make our response more effective. [emphasis added][51]

In 2001, the Vajpayee government admitted that the HIV/AIDS problem is "one of the most serious public health problems in the country".[52] One year later, the prime minister launched another attempt to securitize HIV/AIDS, which was once perceived as a mere public health problem that should be tackled by state governments only, by uttering positive speech acts showing the continuous political will to securitize HIV/AIDS in subsequent years by stating that:

> Our preoccupation with terrorism should not dilute our commitment to tackle the **non-military threats** to **human and international security**. We have to sustain the fight against...the pandemic of **HIV/AIDS**...Food security, energy security, and **health security** are important goals. [emphasis added][53]

Aside from positive speech acts, legislative formulation was also observed. On top of the National AIDS Prevention and Control Policy in 2001, two other HIV/AIDS-related legislations, including the *National Blood Policy* and *An Action Plan for Blood Safety*, were enacted in 2000 and 2003, respectively. Regarding policy measures and budgetary allocation in dealing with HIV/AIDS, the second phase of NACP (NACP-II) was launched between November 1999 and 2006.[54] The total expenditure of the NACP-II was Rs. 14,315.66 million (US$313.94 million). The central and state government contributed Rs. 1,769.3 million (US$38.8 million),[55] while the remaining budget (Rs. 12,546.36 million or US$275.14 million) was funded by three international organizations, namely the International Development Association (IDA) of the World Bank and the United States Agency for International Development (USAID) in conjunction with the Department for International Development (DFID) of the United Kingdom.[56]

However, budgetary allocation was problematic in terms of ARV drugs provision. In late 2003, the health minister negotiated with the drug industry to lower its prices on ARV drugs, and announced that "women, children below the age of 15 and those patients suffering late-stage AIDS will be provided free antiretroviral drugs in government hospitals from April 1, 2004."[57] Nevertheless, free ARV drug provision was scarce in India; the drugs were only available in eight hospitals in the six high-prevalence states (one hospital each in Andhra Pradesh, Karnataka, Maharashtra, Tamil Nadu, Manipur, and Nagaland) and two in New Delhi.[58] Budget sustainability of the program was barely certain. The ministry's budget was only Rs. 2,280 million (US$50 million), which was insufficient to support the program that costs Rs. 6,065 million (US$133 million) annually.[59] More devastatingly, the cost reduction negotiation initiated by the health minister with pharmaceutical manufacturers collapsed because the general elections in early 2004 prevented the budget from being finalized.[60]

Given the presence of positive speech acts but the absence of a full set of emergency measures (i.e., the lack of free ARV provision and HIV/AIDS-related institution establishment), the HIV/AIDS securitizing move was solely rhetorical under the Vajpayee government. Compared to the previous stage, statements of support (positive speech acts) from the prime minister palpably increased. However, skepticism about the scope of HIV/AIDS continued among the high-level government officials.[61]

Their denial was recorded on several occasions. In 2002, the National Intelligence Council (NIC) predicted that about 20–25 million people in India would be infected with HIV/AIDS by 2010.[62] Nevertheless, health minister Shatrughan Sinha dismissed the prediction as "completely inaccurate."[63] Sinha also criticized United States Ambassador Robert Blackwill and Bill Gates for "spreading panic" when they cited the NIC prediction in their public speeches.[64] Similar to Sinha's standpoint, human resource minister Murli Manohar Joshi asserted that the figure (25 million HIV/AIDS infected population in India) is highly exaggerated.[65] Prime Minister Vajpayee even cancelled a scheduled meeting with Gates because he was deeply unsatisfied with the epidemiological prediction.[66]

Downplaying the HIV/AIDS preventive methods prevailed in other places in India at that time. Human resource minister Joshi asserted that sex education in schools would create an "immoral society" and a "growth in single parent families."[67] Furthermore, health minister Sushma Swaraj was a critic of condom promotion as a prevention strategy.[68] Swaraj promoted in a condom advertisement that abstinence and monogamy are far more important than condom use.[69] However, with over 85 percent of HIV/AIDS infections attributed to sexual transmission, condom promotion should be considered the most significant and effective intervention especially in India.[70]

Taken together, the effectiveness of rhetorical securitizing move was in doubt. This outcome was partly proved by the upsurge in the number of infected cases in the country, from 3.5 million in 1998 to over 5 million in 2003,[71] which accounted for over a 40 percent increase in the second phase of the program.

Full Securitizing Move (2004–2009)

> [HIV/]AIDS is **no longer just a public health issue**, but it has [also] become **one of the most serious** socio-economic and developmental concerns... We have **no choice but to act**, and act with **firmness**, with **urgency** and with **utmost seriousness**. [emphasis added][72]
>
> Given the scale of suffering wrought by the HIV/AIDS epidemic, it is to be expected that **doomsday scenarios of its spread** are commonplace. My country [India] figures prominently in all these projections. [emphasis added][73]

Under the new leadership of Prime Minister Manmohan Singh and party president Sonia Gandhi in May 2004, the HIV/AIDS securitizing move shifted into a positive development with positive speech acts and a full set of emergency measures. The commitment of the new government to HIV/AIDS issues was also realized in the National Common Minimum Program (NCMP) of the ruling party in May 2004, stating that the party will allocate financial resources to contain all communicable diseases and provide leadership to the national HIV/AIDS programs.[74] In addition to positive speech acts, subcategories of emergency measures have all been identified since 2004, as illuminated in the following sections.

Budgetary Allocation

Along with the commitments stated, HIV/AIDS-related funding surged from Rs. 2,334 million (US$50.7 million) in 2003 to Rs. 4,260 million (US$92.6 million) in 2004. This 82.52 percent increase in the HIV/AIDS budget reflected an obvious shift of budget toward the HIV/AIDS control and prevention undertaking.

Policy and Institutional Arrangement

With respect to the pertinent policy and institutional arrangement, the government has strikingly incorporated media as one of the core components of the HIV/AIDS intervention program since 2004.[75] The first Bollywood movie related to HIV/AIDS, *Phir Milenge* (We'll Meet Again), was shown in mainstream Indian cinemas in August 2004 to change the perception of Indian people toward HIV/AIDS and the people living under the epidemic.[76] This reaction was believed to break the silence and misunderstanding of HIV/AIDS that persist in Indian society. In addition, the national broadcaster Doordarshan, who could reach out to 400 million people in 12 local languages,[77] started airing a daily half-hour show on HIV/AIDS issues in 2005.[78]

Aside from the breakthrough in broadcasting HIV/AIDS-related films and TV shows, the MoHFW reversed the previous National Democratic Alliance Government's decision on banning condom advertisements by negotiating with the Ministry of Information and Broadcasting.[79] This policy decision facilitated condom promotion and the overall HIV/AIDS interventions in India, given that over 80 percent of HIV/AIDS infections resulted from unprotected sexual contact.

Regarding the HIV/AIDS-related institutional arrangement, the National Council on AIDS (NCA) was constituted in 2005, aiming to lead the national HIV/AIDS control efforts as pledged in the NCMP. The council is chaired by the prime minister and composed of 31 ministries, seven chief ministers, civil society representatives, positive people's network, and private sector organizations.[80] Subsequent to the establishment of NCA, State Councils of AIDS (SCA) were also formulated in 25 Indian states.[81] Most importantly, the chairmanship of the prime minister in this council is a reflection of the highest level of commitment of the Indian government in containing HIV/AIDS.[82]

Aside from the establishment of NCA and SCAs, a new department specified for HIV/AIDS—Department of AIDS Control—was formulated under the MoHFW in 2008. Previously, NACO was one of the administrative bodies under the Department of Health. After the formulation of Department of AIDS Control, NACO is now operating underneath the HIV/AIDS-focused department.[83] This institutional arrangement implies the exclusiveness of HIV/AIDS issues among other health care and disease control programs, as well as the extended commitment toward HIV/AIDS response within the Indian government.

Legislation Amendment and Formulation

A prominent law amendment related to anti-HIV/AIDS measures in India is the scrapping of Section 377 of the Indian Penal Code (IPC), a 150-year-old law enforced in 1860 by India's British rulers.[84] Section 377 stated that a person would be imprisoned for up to ten years if he "voluntarily has carnal intercourse against the order of nature with any man, woman or animal."[85] Simply put, homosexuality is illegal and strongly considered a taboo in India. Hence, MSM are reluctant to identify their status publicly or seek any HIV/AIDS test or treatment.

In addition, the law has been frequently misused by the police to harass MSM and NGO activists working for MSM communities.[86] For example, four activists of The Naz Foundation (India) Trust and Bharosa Trust who were accused of promoting homosexuality were imprisoned in Lucknow, Uttar Pradesh.[87] Serious incidents of police abuse against NGO staff have also been reported in Mumbai, Chennai, Sangli, Bangalore, and New Delhi.[88]

The High Court eventually decriminalized homosexuality on July 2, 2009, which was viewed as an improvement on the social acceptability of homosexuality that was once condemned by the Indian government and the public. Activists working for homosexual groups revealed a significant decline in the police harassment of MSM after the decriminalization of homosexuality.[89] Dr. M. K. Nabeel, research associate of UNAIDS India Office, asserted that "legislation does influence HIV/AIDS programs. For example, after the write down of Section 377, the HIV/AIDS workers feel they have more freedom to work for MSM population."[90]

Emerging Issue: Fading-Out of Full HIV/AIDS Securitizing Moves (2010 Onward)

Unlike China, the effect of the post-2004 full securitizing move has dwindled since 2010 despite the implementation of several emergency measures in recent years, such as the removal of travel and residency bans for HIV/AIDS-infected individuals entering India by the External Affairs Ministry in late 2010,[91] and the release of the fourth phase of NACP in 2012.[92] It is anticipated that the emergency measures related to institutional arrangement and HIV/AIDS-specific legislation are deemed to fade out in India.

The HIV/AIDS Bill, which aims to obligate the Indian government to provide complete ARV treatment, diagnostics, and nutritional supplements to HIV/AIDS-infected individuals, was prepared in 2005.[93] However, the bill has been pending within the Ministry of Health since 2010, and is yet to be introduced to the Indian parliament.[94] A government official [R39] explained the pending status of the bill in an interview: "It is because people are debating with different issues. Some people argue why it should be an AIDS Bill. Why not have a bill for all the diseases, for we have many other diseases in India."[95] In July 2011, health minister Ghulam Nabi Azad announced that the government intends to remove from the bill the chapter on the provision of HIV/AIDS-related treatment.[96] The treatment chapter mandates the government to provide free treatment and preventive services for people living with HIV/AIDS.[97] This incident implies that the commitment of the national government toward HIV/AIDS legislation is apparently in doubt.

On top of the resistance to pass the HIV/AIDS Bill, the existence of the stand-alone HIV/AIDS institution and program is subject to challenge. Since 2005, previously stand-alone National Disease Control Programs such as malaria, TB, Kala Azar, Filaria, Blindness, and Iodine Deficiency have already been incorporated into the NRHM.[98]

NRHM is an articulation of the government commitment under the NCMP to increase public spending on health from a GDP of 0.9 percent to 2–3 percent.[99] The NRHM aims to provide integrated comprehensive primary health care for the rural population in the entire country, especially by giving special attention to 18 states with weak public health indicators and/or fragile health infrastructure compared to the rest of the Indian states.[100] These are the eight northeastern states (Arunachal Pradesh, Nagaland, Manipur, Mizoram, Assam, Meghalaya, Sikkim, and Tripura), as well as the eight Empowered Action Group (EAG) states (Uttar Pradesh, Bihar, Madhya Pradesh, Orissa, Jharkhand, Uttarakhand, Rajasthan, and Chhattisgarh), Jammu, Kashmir, and Himachal Pradesh.[101] The portion of the budget allocated to the NRHM surged over 60 percent of the total health budget as a result of the special attention given toward the primary health care provision. In addition, the program is likely to get an extension until 2020.[102]

Budgetary allocation to HIV/AIDS interventions has been continuously augmented. However, compared to the portion of health budget dispensed to NRHM, the vast majority of the government health funding has been allocated to NRHM, as shown in table 7.1. This budget allocation suggests that the Indian government is more concerned with primary health care in general than with HIV/AIDS.[103] In other words, HIV/AIDS was no longer treated as the single most serious problem; rather, it was simply considered as one of the many health problems in India.

Aside from the continuous increase in the financial resources of the NRHM, budgets for HIV/AIDS interventions have been reallocated into the NRHM to enhance the quality of the public health system.[104] In 2010, six components of the NACP-III have been merged with the NRHM,[105] namely Integrated Counselling and Testing Centres (ICTC); prevention of parent-to-child transmission (PPTCT); blood safety; sexually transmitted infections (STI) services; condom programming; together with ART.[106] The convergence of NACP into NRHM can also be observed in the participation of the NRHM in Red Ribbon Express-II, which was not included in the first phase.[107] Aside from the exhibitions of HIV/AIDS provided by NACO, information on other diseases and general health services such as

Table 7.1 Health Budget Allocated to the NRHM and HIV/AIDS (2005–2011)

Year	Total Health Budget (in Rs. million)	NRHM Budget (in Rs. million)	HIV/AIDS Budget (in Rs. million)	Health Expenditure on NRHM (%)	Health Expenditure on HIV/AIDS (%)
2005–2006	100,400	69,700	5,335	69	5.3
2006–2007	117,580	82,500	7,056.7	70	5.9
2007–2008	149,740	110,310	9,433.4	74	6.2
2008–2009	179,090	124,840	11,233.6	70	6.2
2009–2010	210,800	140,180	9,801.5	66	4.6
2010–2011	244,940	162,190	14,002.2	66	5.7

Sources: "Finance Minister P. Chidambaram's Budget Speech," "Annual Report 2008–2009," "UNGASS Country Progress Report 2010: India," and "Annual Report 2010–2011."

H1N1, tuberculosis, malaria, reproductive and child health services, and general health and hygiene were also found in an entire training provided by the NRHM.[108]

Taking the integrated approach toward HIV/AIDS programs, the Indian government has reacted to the HIV/AIDS problems within a *nonemergency mode* since 2010. The convergence was unequivocally guaranteed in an official document released in 2010, stating that "the DAPCU works seamlessly with the district administration and programs provided under the NRHM with which the NACP will eventually be merged."[109] A government official [R48] confirmed the convergence trend in an interview in March 2011, claiming that "the government is trying to merge separate malaria, TB, and HIV/AIDS programs into the NRHM."[110]

Several respondents also remarked on the convergence trend during the interview. For instance, Amita Chebbi, country director of the Clinton Health Access Initiative, contended that "HIV/AIDS has been treated as a separate disease from other diseases as HIV/AIDS is tackled by the NACO... However, the future trend would be the integration of the existing HIV/AIDS program into the public health system... NACO will be under the NRHM as a separate division."[111] S. Samraj also believed that the "mainstreaming of health programs is ongoing in India. The government pulls back the past stand-alone HIV/AIDS programs to the general health care system."[112]

In an attempt to reverse the full HIV/AIDS securitizing move, the Indian government is integrating stand-alone national HIV/AIDS programs into the NRHM. The attempt of the Indian government to reverse the full securitizing move is supported by a number of respondents. For example, Padma Buggineni, program manager of the International HIV/AIDS Alliance, believed that "it is better for NACP to incorporate into the NRHM, since it can reduce the burden of government on public health expenses. Also, other health workers can be equipped with HIV/AIDS knowledge in the converging program."[113] Holding a similar viewpoint, Dr. I. S. Gilada, managing director and consultant in Skin, STDs and HIV/AIDS of Unison Medicare and Research Care Pvt Ltd, remarked that "it is a good idea. When a new problem comes up, we will see it as a big problem. For cost effectiveness, it is better for HIV/AIDS to be integrated."[114]

Despite these opinions on treating HIV/AIDS in a nonemergency manner, the attempt to pull back emergency measures has received fierce opposition from HIV/AIDS practitioners. Loon Gangte, executive director of Delhi Network for People Living with HIV/AIDS, expressed his worries about the level of HIV/AIDS funding: "NRHM will do many things, not only HIV/AIDS. In that sense, funding [for HIV/AIDS] will be diluted."[115] Sujit Kumar Sahu, HIV and AIDS program coordinator of EFICOR, raised his doubt on the priority of HIV/AIDS issues on the government agenda: "It is a good idea for the NRHM to put money on maternal and child health care, but how about the HIV/AIDS programs? I am afraid that NACP may become a small and not a high priority [program] in the NRHM. It is better to keep NRHM and NACP separate."[116]

Vinod Bhanu, executive director of the Center for Legislative Research and Advocacy, explained the reason for the resistance of institutional change: "They [HIV/AIDS practitioners] are afraid that the government will put less focus on NACP within the NRHM program."[117] To understand the stance of the Indian government on the future development of national HIV/AIDS institution and program, two government officials were interviewed and commented on this issue. A government official in an HIV/AIDS-related department [R46] claimed, "We are planning for the NACP-IV. NACP will not lose its identity in the NRHM."[118] Dr. Thokchom Meinya, member of parliament (Lok Sabha), asserted that "NRHM combines all the rural health programs together. We have fixed budgets for each health program, so budgets for HIV/AIDS would not be reduced due to the integration."[119] At this stage, concluding whether the Indian government will maintain its national budget for HIV/AIDS is too early. However, the push against full HIV/AIDS securitizing moves in India in recent years has been confirmed. Simply put, HIV/AIDS was no longer perceived as the single most important issue that has to be dealt with; thus, the previous stand-alone programs are being put under the umbrella of public health programs.

The Indian government possibly has a strategic reason for drawing back the full securitizing move. As mentioned in chapter 4 of this book, most of the public health programs in India considerably resort to international or foreign monetary support. Table 7.2 shows that over 85 percent of the budget in the first and second phases of NACP and 75 percent in the third phase were overwhelmingly granted by international funding agencies and bilateral governments. As such, government financial contribution to its national HIV/AIDS program is very limited, and the pertinent budget in the country is prone to alter by the prevailing international health agenda.

Aside from the finite contribution of the national government, a government official mentioned during the interview that the sustainability of the national HIV/AIDS program in India is also problematic because "it is a general phenomenon to mainstream health [at the international level]. In other words, the [international] funding now focuses on the general health care system, like [how] NRHM functions."[120] Gopal Mukherjee, program manager of Family Health International, also pointed out that

Table 7.2 Summary of the Financial Expenditures of the Indian Government and External Agencies on NACPs

	NACP-I (1992–1999)	NACP-II (1999–2006)	NACP-III (2007–2012)
Total expenditure (in million)	Rs. 4,541.8 US$ 99.6	Rs. 14,315.66 US$ 313.94	Rs. 115,850 US$ 2,540.57
Indian government expenditure (in million)[a]	Rs. 643. US$ 14.1	Rs. 1,769.3 US$ 38.8	Rs. 28,610 US$ 627.4
Indian government expenditure to the total expenditure (%)	14.2	12.4	24.7
Major external Aid Component inside the government and direct funding from other donors outside the government	World Bank WHO/GPA	IDA USAID DFID	WB DFID PEPFAR GRATM BMGF Clinton Foundation UN EU
External agencies expenditure (in million)	Rs. 3,898.8 US$ 85.5	Rs. 12,546.36 US$ 275.14	Rs.87,240 US$ 1,913.17
External agencies expenditure to the total expenditure (%)	85.8	87.6	75.3

Sources: "Project Performance Assessment Report"; "World Bank to Give India 191M US Dollars for AIDS Control"; "UNGASS Country Progress Report 2010: India."
[a]Government expenditure with the exclusion of the external aid components inside the government.

"international agencies have shifted their funding priorities from HIV/AIDS to other lifestyle diseases such as tobacco control and cancers."[121] Gopal further clarified: "In other words, the international priority has been changed from one specific disease to more general public health problems. In this sense, if the national government perceives HIV/AIDS as a general public health problem, funding from the international agencies will be increased, if HIV/AIDS is conceived as a stand-alone program, funding will be reduced."[122]

Given the massive reliance on foreign funds to support its own national HIV/AIDS programs, the Indian government was compelled to change its security frames and strategies to match the international concerns/funding for HIV/AIDS interventions. As such, HIV/AIDS funding is likely to be guaranteed if the future NACPs exist underneath the gigantic public health system instead of a stand-alone program.

Summary

The first HIV/AIDS case in India was detected in Chennai, Tamil Nadu in 1986. Early infections were discovered among FSWs and IDUs in states such as Maharashtra, Tamil Nadu, and Manipur. By the late 1990s, HIV/AIDS infections were reported in all states and union territories. The current epidemiological situation in India is similar to the past. Heterosexual contact has remained the most prominent route of infection, followed by IDU. Heterosexual contact is the primary mode of infection in the southern states of Maharashtra, Karnataka, Tamil Nadu, and Andhra Pradesh, whereas IDU is the primary transmission mode in the northern states of Manipur and Nagaland.

HIV/AIDS-related political responses at the national level in different periods of time were analyzed using the revised securitization framework. Similar to the attitude of the Chinese government toward HIV/AIDS in the early years, HIV/AIDS issues did not gain positive political recognition from top-level leaders in India. Thus, the securitizing move largely failed in the early period. This chapter demonstrated that a full securitizing move to HIV/AIDS has been generated within the Indian government since 2004. Aside from the presence of positive speech acts, a full set of emergency measures, including a significant augmentation in financial resources, formulation of HIV/AIDS-related policies and institutions, and establishment of related legislation, have been observed since 2004.

Arguably, however, the full securitizing move is no longer maintained within the Indian government, that is, HIV/AIDS is no longer perceived as a top-priority issue in the national government agenda. In other words, the continuous budgetary allocation for HIV/AIDS interventions is no longer guaranteed, whereas policy, institution, and legislation related to HIV/AIDS may not exist in a stand-alone manner. Although there has been no denial of the existential threat posed by HIV/AIDS, nor any declaration that the threat has passed, a push against full HIV/AIDS securitizing moves is present. The future NACPs are expected to be presented as a stand-alone program with greater integration with the NRHM, or largely formulated as one of the infectious disease programs under the umbrella program of the NRHM.

Chapter 8

Audience Acceptance in India: Case Studies in New Delhi, Mumbai, and Imphal

Introduction

By applying the securitization framework in the Indian context, the previous chapter revealed that a full HIV/AIDS securitizing move was generated by the Indian government in 2004. However, as argued in chapter 7, the full securitizing move in 2004 was no longer maintained within the Indian government. In other words, HIV/AIDS was no longer framed as the most serious problem or perceived as a top-priority issue in the national government agenda. In this sense, the HIV/AIDS securitizing move in India existed in the failed rather than in full version.

After the latest rhetorical security act was located in 2009, an explicit positive speech act has yet to be identified since 2010. Without any positive utterance toward HIV/AIDS, the form of speech acts in this period is deemed to be negative (-SA). With regard to the political reactions toward HIV/AIDS problems, the Indian government had reacted and was reacting to the problem within a nonemergency mode (-EM). A scale-up effort was recognized in terms of budgetary allocation in this mode of political reaction. However, revised or new HIV/AIDS-specific institution and legislation formulation was largely absent. In contrast, the Indian government decided to integrate the previously stand-alone HIV/AIDS program, the NACP, into the umbrella public health program NRHM. Additionally, the Indian government hitherto deferred the legislation of the HIV/AIDS

Bill that had been drafted in 2005. In other words, the form of HIV/AIDS securitizing move that prevailed in 2011 was simplified as follows:[1]

(−SA) + (−EM) → Failed securitizing move

In accordance with securitization theory, the possibility of a securitizing move produced by a securitizer to turn to securitization was decided by the target audience. "Audience acceptance," which was defined in the revised securitization framework, denoted the *support of the audience toward a particular securitizing move*. "Support" was composed of two dimensions: *moral* and *technical* support. In the case of India, the presence of a strong moral and technical support (+AA) referred to the generation of a failed securitization, whereas the absence of either or both (−AA) denoted failure. This situation was simplified as follows:

Failed securitizing move + (+AA) → Failed securitization

Or

Failed securitizing move + (−AA) → Void failed securitization

This chapter aims to discover the level of audience acceptance (support) in three Indian cities—New Delhi, Mumbai, and Imphal—toward the failed HIV/AIDS securitizing move in India. Similar to the case of China, these three localities were selected to showcase the levels of audience acceptance in different parts of India. Individuals working in HIV/AIDS-focused NGOs comprised the target audience in this study.

A section on the overview of HIV/AIDS situations in these cities is first illustrated to contextualize these case studies. With a view to capturing "what the audience already knows" about the prevailing HIV/AIDS securitizing move in their local contexts,[2] an elaboration of the local understanding of the failed HIV/AIDS securitizing move in each city is provided prior to the audience acceptance section. To uncover the local understanding of the failed securitizing move, NGO respondents were invited to give comments on whether (1) HIV/AIDS was the most serious public health problem in the eyes of the Indian government, and (2) HIV/AIDS was the top-priority issue in the national government agenda. The justifications for their responses were also collected.

The level of moral and technical support of the respondents in the selected cities is compared and contrasted using the interview materials and existing secondary data. The type of HIV/AIDS securitization in India is identified in the last section after the discovery of overall audience acceptance.

Overview of HIV/AIDS Situations and Local Understanding of Failed Securitizing Moves in Selected Cities

New Delhi: Overview of the HIV/AIDS Situation

The first HIV/AIDS case in Delhi was reported in 1988.[3] Defined as a low HIV/AIDS prevalence state (0.25 percent),[4] the estimated number of HIV/AIDS cases in Delhi was 51,818 in 2007.[5] Among the 51 thousands infected individuals in the state, over 32,000 HIV/AIDS-infected people are from New Delhi.[6] However, there are at least one million people in the city who are vulnerable to HIV/AIDS,[7] considering that Delhi state and its capital city have a large and diverse population with a considerable number of migrants, mostly from the less developed states of Bihar and Uttar Pradesh.[8] Nearly 77 percent of the spread of the disease is transmitted through unprotected sexual practices, followed by IDU (8.79 percent) and infected blood transfusion (7.14 percent).[9]

Local Understanding of Failed HIV/AIDS Securitizing Moves

Regarding the local understanding of failed securitizing moves, the majority of the respondents in New Delhi conceived that the Indian government treated HIV/AIDS as only one of the most serious public health problems or not a serious problem at all.[10] Amita Chebbi, country director of the Clinton Health Access Initiative, contended that HIV/AIDS is not the most serious problem, because the national government agenda has been overwhelmingly occupied by "other more serious problems in the country."[11]

Amita's view is fairly shared by other NGO respondents in New Delhi. For instance, Dr. M. K. Nabeel, research associate, Solution Exchange AIDS Community, UNAIDS India Office, stated that "HIV/AIDS is not an emergent issue as there are so many other issues in India that need to be addressed."[12] Sujit Kumar Sahu, HIV and AIDS program coordinator of The Evangelical Fellowship of India Commission Relief, pointed out "other issues" that have been equally raised by other respondents: "The government perceives TB, HIV/AIDS, and mother-and-child health as the most serious public health problems in India."[13]

Only a small portion of the New Delhi respondents staunchly believed that HIV/AIDS was a high priority in the government agenda.[14] For instance, Pallavi Upadhyaya, prevention programs coordinator of AIDS Healthcare Foundation India Cares, noted, "The priority of HIV/AIDS is very high, as the government has granted NACO special powers to work on HIV/AIDS problems. For other diseases, the government deals with these only via the pre-existing health care system."[15] Vinod Bhanu, executive director of the Centre for Legislative Research and Advocacy, upheld a similar view on the HIV/AIDS precedence: "HIV/AIDS is one of the high priority issues in the national government agenda. Some people working on TB and malaria believe that HIV/AIDS has overtaken the government attention as more funds have been allocated to HIV/AIDS interventions."[16]

Taken together, over half of the respondents in the capital city asserted that instead of HIV/AIDS, other issues such as maternal and child health care and rural and national economy should be the top-priority issue in the government agenda.[17] Consider the following selection:

> Given that the HIV/AIDS prevalence is low in India, it cannot be the top priority issue. Issues such as **maternal and child health are more prioritized**. [emphasis added][18]
>
> I don't know what the top priority issue is. I believe **the economy may be the top priority issue** for the government. [emphasis added][19]
>
> HIV/AIDS is not the top priority issue. For developing countries, **economy** is the top priority issue. In many economic superpowers, public health spending is less than 3 percent. Public health is not in the government agenda. **Health issues cannot become national security threats.** [emphasis added][20]

Mumbai: Overview of the HIV/AIDS Situation

Mumbai is a major financial hub and port city in the country. The city is also the most populous conurbation in India and the sixth most populous agglomeration in the world. According to a 2001 census, population in Mumbai increased from 9.93 million in 1991 to 11.91 million in 2001. Some officials in Mumbai estimate that an additional 2–3 million "floating population" also resides in the city.

As previously mentioned, over 80 percent of HIV/AIDS cases in the country are transmitted through heterosexual sex. Mumbai is considered the epicenter of the HIV/AIDS epidemic transmitted via this route because the city is purportedly reported the largest number of brothel-based commercial sex workers in India.[21] In 1990, approximately 100,000–150,000 FSWs in Kamathipura (also known as Falkland Road), Mumbai's red-light district, were located in the southern part of the city.[22]

FSWs in Mumbai come from primarily three "sources": (1) half of the FSW population in Mumbai brothels are Nepalese women smuggled to the city via the northeastern region of India;[23] (2) girls who "married" a temple god (devadasi system) and provided sexual services to priests but ended up in the flesh trade (about 15 percent of the women in Mumbai's red-light district are devadasis);[24] and (3) women from other parts of rural India seeking better job opportunities in the city, but eventually entering the sex trade either voluntarily or involuntarily.[25] These women are especially vulnerable to HIV/AIDS and other sexually transmitted diseases due to language barriers, low social status, and low literacy rate.[26] These factors hinder FSWs from receiving preventive information on HIV/AIDS and negotiating for safer sex with their male clients.

The first case of HIV/AIDS infection in Mumbai was detected in 1986, whereas the first case of late-stage AIDS was reported in 1987.[27] The percentage of FSWs tested for HIV/AIDS in Mumbai's red-light districts rocketed from 1 percent in 1987 to 35 percent in 1992.[28] More than 33 percent of the estimated 100,000–150,000 FSWs may be infected with HIV/AIDS.[29] HIV/AIDS prevalence among this group even reached 60 percent in 2000.[30]

FSWs can be easily recognized in brothels, whereas MSM are diverse and often hard-to-reach in India.[31] Ashok Row Kavi, one of the prominent experts on sexual minority groups in India, estimated that 40–50 million Indian men are MSM.[32] Hence, only 5–10 percent of MSM have been identified in India.[33] This group is usually denoted the "hidden population" because open discussion of MSM is not tolerated in Indian society, albeit the description of same-sex activity in the Indian ancient scripture *Kama Sutra*.[34] MSM who have "come out of the closet" tend to be English-speaking and wealthy, and are concentrated in major Indian cities such as Mumbai.[35]

Same-sex relationship is a strong taboo in Indian society; hence, several homosexual or bisexual men marry women to disguise their status. Additionally, Ashok Row Kavi estimated that 80 percent of MSM in the country are married. As such, the wives of these men are inevitably at high risk of being infected with HIV/AIDS.[36]

Intense political attention has been given to FSWs and IDUs; on the other hand, MSM were previously excluded because Indian scientists insisted that this category did not exist in India.[37] However, HIV/AIDS has taken root within this hidden population, disproving the preceding claims made by scientists. Scientific evidence later revealed that MSM were 19 times more likely to be infected with HIV/AIDS than the general population.[38] Another study conducted by the Humsafar Trust, one of the first community-based organizations (CBOs) working on MSM in India, revealed a 20 percent HIV/AIDS prevalence among MSM.[39] One of the studies conducted between 2002 and 2004 claimed that HIV/AIDS prevalence among the MSM community was 14 percent. About 62 percent of the 14 percent prevalence have confirmed STIs.[40] In 2006, HIV/AIDS prevalence among MSM was 7 percent in Mumbai.[41] Based on the research conducted by Kumta et al. in 2010, HIV/AIDS prevalence among MSM in Mumbai was 12.5 percent.[42] Although an upsurge in HIV/AIDS prevalence was seen among MSM, the prevalence of the virus among the general population was reduced to 7.69 percent in May 2010 from 10.65 percent in 2007.[43]

Local Understanding of Failed HIV/AIDS Securitizing Moves

In the course of the interview sessions, less than half of the respondents from Mumbai perceived that HIV/AIDS was the most serious public health problem in the eyes of the Indian government.[44] For instance, Umesh Tandel, project manager of Mukti Sadan Foundation, stated, "HIV/AIDS is a top priority issue in India. Compared to individuals suffering from other diseases, HIV/AIDS-infected patients can receive operations earlier in government hospitals."[45] Notwithstanding the seriousness of the HIV/AIDS perceived in the eyes of the respondents, over half of the respondents in Mumbai believed that instead of HIV/AIDS, the top-priority issue should be rural health, public health care, or economic development.[46] Consider the following selection:

> The priority of the government is to **improve the quality of health of people living in the rural areas**. It is because around 60 to 70 percent of people are living in rural areas in India. Therefore, **rural health is the primary concern of the national government**. [emphasis added][47]
>
> HIV/AIDS is the **second issue** in the eyes of the national government. The government puts **more emphasis on public health**. [emphasis added][48]
>
> HIV/AIDS is **not the first priority** in the government agenda. The government did not recognize the seriousness of HIV/AIDS in India, in which the disease can destroy the next generation. The **top priority in the national government agenda should be economic development**. [emphasis added][49]

Imphal: Overview of the HIV/AIDS Situation

The Northeastern (NE) Region of India comprises eight states, namely Assam, Arunachal Pradesh, Manipur, Meghalaya, Mizoram, Nagaland,

Tripura, and Sikkim (included later by the Northeastern Council).[50] With a 358 km-long international border with Myanmar, Manipur is one of the major routes for illegal international drug trafficking for Myanmar heroin (also known as No. 4) since the early 1980s.[51] Heroin transportation is facilitated by the National Highway 39, which starts at Moreh,[52] a town in Churachandpur District close to the Myanmar border, runs north through Manipur, to Nagaland, and then to Dimapur via Kohima (capital of Nagaland), and to Guwahati and the core part of India.[53]

The first HIV/AIDS case in Manipur was reported in February 1990, which was discovered from the blood samples of six imprisoned IDUs.[54] HIV/AIDS prevalence among IDUs surged rampantly from 0 percent to 50 percent within six months after the discovery of the initial cases in early 1990.[55] In April 1998, health department officials reported that 94 people died from late-stage AIDS, whereas 6,194 were HIV-positive in Manipur at that time.[56] As of January 2011, the total numbers of HIV-positive cases in Manipur were 38,016.[57] However, as Dipak put it, "The figure of HIV-positive people in the state can be just the tip of the iceberg as many people try to conceal their positive status due to the stigma attached to the disease."[58]

In recent years, however, HIV/AIDS in Manipur is no longer confined among the IDU population; rather, the disease has been increasingly driven by homosexual or heterosexual transmission.[59] According to the sentinel surveillance report released by the Manipur State AIDS Control Society (MSACS) in 2009, HIV/AIDS prevalence among IDUs was decreased to 17.9 percent, whereas prevalence among MSM and FSWs increased to 16.4 percent and 12.9 percent in 2007,[60] that is, from 12.4 percent and 11.6 percent in 2006, respectively.[61] Nevertheless, the current epidemiological pattern in Manipur still contrasts with the rest of India, where heterosexual contact is the major mode of HIV/AIDS transmission in most parts of the country (87 percent).[62]

Imphal is the capital city of Manipur. Among the cities and districts in the state, Imphal has the highest HIV/AIDS prevalence throughout the decades. Out of the 629 late-stage AIDS cases found in Manipur in 1990, 279 cases (44.36 percent) were from Imphal, followed by 69 cases from Churachandpur (10.97 percent), and 41 cases from Chandel (6.52 percent).[63] As of October 2002, 14,097 HIV-positive cases and 1,532 late-stage AIDS cases were reported in Manipur; 69 percent of these are from Imphal.[64] Accordingly, in a district-wise surveillance in 2007, Imphal was rated as the district with the highest number of HIV-positive cases (57.23 percent), while the remaining 42.77 percent were scattered in other districts of Manipur.[65]

Aside from the mode of HIV/AIDS transmission, which is mainly IDU, HIV/AIDS-hepatitis C coinfection is another distinctive issue particularly prevalent in Manipur. During the interviews, several respondents in Imphal expressed their concerns regarding the coinfection of HIV/AIDS–hepatitis C especially found in HIV/AIDS-infected people in Manipur. A high-ranking official in the Manipur State AIDS Control Society [R64] acknowledged that the coinfection problem was severe in HIV/AIDS-infected individuals in the state because of the needle-sharing habit.[66]

In an interview with Dr. K. Priyokumar Singh, a physician working in Jawaharlal Nehru Hospital in Imphal, he further confirmed the HIV/AIDS–hepatitis C coinfection issue: "HIV/AIDS–hepatitis C coinfection problem is serious in Manipur. Approximately 90 percent of people having HIV/AIDS–hepatitis C coinfection in India live in Manipur."[67] A recent survey also showed that over 90 percent of HIV/AIDS-infected individuals in Imphal were infected with hepatitis C.[68] However, Dr. K. Priyokumar Singh lamented that "while other countries are prepared to provide treatment for people with HIV/AIDS–hepatitis C coinfection, no free hepatitis C treatment is available in government hospitals...the cost for hepatitis C drugs is about Rs. 80,000."[69] Many patients cannot afford hepatitis C treatment as it is extremely costly at the individual level.[70] Without an affordable treatment available, hepatitis C has become the main cause of mortality of HIV/AIDS-infected people in Imphal and Manipur.[71]

Together with the medical problem of the coinfection of HIV/AIDS–hepatitis C, political and social instability in Imphal and Manipur are other daunting problems that are yet to be resolved, thwarting HIV/AIDS interventions in the state. Persistent insurgency is one of the major problems faced in the NE states. The region is home to various rebel and insurgent groups that represent different communities struggling for independence after the transition from the British colonial system to the Indian state. Given its unstable circumstance, the Indian government declared several parts of this region as "disturbed areas," including Manipur, Assam, Nagaland, and some parts of Arunachal Pradesh, and Tripura.[72]

R. K. Gyanandra Singh, program officer of Catholic Relief Services, pinpointed the impacts of the insurgent groups on the local people:"insurgent groups [in Manipur] are powerful in a way they claim themselves as the second local government in Manipur. There are limited livelihoods in Manipur as the insurgent groups ban all Indian movies showing in local cinemas. Public facilities are mostly unavailable for people."[73] In addition to insurgency, underdevelopment, and police corruption, R. K. Gyanandra Singh further mentioned other social issues in Manipur: "unemployment rate is high...In Manipur, people are well-educated, but they cannot get jobs in the state...If they want to get a job in a government department, they need to give bribes in order to get a job...Thus, many youngsters and educated people have chosen to leave the state to seek a better livelihood.

People remaining in the state are mostly unemployed, and they start taking drugs."[74]

Local Understanding of Failed HIV/AIDS Securitizing Moves

In contrast to the failed securitizing moves, half of the respondents from Imphal believed that HIV/AIDS was the most serious problem in India.[75] Consider the following responses:

> The Indian government is said to have **taken HIV/AIDS as a serious public health problem**. HIV/AIDS detecting measures are integrated with all maternal and child health care and other treatment facilities in public health sectors. Adequate concern is given to awareness on marital and rights issues. Political commitments [toward HIV/AIDS] are also reflected in political agenda and public policy. [emphasis added][76]
>
> While other health problems are tackled within the general health programs, NACO is a separate department. In the NACP-III, we can see an increase in [HIV/AIDS-related] funding, capacity building and training. The government is **concerned about HIV/AIDS more than other public health problems**. [emphasis added][77]

Concurrently, half of the respondents considered HIV/AIDS as a top-priority issue in the government agenda.[78] For example, R. K. Gyanandra Singh noted that "HIV/AIDS is a top-priority issue in both the national and Manipur government agenda."[79] Amun Leivon, director of Calvary Counseling Centre, also commented on the priority of HIV/AIDS: "HIV/AIDS issue is a top priority issue in the government agenda because a national HIV/AIDS policy, political commitment, and a sizable budget are present. In addition, the HIV/AIDS issue is included in the election manifesto [of the current national government]."[80]

Semi-Summary

To conclude, unprotected heterosexual contact is the major HIV/AIDS transmission mode in New Delhi and Mumbai (the core part of India). In contrast to the core areas, IDU is the prime mode of HIV/AIDS transmission in Imphal (the peripheral part of the country).

In line with the existing failed securitizing move, majority of the respondents in New Delhi and Mumbai perceived that Indian authorities did not treat HIV/AIDS as the most serious public health problem in the country and as the top-priority issue in the national government agenda. Unlike New Delhi and Mumbai, half of the respondents in Imphal believed that Indian political leaders treated HIV/AIDS as the most serious problem and as a top-priority issue in the government agenda. Hence, the level of understanding toward failed securitizing moves was higher among NGO respondents in New Delhi and Mumbai, and lower among respondents in Imphal.

Having understood the HIV/AIDS securitizing moves in three local contexts, the following sections demonstrate the level of moral and technical support of the respondents toward failed HIV/AIDS securitizing moves in New Delhi, Mumbai, and Imphal in comparative perspectives. An analysis of the moral and technical support observed in the cases is also provided. The last section discusses the overall audience acceptance and the type of HIV/AIDS securitization in India.

Audience Acceptance Toward Failed HIV/AIDS Securitizing Moves

Level of Moral Support

Respondents were asked during the face-to-face interviews whether they agree with the stance that "HIV/AIDS is the most serious public health problem in India in comparison to other public health problems." The following sections demonstrate the similarities and differences of interviewee responses and the justifications for their views.

Similarities

Over half of the respondents from Mumbai and Imphal recognized HIV/AIDS as the single most serious public health problem in India.[81] Consider the following responses:

> Regarding the required amount of prevention, treatment, care and support, HIV/AIDS is a serious public health problem.[82]
>
> HIV/AIDS is not only a problem in India; it is [also] a problem of the world. If you consider the HIV/AIDS prevalence in India, the number is small. Yet, when you consider the number of people being infected in India, the number is great. When you consider 40 percent of our population is [composed of] young people, HIV/AIDS should be a major concern in India. If we do not address the HIV/AIDS problem, we may lose the youth and they may become a big burden for the country, as it would affect the productivity of this group.[83]

Differences

Unlike the prevailing view among the respondents from Mumbai and Imphal, less than half of the respondents from New Delhi believed that HIV/AIDS was the *single* most serious public health problem in India.[84] In terms of the number of infections, Anuradha Mukherjee, programs manager of The Naz Foundation (India) Trust, perceived HIV/AIDS as the most serious public health problem in India: "There are 2.3 million people living [with] HIV/AIDS, which is a huge number in terms of the number of infections."[85]

Gopal also explained the severity of the HIV/AIDS problem in India, especially in the rural areas, stating that:

> Although the HIV/AIDS prevalence is low in India, the number of HIV/AIDS infections is huge considering the size of the population. The disease is controlled well in cities, but not in rural areas. A massive flow of migration from rural to cities…when the men have sexual contact with HIV/AIDS infected female sex workers, these men will bring the disease back to their wives, and then to children living in the village.[86]

However, over half of the respondents in New Delhi conceived HIV/AIDS as *only one of the most serious* public health problems in the country, in comparison to other public health issues or diseases. A project director of a national NGO [R54] stated, "I won't say HIV/AIDS is the most serious problem; it is only one of the serious problems in India."[87] Instead of HIV/AIDS, Kajal Bhardwaj, an independent HIV/AIDS-related legal researcher, contended that "HIV/AIDS is one of the top issues along with cancer and TB."[88] Additionally, several respondents believed that HIV/AIDS was a serious problem only among women and marginalized communities. Consider the following views:

> HIV/AIDS is one of the most serious problems in India. It is linked with many other issues [such as] women sexual health and marginalized community.[89]
>
> HIV/AIDS is not the most serious problem. It is only serious such that it affects mostly the marginalized and powerless people, as stigma and discrimination [are] attached to the disease.[90]
>
> HIV/AIDS is not the most serious public health problem compared to maternal health, child mortality and TB. However, HIV/AIDS is a serious problem among migrant population and women.[91]

Taken together, majority of the respondents from Mumbai and Imphal perceived HIV/AIDS as the *single* most serious public health problem in India. Meanwhile, more respondents in New Delhi debated that HIV/

AIDS was not the single most serious public health problem in the country; the problem was severe only in some pockets of the population such as women and marginalized communities.

Level of Technical Support

The level of technical support was reflected in the extent to which NGOs were involved in the HIV/AIDS-related political measures. During the interview sessions, respondents were invited to comment on NGO involvement in the national HIV/AIDS control and prevention programs. The following sections illustrate the similarities and differences of the responses collected in selected cities.

Similarities

An overwhelming majority of the NGO respondents in New Delhi,[92] Mumbai,[93] and Imphal[94] recognized the engagement of the national government via policy implementation, such as HIV/AIDS-related advocacy, education, treatment provision, as well as care and support programs in their respective cities, districts, and subdistricts. Consider the following views:

> We have a good relationship with the government... We work closely with NACO, and we run 10 programs with the SACS.[95]
>
> We have a good relationship with the national government. The programs funded by the Global Fund are part of the government policy. Every program that we plan to launch in the country should confer with the consultant of NACO in advance.[96]
>
> We have a reciprocal relationship with the government. Our center focuses on media. We have worked with UNAIDS and NACO. We educate people working in the media at the district and subdistrict levels.[97]
>
> We have cooperated with different government departments such as MDACS [Mumbai District AIDS Control Society], MACD [Maharashtra AIDS Control Society] and government hospitals. We also have cooperated with the police in Mumbai. We have an advocacy meeting with the police and tell them the reason why these people end up on the streets. In the past, when the police saw IDUs on the streets, they would just throw them away.[98]
>
> In recent years, the government has realized our work in the community. We have a program in Thane that is funded by the government via NACO. Through this program, a community care center and a hospital were established in Thane. [a district in Mumbai][99]

There are ART linkage centers operated by my organization and the government.[100]

Differences

However, only the respondents from New Delhi highlighted the involvement of the national government in HIV/AIDS-focused NGOs in the policy-making processes of NACP-III. Consider the following responses:

> NACO has involved more civil society members in the [policy] consultation.[101]
> NACP-III is a more comprehensive program as more people [NGOs] have been consulted in the program.[102]
> NACP-III involved a lot of civil societies in the consultation processes.[103]
> There is increased and sustainable involvement of civil society groups in the national HIV/AIDS policy.[104]

To conclude, majority of the respondents in the selected cities agreed that the government engaged NGOs in its national HIV/AIDS programs in terms of policy implementation. However, only the respondents from New Delhi mentioned their involvement in the policy consultation of NACP-III.

Using the language in the revised securitization framework, the level of moral support toward the failed HIV/AIDS securitizing move was relatively *stronger* in New Delhi and Mumbai than that in Imphal. Empirical data also showed that technical support was *strong* in all selected cities, with a majority of respondents in all selected cities recognizing NGO involvement in national HIV/AIDS programs.

Analysis of the Audience Acceptance of Failed HIV/AIDS Securitizing Moves

Moral Support

The previous section illuminated the moral support of individuals working in HIV/AIDS-related NGOs toward failed HIV/AIDS securitizing moves. In comparison to three selected cities, majority of the respondents from Mumbai and Imphal perceived HIV/AIDS as the *single* most serious public health problem in India; meanwhile, majority of the respondents from New Delhi debated that HIV/AIDS was *only one of the most serious* public health problems in the country.

As a matter of fact, the estimated number of HIV/AIDS-infected people in India is the highest in Asia[105] and the third highest globally after South Africa and Nigeria.[106] However, aside from HIV/AIDS, India concurrently encounters other threatening public health issues. Of the other two Global Fund diseases (TB and malaria), India is greatly burdened by TB, which bears one-fourth of the total TB problems in the world.[107] In addition, approximately 63,000 cases of multidrug resistant tuberculosis (MDR-TB) were reported in India in 2010, which is the highest among countries in Southeast Asia.[108]

Aside from TB, India is one of the major endemic centers of malaria in Southeast Asia, along with Bangladesh, Indonesia, and Myanmar.[109] Latest figures revealed that over 70 percent of the Indian population faces the risk of malaria infection,[110] whereas infection cases are primarily concentrated in the northeastern states of India.[111] Lincoln Choudhury, a UNAIDS representative, added that "in the northeast region, the most serious public health problem is malaria, [followed by] TB and HIV/AIDS."[112]

Several NGO respondents asserted that the multitude of public health problems in India is primarily caused by poverty. Dr. M. K. Nabeel, research associate at the Solution Exchange AIDS Community, UNAIDS India Office, commented, "I won't say either HIV/AIDS or TB. Poverty is the most serious public health problem in India."[113] Timothy Gaikwad, project manager of a Mumbai-based NGO, believed that poverty is the main cause of HIV/AIDS: "We cannot look at HIV/AIDS in isolation, as it is so closely related to poverty. More than 300 million people, [or] about one in four Indians, live below the poverty line. A vast population lives in abject poverty on less than US$1 per day."[114]

Most seriously, as discussed in chapter 4 of this book, primary health care provision remains one of the most neglected aspects of development in India.[115] A campaign coordinator of an INGO [R69] gave a vivid description of the poor condition of health care provision, especially in HIV/AIDS-related treatment in India:

> In fact, in India the quality of basic health care is poor. For example, in ARV centers, there is no vaccine to prevent STI and hepatitis B. There is no treatment for OIs as well. Overall, the basic things are missing. The DOT [Directly Observed Therapy] program for TB treatment is worse than the HV/AIDS treatment. For HIV/AIDS treatment, there are more counselling and support, while these are absent in TB treatment. In the DOT, patients just go and take their medicines without being provided with information related to the disease and medicines taken.[116]

Poor health quality is attributed to low public expenditure, which is less than 2 percent (around 1.2 percent) of GDP.[117] Michel Kazatchkine, executive director of Global Fund, stressed, "Clearly India is one of the countries with the smallest percentage of health budget of its overall budget going into health, and this is an issue."[118] Additionally, the issue was rarely an important topic in the election campaign except in 2004 when the ruling government pledged to raise health care expenditure from 0.8 percent to 3 percent of GDP.[119] Despite the pledge to boost the health budget, Siddhartha Vatsysyan, director of AIDS Awareness Group, criticized that "the increase cannot catch up with the inflation in the medical cost."[120]

The respondents did not easily realize "AIDS exceptionalism" in India despite the great number of HIV/AIDS cases in Asia and globally due to the great variety of public health problems in the country. Of the responses collected in New Delhi, only a few respondents stated that compared to TB and malaria, HIV/AIDS was the single most serious public health problem in India due to the stigmatized condition of the disease.[121] Consider the following views:

> HIV/AIDS [is the most serious public health problem in India]. It is because HIV/AIDS is **stigmatized**, while the same situation does not exist in TB and malaria [emphasis added].[122]

> HIV/AIDS [is the most serious public health problem in India]. HIV/AIDS is concentrated among high-risk groups that are hard to reach. With **stigma and discrimination**, they are reluctant to disclose their positive statuses. MSM are especially in a complicated situation and not likely to disclose their statuses... they may not be homosexual, but bi-sexual as well. [emphasis added][123]

Notwithstanding the recognition of the severity of HIV/AIDS, Sujit Kumar Sahu, HIV/AIDS program coordinator of The Evangelical Fellowship of India Commission Relief, conceived other threatening issues such as maternal and child health as the most serious public health problem in India,[124] cited, "HIV/AIDS is not the most serious public health problem compared to maternal health, child mortality, and TB. However, HIV/AIDS is a serious problem among migrant population and women... I would say maternal and child health is the most serious problem, followed by TB and HIV/AIDS."[125]

Instead of HIV/AIDS, several respondents from New Delhi believed that TB was the single most serious problem in the country.[126] For instance, Pallavi Upadhyaya, prevention program coordinator of AIDS Healthcare Foundation—India Cares, asserted, "TB is the most serious public health problem among the three... In fact, India is one of the countries having the largest number of TB infections in the world."[127] Amita Chebbi, country director of the Clinton Health Access Initiative, further added, "In the public health perspective, TB is the most serious problem among the three. Also, HIV–TB coinfection cases are increasing; thus, many HIV/AIDS patients are prone to be infected with TB."[128]

In contrast, some respondents in New Delhi did not single out a disease as the most serious public health problem, but they believed that HIV/AIDS, TB, and malaria were all equally threatening public health problems in India.[129] Consider the following responses:

> All [HIV/AIDS, TB and malaria] are serious in India. For TB, we target people in the factories and slum areas. For malaria, geographic location is a factor for the spread of the disease. For HIV/AIDS, it possesses vulnerable factors. HIV/AIDS patients are invisible. It is a silent disease. HIV/AIDS people are stigmatized by the public. [emphasis added][130]
>
> All three diseases are serious and they are top priority issues in India. The number of cases of drug resistance among TB patients is increasing in India. For malaria, the disease is concentrated in the southern part of India; it has then spread to the central and the northeastern parts of India. [emphasis added][131]
>
> The number of malaria and TB infections is high. But HIV/AIDS is a life-threatening disease. Overall, **all three diseases threaten people's life in a similar level.** [emphasis added][132]

Given the multitude of diseases and public health problems in India, the national government launched the NRHM program to integrate all previously separated infectious diseases programs under a single program since 2005.[133] Among the respondents in the selected cities, nearly half of the respondents in New Delhi believed that the stand-alone NACPs should be incorporated into the NRHM program.[134] Consider the following views:

> HIV/AIDS issues are also related to other social issues; thus, the disease cannot be isolated and tackled alone...NRHM can better reach targeted groups at the grassroots level. The manner of the NRHM [is such that it] will not look at one program in isolation.[135]
>
> HIV/AIDS cannot be a stand-alone program, since there are many other issues such as the management of OIs, TB, and HIV/AIDS–hepatitis C coinfection, which should be dealt with in other [health-related] programs."[136]

Although the other half of the respondents from New Delhi realized the necessity of the NRHM program, they argued that the NACP should not be incorporated into NRHM program because the national HIV/AIDS program would be destroyed in the course of convergence.[137] Consider the following responses:

> What I mean by convergence is that we have to find out where programs with similar objectives can work together. For example, the maternal health in NRHM and the program of PMTCT [Prevention of Mother-To-Child Transmission] in HIV/AIDS programs can work together. However, convergence can only work at the local level. HIV/AIDS programs will lose their focus if convergence happens at the national level. In other words, the NACP will lose its focus if the program is incorporated into NRHM. Thus, NACPs should not be integrated into NRHM.[138]
>
> There are problems if HIV/AIDS is a complete vertical and separate program. Other diseases such as TB and malaria cannot be addressed in HIV/AIDS measures. However, the HIV/AIDS program may be destroyed if NACP is integrated into the NRHM. For instance, Africa destroyed its national HIV/AIDS program when the program was integrated into the public health system. Thus, it is inapplicable to put NACP under a one-roof program.[139]
>
> NRHM is a successful program. In NRHM, 18 states are the priority states; thus, other states will be sidelined. For NACP-IV, all states are the priority states regardless of the prevalence rate. It is a good idea for the NRHM to put money on maternal and child care, but how about the HIV/AIDS program? I am afraid that NACP may become a small program and may not be a high priority in the NRHM. Thus, it is better to keep NRHM and NACP separate.[140]

Unlike the responses of New Delhi interviewees, over half of the Imphal respondents strongly disagreed with the mainstreaming of the NACPs,[141] as they doubted the effectiveness of the HIV/AIDS programs after integration. For instance, R. K. Gyanandra Singh, program officer of Catholic Relief Services argued that "everything will start from scratch. We will lose a few years to train the staff to work for HIV/AIDS. I will ask how effective can the program [NACP] run in the NRHM and whether people can access the service."[142] Dr. K. Priyokumar Singh, physician and nodal officer of Jawaharlal Nehru Hospital, strongly disagreed with the idea of integration: "I don't agree with NRHM. I think it is a big joke. How can a grassroots doctor without proper training treat people?."[143]

Empirical data on audience perception toward HIV/AIDS as well as the integration of HIV/AIDS programs in the NRHM showed that negative rhetorical security moves had been diffused and shared among audiences in selected cities with various intensities. Imphal respondents tended to perceive HIV/AIDS as the single most serious problem and thus preferred to treat HIV/AIDS as a separate issue; meanwhile, respondents from New Delhi and Mumbai believed that HIV/AIDS was simply one of the many public health problems, and it should be dealt with in an integrated manner. Thus, the level of moral support toward failed securitizing moves was relatively *stronger* in New Delhi and Mumbai, whereas it was *weaker* among the audience in Imphal.

Technical Support

In democratic countries such as India, the financial and social mobilization power of civil society groups is comparatively greater, which allows them to limit the power of political leaders.[144] In other words, by acting as audience in the securitization process, civil society groups can also constrain the power of the securitizer to engage in or remove the securitizing effort of particular issues. The bottom-up pressure from civil society groups played a very critical role in moving governmental policy decision and legislative reform in India. For example, the HIV/AIDS-focused NGOs in India actively participated in the HIV/AIDS securitization process on several occasions in the past years. The director of the Naz Foundation and other homosexual activists and domestic NGOs initiated the legalization of same-sex relationship in India in 2001. Ultimately, the Delhi High Court heeded the plea of homosexual activists and legalized homosexuality in 2009.

The rotation of party seats via regular election, which is guaranteed by the political system, allows securitizers to maintain a considerable relationship with their targeted individuals or groups to secure their positions in the government for the next term. Unlike its Chinese counterpart, securitizers are thus more willing to engage civil society groups in policy formulation, implementation, and evaluation to win "moral" and "formal" support from the audience.[145] Civil society groups are thereby in a position to become partners of the state.[146]

NGOs have been involved in various HIV/AIDS-related issues such as HIV/AIDS-specific legislative formulation. For example, the national government invited the NGO Lawyers Collective to draft an HIV/AIDS Bill in 2005. Kajal Bhardwaj, an independent legal researcher who participated in drafting the bill, mentioned the drafting process in the interview:

> In the past years, the anti-discrimination law regarding HIV/AIDS did not cover discrimination cases in the private sector, hospitals, and schools. The government initiated the draft of an HIV/AIDS Bill, and the government

invited the Lawyers Collective to do that draft. Since then, the Lawyers Collective has held 14 meetings and consultations in India, and special meetings for many groups (children/MSM/FSW) to go through the drafted Bill.[147]

The engagement of HIV/AIDS-related NGOs mushroomed especially in NACP-III. As stated in the official document, "the National AIDS Control Program Phase III aims to closely work with NGOs, CBOs and Networks of People Living with HIV/AIDS (PLHAs)."[148] A government official working in an HIV/AIDS-related department [R47] also stated that "CBOs and NGOs are important implementers in the Targeted Interventions (TIs) program [in the NACP-III]. Street-level representatives such as PLHAs are also highly involved by the government."[149]

The TIs program, which is the main strategy in NACP-III, aims to provide comprehensive HIV/AIDS preventive services for HRGs.[150] Based on NACP-III, HRGs include FSWs, MSM, transgenders (TGs), and IDUs.[151] NGOs often have a unique access to HRGs such as FSWs and IDUs,[152] whereas CBOs are the affected communities targeted by the government. Therefore, NGOs and CBOs are engaged in the government policy-making process.[153] Civil society involvement is also recognized by several NGO respondents, as follows:

> The government works through both CBOs and NGOs. The government actively cooperates with INP+ [Indian Network for People living with HIV/AIDS] by supporting their programs.[154]
>
> The design of NACP-III is very good. The process involved several civil society groups. Lots of consultations have been done... In NACP-III, the government has recognized some communities working on HIV/AIDS, which is important for the community involvement.[155]
>
> HIV/AIDS patients are [greatly] involved in HIV/AIDS programs. Also, civil society groups such as Lawyers Collective and HIV/AIDS Network for Positive People work closely with the government. The HIV/AIDS patient group is the first patient group to be involved in the decision-making process in the government. Many civil right groups have also worked on public health/HIV/AIDS issues. They realized and debated that it is a right for HIV/AIDS patients to receive treatment.[156]

Contrasting with the Chinese counterparts, several respondents claimed that the Indian government even prefers CBOs to NGOs in leading the TIs programs. Dr. M. K. Nabeel, research associate, Solution Exchange AIDS Community of UNAIDS India Office, asserted that "the government prefers to work with CBOs as the policy stated."[157] Several respondents also acknowledged the Indian government's preference for CBOs over NGOs:

> In terms of sustainability, CBOs model should be better as it is closer to the ground.[158]
>
> The government prefers CBOs to NGOs [because] the government can directly fund the CBOs, and these people can easily reach the targeted community. [Moreover], the administrative cost is lower for CBOs. The government also shows more interest in working with NGOs that focus their work on India.[159]
>
> The government prefers to work with CBOs rather than NGOs. It is because the CBOs have more flexibility to work, and their work can meet the expectations of the government.[160]
>
> It depends on different cases. For programs targeting high risk groups, the government prefers to work with CBOs. It is because CBOs are closer to the community, but NGOs are [comparatively] far away from the community.[161]
>
> The government prefers to work with CBOs since they believe people working in the CBOs are more responsible and active, and the work is more sustainable. Of course, technical support is needed for CBOs. However, in terms of commitment, it is higher among CBO people than in those from NGOs. Also, they can easily identify the targeted groups, and people are more willing to seek CBOs' help as they are one of them.[162]

Aside from NACP-III, the Global Fund financing to India also contributed to the enhancement of civil society engagement in the national HIV/AIDS prevention and control undertaking. Government agencies in India such as the NACO and the MoHFW (Rounds 2, 4, 6, and 7) are not the only ones eligible to be the PRs; five civil society groups have also acted as the PRs of the grants, including IL&FS Education and Technology Services Ltd. (Round 2), India HIV/AIDS Alliance (Rounds 6 and 9), Tata Institute of Social Sciences (Round 7), Indian Nursing Council (Round 7), and the Emmanuel Hospital Association (Round 9).[163]

Taking India HIV/AIDS Alliance as an example, the Alliance acted as the civil society PR of the Global Fund in Round 6 to roll out the HIV/AIDS-related program named as CHAHA, which is an expanded child-centered home and community-based care and support program,[164] from June 1, 2007 to March 31, 2011.[165] Along with nine sub-recipient NGOs/CBOs, CHAHA was carried out in Manipur, Andhra Pradesh, Tamil Nadu, and Maharashtra.[166] By December 2009, 35,947 children living with and/or affected by HIV/AIDS and their families were reached by the program.[167]

The involvement of HIV/AIDS-focused CBOs was even bolstered in Round 9 of the Global Fund. The focus of Round 9 was to prevent the spread of HIV/AIDS among the most hard-to-reach groups, namely the MSM, TG, and Hijra (MSM/TG/Hijra) populations in India.[168] Again acting as the civil society PR in the country, the Indian HIV/AIDS Alliance proposed that the prevention programs for MSM/TG/Hijra should be led by CBOs. Thus, the Alliance strengthened both new and existing CBOs by building their institutional capacity and work toward policy development and advocacy.[169]

The detailed development processes of the HIV/AIDS-focused CBO in Round 9 are given as follows: (1) establishing 110 new CBOs in 14 states of India reaching 147,250 new MSM/TG/Hijra populations; (2) strengthening 90 existing CBOs across 13 states by expanding the ongoing TIs programs of the CBOs; (3) providing organizational development support (for example, institutional building, CBO management, leadership development, relationship with SACS, DAPCU, and local political leaders, and CBO registration) for all 200 CBOs across 17 states,[170] reaching more than 450,000 MSM, Hijras, and TG in India.[171] The proliferation of civil society involvement in national HIV/AIDS programs is thoroughly illustrated in this point.

Type of HIV/AIDS Securitization in India

Failed HIV/AIDS Securitization

A comprehensive picture of the type of HIV/AIDS securitization in India could be generated by identifying the level of moral and technical support among the NGO respondents in the three selected cities. Of the 28 total NGO respondents in the three selected cities, over half of the respondents believed that HIV/AIDS was simply one of the most serious problems or not a serious problem in India at all. On the level of technical support, a vast majority of respondents confirmed that NGOs were involved in national HIV/AIDS interventions, whereas a few respondents disagreed with the stance. This result suggests a *failed HIV/AIDS securitization tended to develop in India*, with a relatively stronger moral and technical support toward failed HIV/AIDS securitizing moves.

Summary

In this chapter, the level of moral and technical support of individuals working in HIV/AIDS-related NGOs in New Delhi, Mumbai, and

Imphal toward failed HIV/AIDS securitizing moves was demonstrated. Having uncovered the level of moral and technical support in selected cities, a generalized picture of the overall level of audience acceptance and the type of HIV/AIDS securitization was identified in India.

The findings showed that a *failed HIV/AIDS securitization* is believed to be developed in India, with an overall high-level moral and technical support toward failed HIV/AIDS securitizing moves among the respondents in New Delhi, Mumbai, and Imphal. Over half of the respondents in selected cities believed that HIV/AIDS was only one of the most serious problems/not a serious problem because of the multitude of other health-related problems that were yet to be resolved in India. Therefore, for the respondents, conceiving HIV/AIDS as a single overwhelmingly threatening issue in the country was more challenging, albeit the huge number of HIV/AIDS cases in Asia and globally. Majority of the respondents believed that NGOs were widely involved in the national HIV/AIDS programs. The involvement of NGOs and CBOs was obvious in NACP-III, as the government needed these organizations to reach HRGs in the TIs programs. Additionally, the Global Fund unequivocally played an imperative role in facilitating the participation of NGOs and CBOs in national HIV/AIDS programs.

Chapter 9

Conclusion: Reconsidering HIV/AIDS Securitization

Introduction

This book set out to develop an alternative securitization framework to help resolve the shortcomings in the original framework. Throughout the reexploration of existing debates on securitization theory, the major shortcomings of the theory were repackaged, including the lack of operationalization and differentiation, together with the presence of Eurocentrism of securitization theory in general, and the three core elements, namely "speech acts," "emergency measures," and "audience acceptance," in particular.[1] By suggesting a modified securitization model, this book also aims to understand the operation of securitization in real-world public policy-making processes by investigating HIV/AIDS securitization in two non-European countries, China and India, in a comparative perspective.

The evolution of security acts and related political measures on HIV/AIDS in China and India was chronologically illustrated using secondary data. Three cities were selected from each country—Beijing, Shanghai, and Kunming in China, and New Delhi, Mumbai, and Imphal in India—for empirical analysis. Semi-structured interviews were conducted with individuals working in HIV/AIDS-focused NGOs and with officials working in government agencies in the selected six city-level cases. The major theoretical and empirical contributions of the book are summarized in this concluding chapter.

Theoretical Revision of the Securitization Framework: A Typology of Securitization

Reoperationalized: The Securitizer and Audience Involvement in the Securitization Process

To achieve the aims, the concepts of "securitizing actors" and "audience," together with the core elements of the theory, are modified and differentiated in the revised securitization framework. This book argues that not everyone has equal political opportunity and capability to utter speech acts or accept the utterances under different political or societal contexts. In this regard, the revised framework assumes that *statesmen or the top-level leaders* of a country are the securitizing agents, because they are politically capable of uttering speech acts.

In relation to the audience involved in accepting security statements, the revised model identifies three groups of audience: (1) audience involved in policy formulation and decision making (e.g., high-level politicians, congress, parliament, or cabinet members); (2) audience involved in policy implementation, (e.g., street-level bureaucrats, provincial and local government officials); and (3) audience involved in policy evaluation (e.g., civil society groups, think-tank members, academic members, public policy scholars, and businessmen). The research singles out *civil society groups, particularly HIV/AIDS-focused NGOs,* as the target audience.

In the revised framework, civil society groups were studied in general and NGOs in particular because they were the only non-state "audience" (actors) involved in the securitization process. Therefore, the state-centric nature of the original version of the securitization theory could be improved by including NGOs in the securitization process. Compared to individual citizens, civil society groups were more organized and thus possessed more political and societal powers and resources to accept or reject the speech acts put forth by political leaders. On the other hand, NGOs played a significant role in the securitization process.[2] Their role was even more significant in developing countries where political leaders were often unable or unwilling to adequately address the problem due to unawareness of the potential threat of the new issue, financial constraint of the government, or political sensitivity of the problem.

Differentiated Core Elements in the Securitization Framework

A trilogy is at the heart of the refined securitization framework: (1) speech acts, or the political statements uttered by the securitizing actors; (2) emergency measures, or the modes of political reactions formulated by the securitizers; and (3) audience acceptance, or the adoption or rejection of the target audience toward a securitizing move developed by the securitizing actors. Regardless of its type, a securitizing move is generated with the presence of (1) and (2), whereas a securitization is composed of (1), (2), and (3).

The concept of speech acts is differentiated into positive and negative notions. A speech act is coded as positive when the actors recognize the problem by uttering "security words," whereas a negative speech act indicates the absence of "security words" or public speeches and texts contracting the positive speech acts. In this book, the notion of negative speech acts attempts to resolve Hansen's question on "the silent security dilemma,"[3] which happens when the possibility of uttering "security" is missing or limited.[4]

However, the speech act alone does not necessarily guarantee subsequent security practices in the real-world political environment. In other words, discrepancies exist between the verbal and physical acts of the securitizer; an empirical loophole that has not been fully addressed by securitization theory. Hence, instead of relying on the illocutionary nature of speech acts alone, an investigation of the actual political reaction enacted by the securitizers should also be emphasized. This book differentiates the three subcategories of emergency measures: (i) *budgetary allocation*; (ii) *policy and institutional arrangement*; and (iii) *legislation amendment and formulation*. This revision can determine whether "the rhetoric of the speech act is matched by subsequent security practices."[5]

In the revised securitization framework, audience acceptance refers to the moral and technical support of the target audience toward a securitizing move, based on their knowledge about the issue. Moral support is indicated by the extent to which the audience holds the same perceptions as the securitizer, whereas technical support is indicated by the extent to which the audience has been involved in the national policies enacted by the securitizer. The presence of both moral and technical support denotes a high level of audience acceptance, whereas the absence of either or both forms of support means a low level of audience acceptance. The division of moral and technical support attempts to cater to the *normative* and *pragmatic* concerns of securitization, regardless of its type. Accordingly, without a strong moral support obtained from the audience, the securitization is said to be "immoral" in form. Following the same logic, the lack of a strong technical support from the audience generates an "ineffective" securitization.

In short, the three core elements underwent the following operationalization and differentiation to make the theoretical framework applicable to empirical studies: (1) the nature of security acts uttered by the securitizer (positive or negative speech acts); (2) the presence or absence of the three subcategories of emergency measures (budget allocation, policy and institutional arrangement, and legislation amendment or formulation) that defines the mode of political reaction toward the perceived threat (emergency or nonemergency modes); and (3) the moral and technical support obtained from the target audience (high or low level of audience acceptance).

Four Types of Securitizing Moves

By differentiating speech acts into positive and negative notions, and political measures into emergency and nonemergency modes, a matrix of four types of securitizing moves, embracing full, rhetorical, performative, and failed securitizing moves was constructed in this book. Thus, a securitizing move is composed of two dimensions: rhetorical (speech acts) and performative (political responses) components. In other words, a *complete* securitizing move does not exist at the point of the speech act (what the original theory defines), but only when a relevant actor changes his or her own behaviors in response to the existential threat justification.[6]

The construction of the four different types of securitizing moves attempts to highlight the nonhomogeneous result of a securitizing move, as debated by McInnes and Rushton.[7] These securitizing moves also respond to Wæver's suggestion for a deliberated study of specific securitizing moves, including "some that fail, and possibly some that succeed only partially."[8]

Typology of Securitization

A typology with eight branches of securitization was constructed by combining the four types of securitizing moves with the two dimensions (high or low level) of audience acceptance. These branches of securitization include full, void full, rhetorical, void rhetorical, void performative, performative, void failed, and failed securitization.

Full securitization, which is an ideal form of securitization, happens when top-level political leaders do what they call for in their public speeches, and the audience morally and technically supports the security move in its strongest sense. *Void full securitization* is the incomplete form of full securitization, in which the audience does not support the threat perception or political reactions toward the perceived threat. *Rhetorical securitization* lacks a full set of emergency measures along with positive speech acts, but the security move receives strong moral and technical support from the target audience. *Void rhetorical securitization* is an incomplete form of rhetorical securitization that is observed when a full set of emergency measures does not follow the utterance of positive speech acts, and the audience does not morally or technically support the threat perception and policies in response to that issue.

Void performative securitization can be observed when audience support cannot be gained easily due to the nature of the issue. This type of securitization can be new (or newly discovered) and/or controversial.[9] Political leaders may choose not to frame the problem as a "security threat" due to the nature of such problem. *Performative securitization* implies the institutionalization of securitization. In short, political measures related to the problem have become inseparably intertwined with the daily national policies and practices. For instance, if HIV/AIDS is securitized, the issue will automatically receive specific attention and continuous resources even in the absence of positive speech acts uttered by political leaders.

Void failed securitization is designed to capture the incomplete form of the failed securitization, in which the audience does not support the absent or negative rhetorical act and/or the related policy measures. *Failed securitization* occurs when (1) an issue is low priority in the government agenda and handled in a nonemergency mode by national authorities, or (2) an issue never existed in the country and therefore does not appear in the national government agenda. By differentiating securitization into eight various types, this book also aims to specifically respond to the argument put forth by Vuori, and McInnes and Rushton that the result of securitization is not a binary division, and there can be a continuum of success and failure.[10]

This book synthesizes securitization and the policy process model with a view to addressing securitization operation in the public policy domain. Based on the revised securitization model, the formulation of the securitizing move (speech acts and political reactions) is similar to the stage of policy formulation and decision-making, in which the securitizing agents decide the policy. Audience acceptance, on the other hand, resembles the stage of policy evaluation, in which the audience acts as the policy evaluators.

This synthesis has a threefold advantage. First, it facilitates the conceptualization of "securitizing actors" and "audience" embedded in the theory, referring to the top-level leaders and the civil society groups, respectively, in the revised framework. Second, the synthesis improves the operationalization of the concepts of "speech acts," "emergency measures," and "audience acceptance." Based on the revised model, "speech acts" and "emergency measures" (securitizing moves) can be found in the policy-making stage, whereas the component of "audience acceptance" is situated at the policy evaluation stage. Third, the synthesis facilitates the understanding of securitization in the real-world policy-making process, thereby enhancing the analytical capability of the theory.

By differentiating securitization into eight types and synthesizing the securitization and public policy process models, securitization can be used as a *post-facto* analytical tool for understanding the securitization process in the day-to-day policy-making process. The revised framework also allows numerous case studies and comparative studies in different stages to be empirically investigated and analyzed in both Western and non-Western contexts. The reason is that the key actors involved in the process of "securitizing actors" and "audience" have been reconceptualized, and two of the core elements— "speech acts" and "audience acceptance"—have been reoperationalized. These revisions can remove the "liberal democratic" or "western" assumptions embedded in the original theory.

Empirically Testing the Revised Framework: HIV/AIDS Securitization in China and India

To test the analytical ability in conducting empirical research, the revised framework is applied to investigate the securitization process of HIV/AIDS in two Asian countries, China and India. Based on the responses of the national governments and civil society groups toward the problem of HIV/AIDS using the securitization lens, the book shows how the health issue of HIV/AIDS has been framed as a security issue via speech acts and responded to via HIV/AIDS-related policies enacted by the national governments. This book also examines the extent to which HIV/AIDS securitizing moves are morally and technically supported by individuals working in NGOs in Beijing, Shanghai, and Kunming in China, and in New Delhi, Mumbai, and Imphal in India, as well as the type of HIV/AIDS securitization in the respective countries.

HIV/AIDS Securitizing Moves in China and India

By applying the framework in the Chinese and Indian context, a similar trend of the development of HIV/AIDS securitizing move was observed within both national governments. The development of HIV/AIDS securitizing moves in China was separated into four phases: failed securitizing move (1985–1994); performative securitizing move (1995–1999); rhetorical securitizing move (2000–2003); and full securitizing move (from 2004 onward). Four phases of HIV/AIDS securitizing moves were also identified in India: failed securitizing move (1986–1991); performative securitizing move (1992–1997); rhetorical securitizing move (1998–2003); and full securitizing move (2004–2009).

Based on the findings, a full HIV/AIDS securitizing move was identified in China and India in 2004. Thus, the study showed that both countries had positive responses toward the HIV/AIDS securitizing move generated since 2000 at the UNSC. However, as demonstrated in chapter 3, the international HIV/AIDS securitizing move in 2000 had started to fade out. Focus on HIV/AIDS had shifted to general public health issues, such as maternal and child health and the establishment of the primary health care system. Hence, the amount of international funding specific for HIV/AIDS had been reduced or redirected to other public health issues. Moreover, due to the continuous economic boom in both China and India, international funding agencies and governments argued that these countries should be the donors instead of recipients of international HIV/AIDS-specific grants and loans.

The study revealed that the national leaders in both countries had reacted differently to the changes in the international health threat priority and HIV/AIDS-related funding level in recent years. The presence of positive speech acts and a full set of emergency measures suggested that the 2004 HIV/AIDS securitizing move had been continued within the Chinese government to date. However, unlike its Chinese counterpart, the 2004 full securitizing move is no longer maintained in the Indian government. In this sense, the HIV/AIDS securitizing move in India at present tends to exist in a failed rather than in a full version (failed HIV/AIDS securitizing move from 2010 onward).

The 2004 full securitizing move in China could be sustained because the Chinese government provided sustainable funds for HIV/AIDS programs in the country. As a result, the HIV/AIDS program in China remained a stand-alone program separated from other public health issues. The 2004 full securitizing move in India changed into a failed form. The Indian government has to change the security frames or strategies to match the prevailing international concerns/funding. The reason is that the funding offered by international agencies has been shifted from a HIV/AIDS-disease-specific to health-integrated approach. As a result, many of its components in NACP-IV have been mainstreamed under the umbrella of NRHM in India.

Audience Acceptance of HIV/AIDS Securitizing Moves in Selected Cases

Full HIV/AIDS Securitizing Moves in China

Based on the level of audience acceptance toward full HIV/AIDS securitizing moves in Beijing, Shanghai, and Kunming, majority of NGO respondents in Beijing and Shanghai believed that HIV/AIDS was the most serious public health problem in China, whereas respondents from Kunming did not perceive HIV/AIDS as the most serious problem. In other words, a stronger moral support prevailed in Beijing and Shanghai, whereas moral support was weaker in Kunming. As a matter of fact, the number of TB infections was far greater than HIV/AIDS in China. However, respondents from Beijing and Shanghai considered HIV/AIDS as the most severe public health problem in China because of the stigma and discrimination attached to the disease and to the infected people. This condition makes HIV/AIDS even more complicated and serious than other infectious diseases such as TB and malaria. Thus, they morally supported the threat-framing of HIV/AIDS generated by the national leaders.

On the level of technical support, majority of the respondents in all selected cities agreed that the Chinese government involved HIV/AIDS-focused NGOs in national HIV/AIDS programs. However, respondents, especially from Shanghai and Kunming, regarded such involvement as unreal because NGO activities were largely controlled by the government, or the government was "forced to" involve NGOs in national HIV/AIDS policies due to the political pressure exerted by international governments and funding agents. Beijing respondents believed that the national government was willing to cooperate with NGOs because top-level Chinese leaders have held a more pragmatic view of grassroots NGOs in recent years. NGOs in Beijing were believed to possess a relatively positive and constructive environment in technically supporting the HIV/AIDS-related policies of the government compared to those working in Shanghai and Kunming.

Arguably, the increase in NGO involvement was largely due to the Global Fund financing of China's national HIV/AIDS program. The Chinese government allowed NGO representatives to participate in the HIV/AIDS-related policy-making process in the CCM of the Global

Fund because of the requirement of the Global Fund to the recipient country. On the other hand, as PRs in China, the national government should disburse a designated portion of the grants to HIV/AIDS-related civil society groups operating in the country. Illustrated in chapter 6 of this book, NGO involvement is deemed to be more obvious in Round 6 of the Global Fund, which aims to "mobilize and support civil society and NGOs' participation in scaling up China's HIV/AIDS prevention and control activities."[11]

Nevertheless, several grassroots NGOs in China have limited financial resources and political ties with the government, creating difficulty in terms of getting registered. The unregistered status of grassroots NGOs creates difficulty in receiving financial support from the central government through the Social Mobilization Program and the Global Fund grants to the Chinese government. Without direct and continuous financial support from the government, some grassroots NGOs are often financially dependent on funds offered by international funding agencies.[12] However, the reliance of NGOs on foreign funding in the absence of domestic support fuels government suspicion.[13] In addition, the audience who challenges the security/nonsecurity frame produced by the securitizers may be pinpointed as threats to national security at best, and subjected to imprisonment at worst.[14] Hence, authorities have suppressed a number of HIV/AIDS activists, either through imprisonment, house arrest, or assault.

Failed HIV/AIDS Securitizing Moves in India

With regard to the level of audience acceptance toward failed HIV/AIDS securitizing moves among the NGO respondents from New Delhi, Mumbai, and Imphal, majority of the respondents from Mumbai and Imphal viewed HIV/AIDS as the most serious public health problem in India. On the contrary, respondents from New Delhi believed that HIV/AIDS was not the single most serious problem, as there were many other burning issues in the country, such as maternal and child health and TB. In this sense, the level of moral support was stronger in New Delhi, and weaker among respondents in Mumbai and Imphal.

Based on the findings, the level of technical support was strong in all selected Indian cities. Respondents from New Delhi, Mumbai, and Imphal reported their involvement in national policy implementation in their respective cities, districts, and subdistricts. Additionally, respondents in New Delhi expressed that the national government had also involved NGOs in the policy consultation of NACP-III.

The Indian government had a positive attitude toward NGOs as these groups were conceived as partners of the securitizer. Thus, the government largely involved NGOs and CBOs in the consultation and implementation of the existing national HIV/AIDS program (NACP-III), as well as in the discussion of the development of the coming NACP-IV. The level of technical support among HIV/AIDS-focused NGOs have been further strengthened by the participation of the Global Fund in Indian HIV/AIDS programs. Five NGOs in India have acted as the PRs of the grants, whereas numerous CBOs have been established and equipped with technical capacities in Round 9 of the Global Fund.

Comparing Overall Audience Acceptance Levels and Types of Securitization

With respect to the overall audience acceptance among the respondents working in HIV/AIDS-related NGOs and the type of securitization, out of the 30 NGO respondents in China, over half of the respondents believed that HIV/AIDS was the most serious public health problem. More than half of the respondents also believed that NGOs were being involved in the national HIV/AIDS programs. Thus, the HIV/AIDS securitization in China at present is believed to be in the form of a *full securitization*. However, as explained in chapter 6 of this book regarding the restriction and suppression of civil societies and HIV/AIDS activists, the full HIV/AIDS securitization generated in China is suspected to be *false securitization*.

Out of the 28 respondents in all selected cities in India, over half of them believed that HIV/AIDS was not the most serious public health problem. Additionally, more than half of the respondents believed that NGOs were involved in the national HIV/AIDS programs. Thus, the HIV/AIDS securitization in India at present is believed to be in the form of a *failed securitization*.

The findings also revealed that the intensity of the acceptance level varied in different cities within a country. The variation was supposed to be larger in big countries such as China and India. The high-level audience acceptance was more likely to be observed in the central area than in the peripheral region of a huge country. To illustrate this point, the level of audience acceptance was the highest in Beijing and New Delhi, which could be attributed to the proximity of the capital city to the central authorities and the abundance of financial, human, and technical resources. In contrast, the level of audience acceptance was comparatively lower in the peripheral cities such as Kunming and Imphal.

Degree of Success

Based on the revised securitization model, a successful securitization, regardless of its type, leads to desecuritization. However, from a biomedical viewpoint, none of the types of securitization efforts can be deemed successful because HIV/AIDS remains incurable to date. However, if success is considered in the form of disease management, raising of social awareness, and the engagement of the government and the civil society in HIV/AIDS interventions, then reaching a more definitive conclusion on this point is a possibility. The findings from this book support the contention of the original model that a full securitization is the most successful type of securitization in managing the HIV/AIDS problem.

Nonetheless, several developed countries over the past decades have fully securitized HIV/AIDS, leading to a dramatic reduction in the HIV/AIDS infection rate among their populations. However, recent global trends showed that HIV/AIDS infection rates have resurged in some developed countries.[15] In addition, despite the overwhelming awareness and implementation of preventive programs in developed countries such as the United States and United Kingdom, about 20–24 percent of the infected individuals in these countries are unaware of their HIV-positive status.[16]

The decline in HIV/AIDS awareness can be attributed to the "burn-out" effect of HIV/AIDS preventive measures and the availability of effective ARV drugs. Marc Cohen, an HIV/AIDS activist, argued that "there is a 'burn-out' factor when it comes to HIV/AIDS prevention. People have heard the safe-sex message for decades and have grown tired of the subject."[17] In addition, David Wilson, an associate professor at the National Centre in HIV Epidemiology and Clinical Research, stressed, "The success of the ARV drugs [has] made HIV/AIDS less frightening to individuals…[thus] condom use had dropped…About a quarter of gay men reported having unprotected sex with casual partners."[18] Based on the earlier illustration, people have in fact *desensitized* HIV/AIDS problems even within the full HIV/AIDS securitization. Thus, the long-term effectiveness of full HIV/AIDS securitization in tackling the disease is problematic in this aspect, which suggests that the temporal aspects of effective securitization responses should also be considered. However, this topic lies outside the scope of this book and could be studied in future research endeavors.

Contributions of the Revised Framework and Comparative Case Studies

Remedied Major Shortcomings in a Single Framework

This book has four major achievements. Its first achievement is that it responds to the fundamental shortcomings of securitization theory by presenting a comprehensive framework. The proposed model differentiates securitization into eight types: full, rhetorical, performative, and failed securitization and the void forms of these four types. In other words, the model revises the simplistic black-and-white notion of "having" or "not having" securitization and replaces it with a continuum of successes and failures. Such differentiation facilitates the empirical study of securitization in real-world situations. Aside from the eight types of securitization, *false securitization* is also addressed in the book to highlight that full securitization can also be falsified. For example, the audience support for the framing and handling of an issue can be a result of their own hidden agenda. The Chinese case in chapter 6 of the book supports this explanation.

Operationalized: The "Role of Audience" and Its Implications to State–Civil Society Relations

The book's second achievement is that the revised model facilitates the empirical study of the "role of audience acceptance," which has been neglected by some security scholars. For example, Floyd argues that a securitization process consists of only speech acts and emergency measures, whereas Balzacq claims that securitization can occur without an identifiable audience. A study on the level of audience acceptance among NGO respondents suggests that securitizer–audience/state–civil society relations in China considerably differ from those in India.

The relationship between the state and non-state actors in China is full of distrust and suspicion, which in turn limits the positive development of civil society groups in the country. On the one hand, the Chinese government must include NGO participants in national HIV/AIDS-related programs because of the seriousness of the problem and the demands imposed by the Global Fund on the recipient countries. On the other hand, the government must prevent the growth of non-state organizations by suppressing HIV/AIDS activists and HIV/AIDS-related campaigns. Despite the technical influence of the Global Fund on national policy, the involvement of civil society groups in China is largely limited.

By contrast, the Indian government largely perceives civil society groups as partners rather than enemies, thereby enabling the development of a vibrant civil society in the country. Unlike its Chinese counterpart, the Indian government allows civil society groups to act as the PRs of the Global Fund. The involvement of civil society groups in national HIV/AIDS interventions even becomes increasingly apparent in Round 9 of the Global Fund, in which HIV/AIDS programs are principally led by NGOs and CBOs.

Explored: The Study of Securitization in Non-Western or Nondemocratic Contexts and Its Implications to the Regime Types

The third achievement of the book is that the revised model facilitates the study of securitization, particularly in nondemocratic societies and in the non-western world. The liberal–democratic assumptions in the original theory have been eliminated after the revision. The applicability of the revised model has been tested through a comparison of two non-western countries with different political systems: authoritarian China and democratic India.

Based on research in China and India, it is argued that regime types influence the *level of the moral support* of the audience. In China's context, the relatively restrictive media and internet access limits the opportunities of the audience to learn about contrary arguments or evidence on a particular issue. Thus, it is argued that the level of moral support becomes *increasingly stable with time* because the bottom-up initiative in securitizing a new issue or challenging the existing securitization in China is relatively limited. In addition, the audience may not and cannot challenge an established way of thinking of securitizers because of political and financial constraints. Thus, certain civil society groups opt for the government's support at the expense of their opinions and judgments. A high level of moral support for the government's thinking can be possibly maintained in authoritarian states. In India, the freedom of the press and speech, as guaranteed by their democratic system, exposes the audience to different arguments on an issue, whether pro-government or anti-government. Thus, the level of moral support *changes frequently* in a democratic system. Aside from regime type, further comparative research can also be conducted on the effect of the level of development of the country on the securitization model, such as China and Singapore or India and the United States.

Advanced: The Applicability of the Securitization Process in the Public Policy Domain

The fourth achievement of the book is that the revised model shifts the study of securitization from discourse (speech acts) to the policy-making process. The synthesis advances securitization theory such that the element of the "feedback loop" in the policy process model complements the securitization process.

Original securitization theory states that a successful securitization leads to desecuritization, which means that the issue is no longer framed as a security threat and no longer results in emergency political measures. In other words, the issue is handled by a normal policy-making process rather than by a securitization process. However, the theory does not mention the subsequent steps that must be taken once the security frames or policies cannot address or remove the threat.

To fill this theoretical gap, the "feedback loop" is included in the new securitization model to indicate that unsuccessful securitization loops back to the earlier stages of the securitization process. Thus, the securitizers can modify the threat-framing or political measures for the problem. Chapters 5 and 7 of the book empirically showed how the "feedback loop" worked in reconceptualizing national HIV/AIDS policies in China and India from the 1980s to 2011. The present work therefore contributes to existing securitization theory by emphasizing that the securitization process is not linear but cyclical.

Summary

Eight branches of securitization have emerged in this book after reviewing the major shortcomings that prevailed in the original framework. The construction of this revised securitization framework is intended to address these original shortcomings, including the lack of operationalization and differentiation, the presence of Eurocentrism in securitization theory in general, and the three core elements, namely "speech acts," "emergency measures," and "audience acceptance," in particular.

Empirical tests of the revised model have been conducted in studying the HIV/AIDS securitization process in China and India in a comparative manner. The findings showed that a full HIV/AIDS securitizing move was generated in 2004 in both countries. The full securitizing move still prevails in China, whereas India has moved away from the approach. The empirical data also revealed that an overall high-level audience acceptance toward the respective form of HIV/AIDS securitizing moves is observed among the respondents in HIV/AIDS-related NGOs in China and India. In this sense, a full HIV/AIDS securitization is present in China, whereas a failed securitization is observed in India.

Despite the strengths of the revised securitization model in addressing political responses to HIV/AIDS in China and India, the revised model is not without its weaknesses. The revised framework cannot explain why the securitizing agent securitizes an issue, nor the process of negotiations and debates between the securitizer and audience. In addition, HIV/AIDS has become desensitized among the individuals even with a full securitization response to the disease in some developed countries. Thus, in contrast with the theoretical assumption of the original and revised frameworks, the full HIV/AIDS securitization may not be the most desirable policy option in a real public policy environment. Therefore, further researches need to be conducted to address the previously mentioned theoretical weaknesses.

In conclusion, the theoretical revision of the securitization framework and the empirical applications toward HIV/AIDS securitization in China and India are conducive to the advancement of the existing knowledge of security studies, the utility of securitization in the public policy domain, and the operation of securitization particularly in the non-Western and nondemocratic world. In practice, the proposed model also serves as a policy matrix for security scholars or public policy scholars and practitioners to understand different aspects of nontraditional security problems in general and of diseases in particular.

Notes

1 INTRODUCTION

1. "Around the World; China Says Argentine Died of AIDS," *New York Times*, July 30, 1985, accessed November 10, 2014, http://www.nytimes.com/1985/07/30/world/around-the-world-china-says-argentine-died-of-aids.html;Z. Y. Wu, et al., "Evolution of China's Response to HIV/AIDS," *The Lancet* 369, no. 9562 (2007): 679.
2. Michael Hamlyn, "Indian AIDS Victim Jailed," *Time*, December 9, 1986, LexisNexis Newspapers.
3. "71 AIDS Cases Recorded in India," *New York Times*, February 15, 1987, LexisNexis Newspapers.
4. Jon Cohen, "Changing Course to Break the HIV-Heroin Connection," *Science* 304, no. 5676 (2004): 1434; Wu et al., "Evolution of China's Response," 679.
5. Mirko D. Gupte, Vidya Ramachandran, and R. K. Mutatkar, "Epidemiological Profile of India: Historical and Contemporary Perspectives," *Journal of Biosciences* 26, no. 4 (2001): 441; Sheela Godbole and Sanjay Mehendale, "HIV/AIDS Epidemic in India: Risk Factors, Risk Behavior and Strategies for Prevention and Control," *Indian Journal of Medical Research* 121, no. 4 (2005): 356; Sonal R. Doshi and Bindi Gandhi, "Women in India: The Context and Impact of HIV/AIDS," *Journal of Human Behavior in the Social Environment* 17, nos. 3–4 (2008): 427.
6. Mark Fineman, "Superstition, Poverty May Bring AIDS Crisis in India," *Los Angeles Times*, May 28, 1990, accessed November 10, 2014, http://articles.latimes.com/1990-05-28/news/mn-51_1_aids-crisis.
7. "HIV/AIDS: China's Titanic Peril," *UNAIDS/WHO*, last modified June 2002, http://www.hivpolicy.org/Library/HPP000056.pdf.
8. "HIV Estimates in India, 1981–2004," *UNAIDS*, last modified March 11, 2010, http://www.unaids.org.in/displaymore.asp?page=17&pagenav=title&subitemkey=439&subchkey=0&itemid=322&chname=HIV%20Epidemic%20in%20India&subchnm=.
9. "Global Report—UNAIDS Report on the Global AIDS Epidemic 2013," *UNAID*, last modified September 2013, http://www.unaids.org

/en/media/unaids/contentassets/documents/epidemiology/2013/gr2013/UNAIDS_Global_Report_2013_en.pdf.
10. "Global Report."
11. "Global Report."
12. Laurie Garrett, "HIV and National Security: Where Are the Links?" *Council on Foreign Relations*, accessed January 4, 2010, http://www.cfr.org/content/publications/attachments/HIV_National_Security.pdf.
13. Carolyn Abraham, "The Smartest Virus in History?" *The Globe and Mail*, last modified April 6, 2009, http://www.theglobeandmail.com/news/national/the-smartest-virus-in-history/article1101945/.
14. Abraham, "The Smartest Virus."
15. S. Young, "Researchers: Toddler Cured of HIV," *CNN*, March 4, 2013, accessed November 8, 2014, http://edition.cnn.com/2013/03/03/health/hiv-toddler-cured/index.html?iref=allsearch.
16. S. Young and J. Wilson, "Virus Detected in Baby 'Cured' of HIV," *CNN*, July 11, 2014, accessed November 8, 2014, http://edition.cnn.com/2014/07/10/health/baby-not-cured-hiv/index.html?iref=allsearch.
17. Young, "Researchers."
18. Young and Wilson, "Virus Detected."
19. Interview with Tony Zheng, chairperson of Shanghai CSW & MSM Center, Shanghai, May 2011; Interview with the director of a national NGO [R35], Beijing, May 2011.
20. Garrett, "HIV and National Security."
21. "UN Security Council Resolution 1308 (2000) on the Responsibility of the Security Council in the Maintenance of International Peace and Security: HIV/AIDS and International Peace-keeping Operations," *United Nation Security Council*, last modified July 17, 2000, http://data.unaids.org/pub/BaseDocument/2000/20000717_un_scresolution_1308_en.pdf.
22. Samantha Kirby, "The Seeker: Should Religiously Devout Be Left Off Ballot?" *Chicago Tribune*, last modified May 23, 2011, http://newsblogs.chicagotribune.com/religion_theseeker/2011/05/should-religiously-devout-be-left-off-ballot.html.
23. See Barry Buzan, Ole Wæver, and Jaap de Wilde, *Security: A New Framework for Analysis* (Boulder, CO: Lynne Rienner Publishers, 1998).
24. Buzan, Wæver, and de Wilde, *Security*, 25.
25. Buzan, Wæver, and de Wilde, *Security*, 26.
26. Buzan, Wæver, and de Wilde, *Security*, 24.
27. Keith Krause and Michael C. Williams, "Broadening the Agenda of Security Studies: Politics and Methods," *Mershon International Studies Review* 40, no. 2 (1996): 243.
28. Maria Julia Trombetta, "Rethinking the Securitization of the Environment: Old Beliefs, New Insights," in *Securitization Theory: How Security Problems Emerge and Dissolve*, ed. Thierry Balzacq (London: Routledge, 2011), 137.
29. Buzan, Wæver, and de Wilde, *Security*, 31.
30. Buzan, Wæver, and de Wilde, *Security*, 25.

31. Emanuel Alder, "Seizing the Middle Ground: Constructivism in World Politics," *European Journal of International Relations* 3, no. 3 (1997): 327.
32. Juha A. Vuori, "A Timely Prophet? The Doomsday Clock as a Visualization of Securitization Moves with a Global Referent Object," *Security Dialogue* 41, no. 3 (2010): 257.
33. Ralf Emmers, "ASEAN and the Securitization of Transnational Crime in Southeast Asia," *The Pacific Review* 16, no. 3 (2003): 419–438.
34. Nicole J. Jackson, "International Organizations, Security Dichotomies and the Trafficking of Persons and Narcotics in Post-Soviet Central Asia: A Critique of the Securitization Framework," *Security Dialogue* 37, no. 3 (2006): 299–317.
35. Carsten Bagge Laustsen and Ole Wæver, "In Defense of Religion: Sacred Referent Objects for Securitization," *Millennium Journal of International Studies* 29, no. 3 (2000): 705–739.
36. Ayse Ceyhan and Anastassia Tsoukala, "The Securitization of Migration in Western Societies: Ambivalent Discourses and Policies," *Alternatives* 27, no. 1 (2002): 21–39.
37. Trombetta, "Rethinking the Securitization of the Environment," 135–149.
38. Sara E. Davies, "Securitizing Infectious Disease," *International Affairs* 84, no. 2 (2008): 295–313.
39. Stefan Elbe, "Should HIV/AIDS Be Securitized? The Ethical Dilemmas of Linking HIV/AIDS and Security," *International Studies Quarterly* 50, no. 1 (2006): 119–144; Colin McInnes and Simon Rushton, "HIV/AIDS and Securitization Theory," *European Journal of International Relations* 19, no. 1 (2013): 115–138 (2012): 1–24; Colleen O'Manique, "The 'Securitization' of HIV/AIDS in Sub-Saharan Africa: A Critical Feminist Lens," *Policy and Society* 24, no. 1 (2005): 24–47; Roxanna Sjöstedt, "Exploring the Construction of Threats: The Securitization of HIV/AIDS in Russia," *Security Dialogue* 39, no. 1 (2008): 7–29; Marco Antonio Vieira, "The Securitization of the HIV/AIDS Epidemic as a Norm: A contribution to Constructivist Scholarship on the Emergence and Diffusion of International Norms," *Brazilian Political Science Review* 1, no. 2 (2007): 137–181.
40. Melissa G. Curley and Jonathan Herington, "The Securitization of Avian Influenza: International Discourses and Domestic Politics in Asia," *Review of International Studies* 37, no. 1 (2011): 141–166.
41. See Ole Wæver, "Securitization: Taking Stock of a Research Program in Security Studies," unpublished draft, 2003, 27–28.
42. Matthew R., Smallman-Raynor, and Andrew D. Cliff, *War Epidemics: An Historical Geography of Infectious Diseases in Military Conflict and Civil Strife, 1850–2000* (New York: Oxford University Press, 2004), 7.
43. "AIDS Toll 'Will Surpass Black Death,'" *BBC News*, January 25, 2002, accessed November 24, 2014, http://news.bbc.co.uk/2/hi/health/1779480.stm.
44. Garrett, "HIV and National Security."
45. Garrett, "HIV and National Security."

46. "AIDS Toll."
47. Stefan Elbe, "Pandemics on the Radar Screen: Health Security, Infectious Disease and the Medicalization of Insecurity," *Political Studies* 59, no. 4 (2011): 850.
48. "UN Security Council Resolution 1308."
49. Colin McInnes and Simon Rushton, "HIV, AIDS and Security: Where Are We Now?" *International Affairs* 86, no. 1 (2010): 230.
50. Simon Rushton, "AIDS and International Security in the United Nations System," *Health Policy and Planning* 25, no. 6 (2010): 497.
51. Varun Gauri and Evan S. Lieberman, "AIDS and the State: The Politics of Government Responses to the Epidemic in Brazil and South Africa" (paper presented at the annual meetings for the American Political Science Association, Chicago, IL, September 2–5, 2004).
52. Tony Barnett, "A Long-Wave Event. HIV/AIDS, Politics, Governance and 'Security': Sundering the Intergenerational Bond?" *International Affairs* 82, no. 2 (2006): 302. In Barnett's definition, a long-wave event means an issue that is likely to have large-scale effects for many decades.
53. Kim Lanegran and Goran Hyden, "Mapping the Politics of AIDS: Illustrations from East Africa," *Population and Environment* 14, no. 3 (1993): 245–263.
54. Robert L. Ostergard, "HIV/AIDS, State Capacity, and the Threat to National and International Security: A Theoretical Overview," in *HIV/AIDS and the Threat to National and International Security*, ed. Robert L. Ostergard (London: Palgrave Macmillan, 2007), 75.
55. Javed Mohammad Iqbal, "AIDS and the State: A Comparison of Brazil, India and South Africa," *South Asian Survey* 16, no. 1 (2009): 131.
56. Gauri and Lieberman, "AIDS and the State," 28.
57. Iqbal, "AIDS and the State," 128.
58. All data in the table are extracted from "Table 6: Command Over Resources, The Rise of the South: Human Progress in a Diverse World," *United Nations Development Program*, last modified March 14, 2013, http://www.undp.org/content/dam/undp/library/corporate/HDR/2013GlobalHDR/English/HDR2013%20Report%20English.pdf.
59. "Table 6: Command Over Resources."
60. Uma Kapila, *Indian Economy: Performance and Policies* (New Delhi: Academic Foundation, 2008–2009), 260.
61. N. J. Kurian, "Financing Healthcare in India," *The Hindu*, January 18, 2010, accessed November 24, 2014, http://www.thehindu.com/opinion/lead/financing-healthcare-in-india/article80956.ece.
62. "Securitization: What Makes Something a Security Threat," *Megalinks in Criminal Justice*, last modified October 25, 2008, http://www.apsu.edu/oconnort/GSS2010/GSS2010lect01a.htm.
63. Curley and Herington, "The Securitization," 146.
64. For the purpose of this research only, Asian region embraces China, Hong Kong Special Administrative Region, Macau Special Administrative Region, Taiwan, Democratic People's Republic of Korea, Japan, Mongolia and

Republic of Korea, Afghanistan, Bangladesh, Bhutan, Brunei Darussalam, Cambodia, India, Indonesia, Islamic Republic of Iran, Lao People's Democratic Republic, Malaysia, Maldives, Myanmar, Nepal, Pakistan, Philippines, Singapore, Sri Lanka, Thailand, Timor-Leste, and Vietnam.

65. Gui-hong Zhang, "China's Peaceful Rise and Sino-Indian Relations," *China Report* 41, no. 2 (2005): 159–171.
66. "Mapping the Global Future: Report of the National Intelligence Council's 2020 Project," *National Intelligence Council*, accessed May 28, 2012, http://www.dni.gov/nic/NIC_globaltrend2020_s2.html.
67. Randeep Ramesh, "India's Growing Pains," *New Economist*, last modified August 2, 2007, http://neweconomist.blogs.com/new_economist/2007/08/randeep-ramesh.html.
68. Ian Buruma, "After America," *The New Yorker*, last modified April 21, 2008, http://www.newyorker.com/arts/critics/atlarge/2008/04/21/080421crat_atlarge_buruma.
69. "Global Report."
70. "Mapping the Global Future."
71. Thomas E. Rotnem and Tinaz Pavri, "The HIV/AIDS Pandemic in Comparative Perspective: The Cases of India and Russia" (paper presented at the Georgia Political Science Association, Conference Proceedings, 2006).
72. Robert Compton, "Dynamics of HIV/AIDS in China and India: Assessing Governmental Response," in *HIV/AIDS and the Threat to National and International Security*, ed. Robert L. Ostergard (London: Palgrave Macmillan, 2007), 234.
73. Stephen M. Walt, "Rigor or Rigor Mortis? Rational Choice and Security Studies," in *Rational Choice and Security Studies: Stephen Walt and His Critics*, ed. Michael Edward Brown et al. (London: The MIT Press, 2000), 8.
74. The East/coastal includes Beijing, Tianjin, Hebei, Liaoning, Shanghai, Jiangsu, Zhejiang, Shandong, Fujian, Guangdong, Guangxi, and Hainan.
75. For the purpose of this study, excluding the eight northeastern states, the rest of the 20 states and the seven Union Territories belong to the central area of India.
76. The central consists of Shanxi, Inner Mongolia, Jilin, Heilongjiang, Anhui, Jiangxi, Henan, Hubei, and Hunan. The West includes Sichuan, Guizhou, Yunnan, Tibet, Shaaxi, Gansu, Qinghai, Ningxia, and Xinjiang.
77. Northeastern region of India comprises eight states, including Assam, Arunachal Pradesh, Manipur, Meghalaya, Mizoram, Nagaland, Tripura, and Sikkim.
78. Other transmission modes include blood transfusion and mother-to-child transmission.
79. Arni S. R. Srinivasa Rao et al., "HIV/AIDS Epidemic in India and Predicting the Impact of the National Response: Mathematical Modeling and Analysis," *Mathematical Biosciences and Engineering* 6, no. 4 (2009): 781.
80. Friedemann Wenzel, Fouad Bendimerad, and Ravi Sinha, "Megacities—Megarisks," *Natural Hazards* 42, no. 3 (2007): 482.

81. "Preventing HIV/AIDS in India," *The World Bank*, last modified June 2005, http://siteresources.worldbank.org/INTINDIA/Resources/HIV-AIDS-brief-June2005-IN.pdf.
82. Martin N. Marshall, "Sampling for Qualitative Research," *Family Practice* 13, no. 6 (1996): 523.
83. Buzan, Wæver, and de Wilde, *Security*, 176.
84. Buzan, Wæver, and de Wilde, *Security*, 177.

2 Security: A Revised Framework for Analysis

1. *Oxford English Dictionary*, s.v. "security."
2. Ole Wæver, "Securitization and Desecuritization," in *On Security*, ed. Ronnie D. Lipschutz (New York: Columbia University Press, 1995), 50.
3. Barry Buzan, *People, States & Fear: An Agenda for International Security Studies in the Post-Cold War Era* (Boulder, CO: Lynne Rienner Great Britain: Hartnolls, 1991), 3–4.
4. Wæver, "Securitization and Desecuritization," 46.
5. See David Chandler, "Review Essay: Human Security: The Dog That Didn't Bark," *Security Dialogue* 39, no. 4 (2008): 427–438.
6. Michael J. Selgelid and Christian Enemark, "Infectious Diseases, Security and Ethics: The Case of HIV/AIDS," *Bioethics* 22, no. 9 (2008): 458.
7. Daniel Deudney, "The Case against Linking Environmental Degradation and National Security," *Millennium Journal of International Studies* 19, no. 3 (1990): 464.
8. Jef Huysmans, "Revisiting Copenhagen: Or, on the Creative Development of a Security Studies Agenda in Europe," *European Journal of International Relations* 4, no. 4 (1998): 491.
9. Stephen M. Walt, "The Renaissance of Security Studies," *International Studies Quarterly* 35, no. 2 (1991): 213.
10. Walt, "The Renaissance," 213.
11. Selgelid and Enemark, "Infectious Diseases," 459.
12. Walt, "The Renaissance," 213.
13. Walt, "The Renaissance," 213.
14. Richard H. Ullman, "Redefining Security," *International Security* 8, no. 1 (1983): 135.
15. Ullman, "Redefining Security," 139.
16. Ullman, "Redefining Security," 139; Jessica Tuchman Mathews, "Redefining Security," *Foreign Affairs* 68, no. 2 (1989): 162.
17. Mathews, "Redefining Security," 162; Buzan, *People*, 369.
18. Buzan, *People*, 363.
19. Ullman, "Redefining Security," 132.
20. Edward Newman, "Human Security and Constructivism," *International Studies Perspectives* 2, no. 3 (2001): 241; Chandler, "Review Essay," 427.

21. "Chapter 2: New Dimension of Human Security," *Human Development Report 1994, United Nations Development Program*, accessed September 27, 2009, http://hdr.undp.org/en/media/hdr_1994_en_chap2.pdf.
22. Laura Neack, *Elusive Security: States First, People Last* (New York: Rowman & Littlefield. 2007), 220.
23. Astri Suhrke, "Human Security and the Interests of States," *Security Dialogue* 30, no. 3 (1999): 275; Mely Caballero-Anthony, "Human Security and Primary Health Care in Asia: Realities and Challenges," in *Global Health Challenges for Human Security*, ed. Lincoln C. Chen, Jennifer Leaning, and Vasant Narasimhan (Cambridge, MA: Global Equity Initiative, Asia Center, Harvard University, 2003), 235; Nicholas Thomas and William T. Tow, "The Utility of Human Security: Sovereignty and Humanitarian Intervention," *Security Dialogue* 33, no. 2 (2002): 177; Chandler, "Review Essay," 428; Edward Newman, "Critical Human Security Studies," *Review of International Studies* 36, no. 1 (2010): 91.
24. Securitization theory is one of the three main lines of security concept developed by the Copenhagen School. The other two lines are sectoral security and as regional security complex theory.
25. Ole Wæver, "Aberystwyth, Paris, Copenhagen: New 'Schools' in Security Theory and Their Origins between Core and Periphery" (paper presented at the annual meeting for the International Studies Association, Montreal, March 17–20, 2004).
26. Ole Wæver, "Security, Insecurity and Asecurity in the West European Non-War Community," in *Security Communities*, eds. Emanuel Adler, and Michael N. Barnett (Cambridge: Cambridge University Press, 1998), 79.
27. Barry Buzan, Ole Wæver, and Jaap de Wilde, *Security: A New Framework for Analysis* (Boulder, CO: Lynne Rienner, 1998), 31; Wæver, "Securitization," 12.
28. Wæver, "Security, Insecurity and Asecurity," 79.
29. Ole Wæver, "The EU as a Security Actor: Reflections from a Pessimistic Constructivist on Post-Sovereign Security Orders," in *International Relations Theory and the Politics of European Integration*, ed. Morten Kelstrup and Michael C. Williams (London: Routledge, 2000), 251.
30. Buzan, Wæver, and de Wilde, *Security*, 26.
31. Referent objects refer to "things that are seen to be existentially threatened and that have a legitimate claim to survival." See Buzan, Wæver, and de Wilde, *Security*, 36.
32. Wæver, "Security, Insecurity and Asecurity," 80.
33. Wæver, "Security, Insecurity and Asecurity," 80.
34. Buzan, Wæver, and de Wilde, *Security*, 40.
35. Ole Wæver, "Securitization: Taking Stock of a Research Program in Security Studies," unpublished draft, 2003, 14.
36. Buzan, Wæver, and de Wilde, *Security*, 31.
37. Buzan, Wæver, and de Wilde, *Security*, 25.
38. Buzan, Wæver, and de Wilde, *Security*, 25.

39. Buzan, Wæver, and de Wilde, *Security*, 31; Wæver, "Securitization," 11; Juha A. Vuori, "Illocutionary Logic and Strands of Securitization: Applying the Theory of Securitization to the Study of Non-Democratic Political Orders," *European Journal of International Relations* 14, no. 1 (2008): 65–99. However, the theory does not consider the fact that the securitizers can use lies and misinformation to deceive the audience. For example, Tony Blair is sometimes alleged to have delivered a 45-minute speech to mislead the British parliament in the run up to the Iraq war.
40. Wæver, "Securitization," 24.
41. Ole Wæver, "Securitizing Sectors? Reply to Eriksson." *Cooperation and Conflict* 34, no. 3 (1999): 337.
42. Wæver, "Securitization," 25.
43. Wæver, "Securitization," 23.
44. "Overview: An Agenda for the Social Summit," *Human Development Report 1994, United Nations Development Program*, accessed September 24, 2009, http://hdr.undp.org/en/media/hdr_1994_en_overview.pdf.
45. Wæver, "Securitization," 20.
46. Melissa G. Curley and Siu-lun Wong, *Security and Migration in Asia: The Dynamics of Securitization* (London: Routledge, 2008), 7–9.
47. Wæver, "Securitization," 27–28.
48. Wæver, "Securitization," 21.
49. See Lene Hansen, "The Little Mermaid's Silent Security Dilemma and the Absence of Gender in the Copenhagen School," *Millennium Journal of International Studies* 29, no. 2 (2000): 285–306; Michael C. Williams, "Words, Images, Enemies: Securitization and International Politics," *International Studies Quarterly* 47, no. 4 (2003): 511–531; Claire Wilkinson, "The Copenhagen School on Tour in Kyrgyzstan: Is Securitization Theory Useable Outside Europe?" *Security Dialogue* 38, no. 1 (2007): 5–25; Frank Möller, "Photographic Interventions in Post-9/11 Security Policy," *Security Dialogue* 38, no. 2 (2007): 179–196; Matt McDonald, "Securitization and the Construction of Security," *European Journal of International Relations* 14, no. 4 (2008): 563–587.
50. Hansen, "The Little Mermaid's," 300.
51. Williams, "Words," 512.
52. Möller, "Photographic Interventions," 179–196.
53. Lene Hansen, "The Politics of Securitization and the Muhammad Cartoon Crisis: A Post-Structuralist Perspective," *Security Dialogue* 42, nos. 4–5 (2011): 357–369.
54. "World Report 2009—China," *Human Rights Watch*, accessed September 24, 2009, http://www.hrw.org/sites/default/files/reports/wr2009_web.pdf.
55. "World Report 2009."
56. Wilkinson, "The Copenhagen School," 12.
57. McDonald, "Securitization and the Construction," 569.
58. John Langshaw Austin, *How to Do Things with Words* (Oxford: Oxford University Press, 1962), 8–9.
59. Hansen, "The Little Mermaid's," 302.

NOTES 185

60. Felix Ciută, "Security and the Problem of Context: A Hermeneutical Critique of Securitization Theory," *Review of International Studies* 35, no. 2 (2009): 316.
61. Roxanna Sjöstedt, "Health Issues and Securitization: The Construction of HIV/AIDS as a US National Security Threat," in *Securitization Theory: How Security Problems Emerge and Dissolve*, ed. Thierry Balzacq (London: Routledge, 2011), 151.
62. Mely Caballero-Anthony and Ralf Emmers, "The Dynamics of Securitization in Asia," in *Studying Non-Traditional Security in Asia: Trends and Issues*, ed. Ralf Emmers, Mely Caballero-Anthony, and Amitav Acharya (Singapore: Marshall Cavendish Academic, 2006b), 25; Wæver, "Securitization," 26.
63. Buzan, Wæver, and de Wilde, *Security*, 24.
64. Buzan, Wæver, and de Wilde, *Security*, 25.
65. Mark B. Salter, "When Securitization Fails: The Hard Case of Counter-Terrorism Programs," in *Securitization Theory: How Security Problems Emerge and Dissolve*, ed. Thierry Balzacq (London: Routledge, 2011), 121.
66. Salter, "When Securitization Fails," 121–122.
67. Buzan, Wæver, and de Wilde, *Security*, 31.
68. Wæver, "Securitization," 26.
69. Wæver, "Securitization," 26.
70. See Jocelyn Vaughn, "The Unlikely Securitizer: Humanitarian Organizations and the Securitization of Indistinctiveness," *Security Dialogue* 40, no. 3 (2009): 263–285.
71. Vaughn, "The Unlikely Securitizer," 275–277.
72. Thierry Balzacq, "The Three Faces of Securitization: Political Agency, Audience and Context," *European Journal of International Relations* 11, no. 2 (2005): 184.
73. Balzacq, "The Three Faces," 184.
74. Holger Stritzel, "Towards a Theory of Securitization: Copenhagen and Beyond," *European Journal of International Relations* 13, no. 3 (2007): 363.
75. Rita Floyd, "Can Securitization Theory Be Used in Normative Analysis? Towards a Just Securitization Theory," *Security Dialogue* 42, nos. 4–5 (2011): 428.
76. Floyd, "Can Securitization Theory," 428.
77. Floyd, "Can Securitization Theory," 429.
78. Floyd, "Can Securitization Theory," 428.
79. Floyd, "Can Securitization Theory," 437.
80. For example, Huysmans, "Revisiting Copenhagen," 499–501; Mely Caballero-Anthony, and Ralf Emmers, "Understanding the Dynamics of Securitizing Non-Traditional Security," in *Non-Traditional Security in Asia: Dilemmas in Securitization*, ed. Mely Caballero-Anthony, Ralf Emmers, and Amitav Acharya (Singapore: Ashgate Publishing Limited, 2006a), 5; Wilkinson, "The Copenhagen School," 5–25; Vuori, "Illocutionary Logic and Strands of Securitization," 65–99; Curley and Herington, "The Securitization," 141–166.
81. Curley and Herington, "The Securitization," 146.

82. Ralf Emmers, Greener B. Barcham, and Nicholas Thomas, "Securitizing Human Trafficking in the Asia-Pacific: Regional Organizations and Response Strategies," in *Security and Migration in Asia: The Dynamics of Securitization*, ed. Melissa G. Curley and Siu-lun Wong (London: Routledge, 2008), 62.
83. Wilkinson, "The Copenhagen School," 5.
84. In-taek Hyun, Sung-han Kim, and Geun Lee, "Bringing Politics Back in: Globalization, Pluralism, and Securitization in East Asia," in *Studying Non-Traditional Security in Asia: Trends and Issues*, ed. Ralf Emmers, Mely Caballero-Anthony, and Amitav Acharya (Singapore: Marshall Cavendish Academic, 2006b), 122.
85. Wæver, "Securitization," 26.
86. Wæver, "Securitization," 26.
87. Wæver, "Securitization," 26.
88. Wæver, "Securitization," 12.
89. Vaughn, "The Unlikely Securitizer," 273.
90. Vuori, "Illocutionary Logic," 72; Colin McInnes and Simon Rushton, "HIV, AIDS and Security: Where Are We Now?" *International Affairs* 86, no. 1 (2010): 244.
91. Wæver, "Securitization," 26.
92. Michael Howlett, M. Ramesh, and Anthony Perl, *Studying Public Policy: Policy Cycles & Policy Subsystems* (Canada: Oxford University Press, 2009), 10.
93. See David Easton, *A Framework for Political Analysis* (Englewood Cliffs: Prentice-Hall, 1965).
94. Easton, *A Framework*, 112.
95. Easton, *A Framework*, 127.
96. Easton, *A Framework*, 126.
97. Easton, *A Framework*, 129.
98. Howlett, Ramesh, and Perl, *Studying Public Policy*, 12.
99. Howlett, Ramesh, and Perl, *Studying Public Policy*, 12.
100. Howlett, Ramesh, and Perl, *Studying Public Policy*, 12.
101. Buzan, Wæver, and de Wilde, *Security*, 26.
102. Hansen, "The Little Mermaid's," 296.
103. Buzan, Wæver, and de Wilde, *Security*, 32.
104. Buzan, Wæver, and de Wilde, *Security*, 32–3.
105. Wæver, "Aberystwyth," 8.
106. Johan Eriksson, "Agendas, Threats and Politics: Securitization in Sweden" (paper presented at the ECPR Joint Sessions, workshop "Redefining Security," Mannheim, March 26–31, 1999).
107. Rita Floyd, "Human Security and the Copenhagen School's Securitization Approach: Conceptualizing Human Security as a Securitizing Move," *Human Security Journal* 5, (2007): 41.
108. Ilavenil Ramiah, "Securitizing the AIDS Issue in Asia," in *Non-Traditional Security in Asia: Dilemmas in Securitization*, ed. Mely Caballero-Anthony, Ralf Emmers, and Amitav Acharya (England: Ashgate Publishing Limited, 2006a), 150; Buzan, Wæver, and de Wilde, *Security*, 29.

Notes

109. Ramiah, "Securitizing the AIDS," 150.
110. "Thailand's Response to HIV/AIDS: Progress and Challenges," *United Nations Development Program*, accessed August 2, 2010, http://www.undp.or.th/download/HIV_AIDS_FullReport_ENG.pdf.
111. Wæver, "Securitization and Desecuritization," 56; Wæver, "Aberystwyth," 9.
112. Hansen, "The Politics of Securitization," 362.
113. Huysmans, "Revisiting Copenhagen," 501.
114. David Matsumoto, *Cultural Influences on Research Methods and Statistics* (Pacific Grove, CA: Brooks/Cole Publishing Company, 1994), 31.
115. Hansen, "The Little Mermaid's," 296.
116. Elizabeth Wishnick, "The Securitization of Chinese Migration to the Russian Far East: Rhetoric and Reality," in *Security and Migration in Asia: The Dynamics of Securitization*, ed. Melissa G. Curley and Siu-lun Wong (London: Routledge, 2008), 91.
117. Catherine Yuk-ping Lo and Nicholas Thomas, "How Is Health a Security Issue? Politics, Responses and Issues," *Health Policy and Planning* 25, no. 6 (2010): 448.
118. Wæver, "Securitization," 27.
119. Michael C. Williams, "The Continuing Evolution of Securitization Theory," in *Securitization Theory: How Security Problems Emerge and Dissolve*, ed. Thierry Balzacq (London: Routledge, 2011), 217.
120. Wæver, "Securitization," 26.
121. Wæver, "Securitization," 27.
122. Javed Mohammad Iqbal, "AIDS and the State: A Comparison of Brazil, India and South Africa," *South Asian Survey* 16, no. 1 (2009): 125.
123. Simon Rushton, "The Development of the HIV/AIDS and Security Discourse: The Role of CSOs" (paper presented at Peter Wall Institute's London Workshop on Civil Society Organizations and Global Health Governance, October 2007).
124. Emmers, Barcham, and Thomas, "Securitizing Human Trafficking," 63.
125. Ramiah, "Securitizing the AIDS," 158.
126. Ramiah, "Securitizing the AIDS," 158.
127. Buzan, Wæver, and de Wilde, *Security*, 25.
128. In Austin's speech act theory, "speech acts" is also named as "performative speech acts," since it is assumed that something is done by the utterance, regardless of any mental reservation. In this thesis the term "performative securitizing move" is christened to highlight the emergency actions performed by the securitizing actors with the absence of speech acts.
129. Floyd, "Can Securitization Theory," 429.
130. Floyd, "Can Securitization Theory," 429.
131. McInnes and Rushton, "HIV, AIDS and Security," 244.
132. Wæver, "Securitization," 23.
133. Rita Floyd, "Towards a Consequentialist Evaluation of Security: Bringing Together the Copenhagen and the Welsh Schools of Security Studies," *Review of International Studies* 33, no. 2 (2007): 329.
134. Buzan, Wæver, and de Wilde, *Security*, 31.

135. Buzan, Wæver, and de Wilde, *Security*, 25.
136. Wæver, "Securitization," 11.
137. Wæver, "Securitization," 26.
138. Rushton, "The Development," 10.
139. Rushton, "The Development," 6.
140. Rushton, "The Development," 7.
141. Pinar Bilgin, "Making Turkey's Transformation Possible: Claiming "Security-Speak"—not Desecuritization!," *Southeast European and Black Sea Studies* 7, no. 4 (2007): 558.
142. "Thailand's Response to HIV/AIDS."
143. Yaowarat Porapakkham et al., "The Evolution of HIV/AIDS Policy in Thailand: 1984–1994," *United States Agency for International Development*, accessed August 2, 2010, http://pdf.usaid.gov/pdf_docs/PNACG546.pdf.
144. Porapakkham et al., "The Evolution of HIV/AIDS Policy in Thailand."
145. Suvam Neupane, "Combating HIV/AIDS: Lesson from Thailand," *nepalnews.com*, July 14, 2011, accessed November 10, 2014, http://www.nepal news.com/archive/2011/others/guestcolumn/jul/guest_columns_04.php.
146. "Act Now: Asia Pacific Leaders Respond to HIV/AIDS," *UNAIDS/Asia Pacific Leadership Forum on HIV/AIDS and Development*, accessed April 14, 2012, http://data.unaids.org/publications/External-Documents/apfl_actnow_en.pdf.
147. "Act Now: Asia Pacific Leaders Respond to HIV/AIDS."
148. "Thailand's Response to HIV/AIDS."
149. Kristina Jönsson, "Issue without Boundaries: HIV/AIDS in Southeast Asia," *Centre for East and South-East Asian Studies, Lund University, Sweden*, accessed August 30, 2010, http://www.lu.se/images/Syd_och_sydostasien studier/working_papers/Jonsson.pdf.
150. "AIDS Prevention and Care in the Workplace: Enhancing the Role of the Private Sector," *World Health Organization*, last modified January 12–13, 1995, http://whqlibdoc.who.int/searo/1994-99/SEA_AIDS_90.pdf.
151. "AIDS Prevention and Care."
152. The Executive branch of the Taiwanese government, headed by the president.
153. "Declaration of Commitment on HIV/AIDS Interventions," *Centers of Disease Control, Republic of China*, last modified December 19, 2001, http://www.cdc.gov.tw/ct.asp?xItem=595&ctNode=1069&mp=220.
154. Steve Hsu-sung Kuo, Su-fen Tsai, and Yen-fang Huang, "Taiwan," in *Fighting a Rising Tide: The Response to AIDS in East Asia*, ed. Tadashi Yamamoto and Satoko Itoh (Tokyo: Japan Center for International Exchange, 2006), 239.
155. Kuo, Tsai, and Huang, "Taiwan," 239.
156. "台爱滋病防治推动委员会成立 斥资 2 亿斗爱滋" [The Establishment of Taiwan Committee for the Promotion of AIDS Prevention and Treatment, with an allocation of 2 billion to fight HIV/AIDS], 北方网 [enorth.com.cn], last modified December 20, 2001, http://news.enorth.com.cn/system /2001/12/20/000222602.shtml.
157. "Declaration of Commitment on HIV/AIDS Interventions."

158. "HIV/AIDS Laws of the World," *Harvard School of Public Health*, last modified February 2, 2010, http://www.hsph.harvard.edu/population/aids/aids.htm.
159. "HIV/AIDS Laws of the World."
160. Vincent Rollet, "Taiwanese NGOs and HIV/AIDS: From the National to the Transnational," *China Perspectives* 60, (2005): 4.
161. AIDS Care Association is operating in Taichung, while Taiwan Love and Hope Association in Kaohsiung. Lourdes Home works in both Taipei and Taichung. The rest of the eight HIV/AIDS-related NGOs are only operating in the capital city Taipei.
162. Rollet, "Taiwanese NGOs," 4.
163. "Indian Premier Seeks Cooperation of Industrial Houses to Contain AIDS," *BBC Monitoring South Asia—Political*, December 1, 2000, LexisNexis Newspapers.
164. "Address by the Prime Minister Stri Atal Bihari Vajpayee at the meeting on National Program for Prevention and Control of HIV/AIDS New Delhi," *Embassy of India*, last modified December 12, 1998, http://www.indianembassy.org/policy/AIDS/prime_minister_AIDS.html.
165. "Indian Premier Calls for Effective Response to HIV/AIDS," *BBC Summary of World Broadcasts*, May 11, 2002, LexisNexis Newspapers.
166. "Business Aid Sought for 4.5 Mln Indian Affected with HIV," *Xinhua*, October 13, 2003, LexisNexis Newspapers.
167. Vladimir Putin, "Opening Remarks at State Council Presidium Meeting on Urgent Measures to Combat the Spread of HIV-AIDS in the Russian Federation," *Official Web Portal: President of Russia*, last modified April 21, 2006, http://archive.kremlin.ru/eng/text/speeches/2006/04/21/2148_type82912type82913_104797.shtml#.
168. Judyth Twigg, "HIV/AIDS in Russia: Commitment, Resources, Momentum, Challenges," *Center for Strategic and International Studies*, last modified October 2007, http://csis.org/files/media/csis/pubs/071016_russiahivaids.pdf.
169. Tom Parfitt, "Sex and Drugs and Russian Roulette," *The Guardian*, September 14, 2010, accessed November 10, 2014, http://www.theguardian.com/global-development/2010/sep/14/mdg6-hiv-aids-russia.
170. "UNAIDS Outlook Report 2010," *UNAIDS*, last modified July 2010, http://data.unaids.org/pub/Outlook/2010/20100713_outlook_report_web_en.pdf.
171. Twigg, "HIV/AIDS in Russia."
172. "Russian Government Commission," *Government of the Russian Federation*, accessed August 30, 2010, http://www.government.ru/eng/gov/agencies/154/.
173. Parfitt, "Sex and Drugs."
174. "HIV and AIDS in Russia, Eastern Europe and Central Asia," *AVERT*, last modified July 23, 2010, http://www.avert.org/aids-russia.htm.
175. Parfitt, "Sex and Drugs."
176. "UNAIDS Outlook Report."

177. Twigg, "HIV/AIDS in Russia."
178. Buzan, Wæver, and de Wilde, *Security*, 29.
179. Buzan, Wæver, and de Wilde, *Security*, 27.
180. Buzan, Wæver, and de Wilde, *Security*, 27.
181. This idea borrows from Vuori's article: Juha A. Vuori, "A Timely Prophet? The Doomsday Clock as a Visualization of Securitization Moves with a Global Referent Object," *Security Dialogue* 41, no. 3 (2010): 259.
182. Howlett, Ramesh, and Perl, *Studying Public Policy*, 191.
183. Eduardo J. Gómez, "The Politics of Government Response to HIV/AIDS in Brazil: Democratization, International Pressures, and the Civic Sources of Institutional Change," Rough draft, July 1, 2008, 30.
184. Varun Gauri and Evan S. Lieberman, "AIDS and the State: The Politics of Government Responses to the Epidemic in Brazil and South Africa" (paper presented at the annual meetings for the American Political Science Association, Chicago, IL, September 2–5, 2004).
185. Gómez, "The Politics," 37.
186. Gómez, "The Politics," 53.
187. The four NGOs include Associação Brasiliera Interdisciplinar de AIDS, Grupo Gay de Bahia, Associção Brasiliera de Entidades de Planejamento Familiar, and Centro Corsini de Investigação Imunológica. Gauri and Lieberman, "AIDS and the State," 12.
188. Drew Forrest, and Barry Streek, "Mbeki in Bizarre AIDS Outburst," *Mail and Guardian*, October 26, 2001, accessed November 24, 2014, http://mg.co.za/article/2001-10-26-mbeki-in-bizarre-aids-outburst.
189. Thabo Mbeki, "Speech of the Opening of the 13th International AIDS Conference, Durban," *JournAIDS*, last modified July 9, 2000, http://www.southafrica-newyork.net/consulate/aidsspeech.htm.
190. "South African Health Minister Must Go, Say Scientists," *The Lancet*, September 30, 2006, LexisNexis Newspapers.
191. Varun Gauri and Evan S. Lieberman, "Boundary Institutions and HIV/AIDS Policy in Brazil and South Africa," *Studies in Comparative International Development* 41, no. 3 (2006): 52.
192. "2003: TAC and Civil Disobedience," *JournAIDS*, accessed August 9, 2010, http://www.journaids.org/index.php/factsheets/the_politics_of_hivaids_in_south_africa/tac_and_civil_disobedience/; Iqbal, "AIDS and The State," 126.
193. Howard Barrell, "President Tells Party Caucus that Western Interests are Seeking to Discredit Him and South Africa," *Mail and Guardian*, October 6, 2000, accessed August 9, 2010, http://www.aegis.org/news/dmg/2000/MG001005.html.
194. "South Africa's Top Twelve AIDS Dissidents," *Democratic Alliance*, last modified August 9, 2010, http://www.da.org.za/docs/612/Top12AIDSDissidents_document.pdf.
195. "AIDS: Open Letter to Thabo Mbeki," *Africa News*, April 9, 2002, LexisNexis Newspapers.
196. "2003: TAC and Civil Disobedience."

197. "China Makes Efforts to Prevent AIDS," *Xinhua*, September 27, 1987, LexisNexis Newspapers.
198. "AIDS Can Be Checked in China—Experts," *Xinhua*, July 22, 1987, LexisNexis Newspapers.
199. Yvonne Preston, "China Sees AIDS as Foreign," *The Age*, November 30, 1991, LexisNexis Newspapers.

3 Health Security and HIV/AIDS

1. Mark P. Friedlander, *Outbreak: Disease Detectives at Work* (New York: Lerner Publications Company, 2000), 16.
2. Diseases such as "plague of Athens" (430–427 BC), smallpox in Japan (735–737), and Black Death (1326–1844) were understood as punishment of gods. For more examples, see J. N. Hays, *Epidemics and Pandemics: Their Impacts on Human History* (Santa Barbara: ABC-CLIO, 2005).
3. "Varro, on Agriculture (1st century BCE)," *Catena: Digital Archive of Historic Gardens Landscapes*, accessed April 11, 2012, http://catena.bgc.bard.edu/texts/varro.htm.
4. Friedlander, *Outbreak*, 31–33.
5. Matthew R. Smallman-Raynor and Andrew D. Cliff, *War Epidemics: An Historical Geography of Infectious Diseases in Military Conflict and Civil Strife, 1850–2000* (New York: Oxford University Press, 2004), 4.
6. Hays, *Epidemics and Pandemics*, preface X.
7. "Global Risks 2009: A Global Risk Network Report," *World Economic Forum*, last modified January 2009, https://members.weforum.org/pdf/globalrisk/2009.pdf.
8. Stefan Elbe, "Pandemics on the Radar Screen: Health Security, Infectious Disease and the Medicalization of Insecurity," *Political Studies* 59, no. 4 (2011): 850.
9. "UN Security Council Resolution 1308 (2000) on the Responsibility of the Security Council in the Maintenance of International Peace and Security: HIV/AIDS and International Peace-keeping Operations," *United Nation Security Council*, last modified July 17, 2000, http://data.unaids.org/pub/BaseDocument/2000/20000717_un_scresolution_1308_en.pdf.
10. See Gwyn Prins, "AIDS and Global Security," *International Affairs* 80, no. 5 (2004): 931–952; Colin McInnes, "HIV/AIDS and Security," *International Affairs* 82, no. 2 (2006): 315–326; Alan Whiteside, Alex de Waal, and Tsadkan Gebre-Tensae, "AIDS, Security and the Military in Africa: A Sober Appraisal," *African Affairs* 105, no. 419 (2006): 201–218; Tony Barnett and Gwyn Prins, "HIV/AIDS and Security: Fact, Fiction, Evidences—A Report to UNAIDS," *International Affairs* 82, no. 2 (2006): 359–368; Pieter Fourie, "The Relationship between the AIDS Pandemic and State Fragility," *Global Change, Peace & Security* 19, no. 3 (2007): 281–300.

11. See Dennis Altman, "AIDS and Security," *International Relations* 17, no. 4 (2003): 417–427; Lindy Heinecken, "Facing a Merciless Enemy: HIV/AIDS and the South African Armed Forces," *Armed Forces & Society* 29, no. 2 (2003): 281–300; David L. Heymann, "Evolving Infectious Disease Threats to National and Global Security," in *Global Health Challenges for Human Security*, ed. Lincoln C. Chen, Jennifer Leaning, and Vasant Narasimhan (Cambridge, MA: Global Equity Initiative, Asia Center, Harvard University, 2003), 108; Alex de Waal, "HIV/AIDS: The Security Issue of a Lifetime," in *Global Health Challenges for Human Security*, ed. Lincoln C. Chen, Jennifer Leaning, and Vasant Narasimhan (Cambridge, MA: Global Equity Initiative, Asia Center, Harvard University, 2003), 125–137; Rachel Girshick, "Adopting Institutional Changes: HIV/AIDS and the Changing Institution of Security" (paper presented at the Annual Conference for the International Studies Association, Montreal, Quebec, March 18, 2004); Colleen O'Manique, "The 'Securitization' of HIV/AIDS in Sub-Saharan Africa: A Critical Feminist Lens," *Policy and Society* 24, no. 1 (2005): 24–47.
12. Colin McInnes and Simon Rushton, "HIV/AIDS and Securitization Theory," *European Journal of International Relations* 19, no. 1 (2013): 122.
13. UN Security Council Resolution 1308 (2000) has dominantly been seen as the key moment in the securitization process.
14. Some scholars debated that the securitization generated in 2000 is not a successful/complete securitization. See Simon Rushton, "Securitizing HIV/AIDS: Pandemics, Politics and SCR 1308" (paper presented at the International Studies Association Convention, Chicago, 2007); Colin McInnes and Simon Rushton, "HIV, AIDS and Security: Where Are We Now?" *International Affairs* 86, no. 1 (2010): 225–245.
15. William H. Stewart, "A Mandate for State Action" (presented at the Association of State and Territorial Health Officers, Washington DC, December 4, 1967), quoted in Brad Spellberg, "Dr. William H. Stewart: Mistaken or Maligned?" *Clinical Infectious Diseases* 47, no. 2 (2008): 294.
16. See "List of Emerging and Re-emerging Diseases," *National Institute of Allergy and Infectious Diseases, National Institutes of Health*, last modified August 8, 2014, http://www.niaid.nih.gov/topics/BiodefenseRelated/Biodefense/Pages/CatA.aspx.
17. Mely Caballero-Anthony, "Combating Infectious Diseases in East Asia: Securitization and Global Public Goods for Health and Human Security," *Journal of International Affairs* 59, no. 2 (2006): 110.
18. "Treatment Resistant Swine Flu Detected in US," *AFP*, August 3, 2009, accessed September 9, 2009, http://www.google.com/hostednews/afp/article/ALeqM5hsS3W74VB3XpDzfh8qD-7Cmq0J0g.
19. Michael Shnayerson and Mark J. Plotkin, *The Killers Within: The Deadly Rise of Drug-Resistant Bacteria* (Boston: Little, Brown and Company, 2002), 35.
20. Shnayerson and Plotkin, *The Killers*, 35.
21. Shnayerson and Plotkin, *The Killers*, 5.

22. "Understanding Vaccines," *National Institute of Allergy and Infectious Diseases, National Institutes of Health*, last modified January 2008, http://www3.niaid.nih.gov/topics/vaccines/PDF/undvacc.pdf.
23. "Emerging and Re-Emerging Infectious Diseases: Introduction and Goals," *National Institute of Allergy and Infectious Diseases, National Institutes of Health*, last modified March 10, 2010, http://www.niaid.nih.gov/topics/emerging/pages/introduction.aspx.
24. Thérèse Murphy and Noel Whitty, "Is Human Rights Prepared? Risk, Rights and Public Health Emergencies," *Medical Law Review* 17, no. 2 (2009): 222.
25. "Constitution of the World Health Organization," *World Health Organization*, accessed September 18, 2009, http://www.who.int/governance/eb/who_constitution_en.pdf. It was adopted by the International Health Conference held in New York from June 19 to July 22, 1946, signed on July 22, 1946 by the representatives of 61 States and entered into force on April 7, 1948.
26. Lynn Thiesmeyer, "Gender, Public Health, and Human Security Policy in Asia," *United Nations: Division for the Advancement of Women*, last modified October 28, 2005, http://www.un.org/womenwatch/daw/egm/enabling-environment2005/docs/EGM-WPD-EE-2005-EP_2_%20L_Thiesmeyer.pdf. Food security is related to readily accessible food and effectiveness in distribution of food. Environmental security refers to the protection of the environment from deforestation and erosion, desertification, pollution, and also the maintainability of sustainable development. Personal security is attained when one can be free from threats from the state (torture), other states (war), other groups of people (ethnic tension) and other individuals or gangs (street crime). Particularly, women can be free from threats of domestic violence and rape; children can be free from threats of child abuse and an individual can be free from threats of drug use and suicide.
27. Thiesmeyer, "Gender."
28. Jonas Gahr StØre, Jonathan Welch, and Lincoln Chen, "Health and Security for a Global Century," in *Global Health Challenges for Human Security*, ed. Lincoln C. Chen, Jennifer Leaning, and Vasant Narasimhan (Cambridge, MA: Global Equity Initiative, Asia Center, Harvard University, 2003), 77.
29. Lincoln C. Chen, "Health as a Human Security Priority for the 21st Century" (paper for Human Security Track III, Helsinki Process, December 7, 2004).
30. Mely Caballero-Anthony, "Human Security and Primary Health Care in Asia: Realities and Challenges," in *Global Health Challenges for Human Security*, ed. Lincoln C. Chen, Jennifer Leaning, and Vasant Narasimhan (Cambridge, MA: Global Equity Initiative, Asia Center, Harvard University, 2003), 242.
31. See Rekha Datta, *Beyond Realism: Human Security in India and Pakistan in the Twenty-First Century* (Lanham: Lexington Books, 2008).
32. David P. Fidler, "A Pathology of Public Health Securitism: Approaching Pandemics as Security Threats," in *Governing Global Health: Challenge,*

Response, Innovation, ed. Andrew F. Cooper, John J. Kirton, and Ted Schrecker (England: Ashgate Publishing Limited, 2007), 42.
33. Colin McInnes and Kelley Lee, "Health, Security and Foreign Policy," *Review of International Studies* 32, no. 1 (2006): 16.
34. Fidler, "A Pathology," 42.
35. James Orbinski, "Global Health, Social Movements, and Governance," in *Governing Global Health: Challenge, Response, Innovation*, ed. Andrew F. Cooper, John J. Kirton, and Ted Schrecker (England: Ashgate Publishing Limited, 2007), 30.
36. Fidler, "A Pathology," 44.
37. Laurie Garrett, "The Return of Infectious Diseases," in *Plagues and Politics*, ed. Andrew T. Price-Smith (London: Palgrave Macmillan, 2001), 185; Chen, "Health as a Human Security Priority," 4.
38. Melissa G. Curley and Nicholas Thomas, "Human Security and Public Health in Southeast Asia: The SARS Outbreak," *Australian Journal of International Affairs* 58, no. 1 (2004): 17.
39. Sara E. Davies, "Securitizing Infectious Disease," *International Affairs* 84, no. 2 (2008): 296.
40. "The Top 10 Causes of Death," *World Health Organization*, last modified May 2014, http://www.who.int/mediacentre/factsheets/fs310/en/.
41. See Mely Caballero-Anthony, "Combating Infectious Diseases in East Asia," 105–127.
42. See Laurie Garrett, "HIV and National Security: Where Are the Links?" *Council on Foreign Relations*, accessed January 4, 2010, http://www.cfr.org/content/publications/attachments/HIV_National_Security.pdf.
43. "Global AIDS Overview," *AIDS.gov*, last modified December 18, 2013. http://www.aids.gov/federal-resources/arounglobal-aidsd-the-world/-overview/.
44. Arno Karlen, *Plague's Progress: A Social History of Man and Disease* (London: Gollancz, 1995), 199–200.
45. Karlen, *Plague's Progress*, 188; Barry E. Zimmerman and David J. Zimmerman, *Killer Germs: Microbes and Diseases That Threaten Humanity* (New York: McGraw-Hill, 2003), 188.
46. Karlen, *Plague's Progress*, 187; Frank Ryan, *Virus X: Tracking the New Killer Plagues: Out of the Present and into the Future* (Boston: Little, Brown and Company, 1997), 250.
47. James Cross Giblin, *When Plague Strikes: The Black Death, Smallpox, AIDS* (New York: HarperCollins Publishers, 1995), 140.
48. Laurie Garrett, *The Coming Plague: Newly Emerging Diseases in a World out of Balance* (New York: Penguin Group, 1994), 284; Giblin, *When Plague Strikes*, 118; Friedlander, *Outbreak*, 90.
49. Ryan, *Virus X*, 277.
50. Phyllis J. Kanki and Myron E. Essex, "Virology," in *The AIDS Pandemic: Impact on Science and Society*, ed. Kenneth H. Mayer and H. F. Pizer (San Diego, CA: Elsevier Academic Press, 2005), 21.
51. Ryan, *Virus X*, 277.

52. Ryan, *Virus X*, 277.
53. Friedlander, *Outbreak*, 30.
54. Garrett, *The Coming Plague*, 293.
55. James Chin, *The AIDS Pandemic: The Collision of Epidemiology with Political Correctness* (Oxford: Radcliffe Publishing Limited, 2007), 46.
56. Garrett, *The Coming Plague*, 283; Zimmerman and Zimmerman, *Killer Germs*, 183.
57. Giblin, *When Plague Strikes*, 118; Karlen, *Plague's Progress*, 185.
58. Garrett, *The Coming Plague*, 284.
59. Garrett, *The Coming Plague*, 284.
60. Zimmerman and Zimmerman, *Killer Germs*, 184.
61. Garrett, *The Coming Plague*, 287; Giblin, *When Plague Strikes*, 120–121.
62. Garrett, *The Coming Plague*, 286.
63. Karlen, *Plague's Progress*, 185.
64. Karlen, *Plague's Progress*, 185.
65. Giblin, *When Plague Strikes*, 120; Karlen, *Plague's Progress*, 185; Hays, *Epidemics and Pandemics*, 427.
66. Giblin, *When Plague Strikes*, 130.
67. Giblin, *When Plague Strikes*, 141.
68. Ryan, *Virus X*, 266.
69. Garrett, *The Coming Plague*, 334; Giblin, *When Plague Strikes*, 142; Zimmerman and Zimmerman, *Killer Germs*, 189.
70. Hays, *Epidemics and Pandemics*, 428.
71. Karlen, *Plague's Progress*, 189; Zimmerman and Zimmerman, *Killer Germs*, 203.
72. Giblin, *When Plague Strikes*, 143; Mark Jerome Walters, *Six Modern Plagues and How We Are Causing Them* (Washington, DC: Island Press/Shearwater Books, 2003), 53.
73. Walters, *Six Modern Plagues*, 59; Hays, *Epidemics and Pandemics*, 431.
74. See Garrett, *The Coming Plague*, 353; Giblin, *When Plague Strikes*, 143; Walters, *Six Modern Plagues*, 52.
75. See Zimmerman and Zimmerman, *Killer Germs*, 199–200.
76. "Race for HIV Cure Overshadows Prevention, Says Expert,' *Aids Cure*, last modified February 19, 2009, http://aidscure-top.blogspot.com/2009/02/race-for-hiv-cure-overshadows.html.
77. Giblin, *When Plague Strikes*, 150.
78. Ryan, *Virus X*, 277.
79. Walters, *Six Modern Plagues*, 54.
80. Zimmerman and Zimmerman, *Killer Germs*, 198.
81. Luc Montagnier, "The Next Steps to Take in Beating AIDS," *Wall Street Journal*, October 21, 2008, accessed November 10, 2014, http://online.wsj.com/articles/SB122455090257552591.
82. Tony Barnett, "HIV/AIDS, a Long Wave Event: Sundering the Intergenerational Bond," in *AIDS and Governance*, ed. Nana K. Poku, Alan Whiteside, and Bjorn Sandkjaer (England: Ashgate Publishing Limited, 2007), 35.

83. Madeline Drexler, *Secret Agents: The Menace of Emerging Infections* (Washington, DC: Joseph Henry Press, 2002), 169.
84. Karlen, *Plague's Progress*, 189.
85. Sodsai Tovanabutra, Deborah L. Birx, and Francine E. McCutchan, "Molecular Epidemiology of HIV in Asia and the Pacific," in *AIDS in Asia*, ed. Lu Yi Chen and Max Essex (New York: Kluwer Academic/Plenum Publishers, 2004), 181; Yu-ching Lan et al., "Molecular Epidemiology of HIV-1 Subtypes and Drug Resistant Strains in Taiwan," *Journal of Medical Virology* 80, no. 2 (2008): 183.
86. Zimmerman and Zimmerman, *Killer Germs*, 203.
87. Karlen, *Plague's Progress*, 190.
88. "About AIDS Vaccines: Why a Vaccine," *International AIDS Vaccine Initiative*, accessed September 10, 2009, http://www.iavi.org/why-a-vaccine/Pages/about-AIDS-vaccine.aspx.
89. Zimmerman and Zimmerman, *Killer Germs*, 197.
90. Anthony Fauci, "Fauci: Why There Is No AIDS Vaccine," *msnbc.com*, last modified March 31, 2009, http://www.msnbc.msn.com/id/29898087/.
91. "Race for HIV Cure."
92. Fauci, "Fauci."
93. Kanki and Essex, "Virology," 25.
94. Karlen, *Plague's Progress*, 190.
95. Hays, *Epidemics and Pandemics*, 447; Akram A. Khan and Nazli Bano, "HIV/AIDS Epidemic in India: A Critical Health and Development Issue," in *Economics of Education and Health in India*, ed. Anil Kumar Thakur and Abdus Salam (New Delhi: The Indian Economic Association, 2008), 472.
96. Barry Buzan, Ole Wæver, and Jaap de Wilde, *Security: A New Framework for Analysis* (Boulder, CO: Lynne Rienner Publishers, 1998), 32.
97. "World Report 2009—India," *Human Rights Watch*, accessed September 24, 2009, http://www.hrw.org/sites/default/files/reports/wr2009_web.pdf.
98. Stefan Elbe, "Should HIV/AIDS Be Securitized? The Ethical Dilemmas of Linking HIV/AIDS and Security," *International Studies Quarterly* 50, no. 1 (2006): 120.
99. Elbe, "Should HIV/AIDS," 120.
100. Lisanne Brown, Kate Macintyre, and Lea Trujillo, "Interventions to Reduce HIV/AIDS Stigma: What Have We Learned?" *AIDS Education and Prevention* 15, no. 1 (2003): 51.
101. Brown, Macintyre, and Trujillo, "Interventions," 51.
102. Mohammad A. Rai et al., "HIV/AIDS in Pakistan: The Battle Begins," *Retrovirology* 4, no. 22 (2007): 3.
103. Pramit Mitra, "India at the Crossroads: Battling the HIV/AIDS Pandemic," *The Washington Quarterly* 27, no. 4 (2004): 99; Peter Piot et al., "A Global Response to AIDS: Lessons Learned, Next Steps," *Science* 304, no. 5679 (2004): 1910; "Act Now: Asia Pacific Leaders Respond to HIV/AIDS," *UNAIDS/Asia Pacific Leadership Forum on HIV/AIDS and Development*, accessed April 14, 2012, http://data.unaids.org/publications/External-Documents/apfl_actnow_en.pdf.

104. "New Hope of a Cure for H.I.V.," *New York Times*, November 28, 2011, http://www.nytimes.com/2011/11/29/health/new-hope-of-a-cure-for-hiv.html?pagewanted=all.
105. Ralf Emmers, Greener B. Barcham, and Nicholas Thomas, "Securitizing Human Trafficking in the Asia-Pacific: Regional Organizations and Response Strategies," in *Security and Migration in Asia: The Dynamics of Securitization*, ed. Melissa G. Curley and Siu-lun Wong (London: Routledge, 2008), 66.
106. Laurie Garrett, "HIV and National Security: Where Are the Links?" *Council on Foreign Relations*, accessed January 4, 2010, http://www.cfr.org/content/publications/attachments/HIV_National_Security.pdf.
107. McInnes and Rushton, "HIV, AIDS and Security," 228.
108. "Declaration on Commitment of HIV/AIDS," *United Nations General Assembly*, last modified August 2, 2011, http://www.un.org/ga/aids/docs/aress262.pdf.
109. "Political Declaration on HIV/AIDS," *United Nations General Assembly*, last modified June 15, 2006, http://data.unaids.org/pub/Report/2006/20060615_hlm_politicaldeclaration_ares60262_en.pdf.
110. "Political Declaration on HIV/AIDS: Intensifying Our Efforts to Eliminate HIV/AIDS," *United Nations General Assembly*, last modified June 8, 2011, http://daccess-dds-ny.un.org/doc/UNDOC/LTD/N11/367/84/PDF/N1136784.pdf?OpenElement.
111. McInnes and Rushton, "HIV/AIDS," 16.
112. "Commentary: Bush Saved 10 Million Lives," *CNN Politics*, January 15, 2009, accessed April 23, 2012, http://articles.cnn.com/2009-01-15/politics/frist.bush_1_antiretrovirals-hiv-george-bush?_s=PM:POLITICS.
113. "Progress on Global Access to HIV Antiretroviral Therapy: A Report on '3 by 5' and Beyond," *WHO/UNAIDS*, last modified March 2006, http://www.who.int/hiv/fullreport_en_highres.pdf.
114. J. Stephen Morrison and Todd Summers, "United to Fight HIV/AIDS?" *The Washington Quarterly*, accessed January 30, 2012, http://www.twq.com/03autumn/docs/03autumn_morrison.pdf.
115. Garrett W. Brown, and Ronald Labonté, "Globalization and its Methodological Discontents: Contextualizing Globalization through the Study of HIV/AIDS," *Globalization and Health* 7, no. 29 (2011): 8.
116. "Core Structures," *The Global Fund to Fight AIDS, Tuberculosis and Malaria*, accessed April 28, 2012, http://www.theglobalfund.org/en/about/structures/.
117. "Core Structures."
118. Ruairí Brugha et al., "The Global Fund: Managing Great Expectations," *The Lancet* 364, no. 9428 (2004): 95.
119. Dong-bao Yu et al., "Investment in HIV/AIDS Programs: Does It Help Strengthen Health Systems in Developing Countries?" *Globalization and Health* 4, no. 8 (2008): 4.
120. "NGO Perspectives on the Global Fund," *International Council of AIDS Service Organizations*, last modified June 2004, http://www.hivpolicy.org/Library/HPP000321.pdf.

121. Sui-lee Wee, "Cutting AIDS Funding to China a Big Mistake: UNAIDS," *Canada.com*, last modified July 11, 2011, http://www2.canada.com/topics/lifestyle/parenting/story.html?id=5083992.
122. "Grant Portfolio: China," *The Global Fund to Fight AIDS, Tuberculosis and Malaria*, last modified January 25, 2012, http://portfolio.theglobalfund.org/en/Country/Index/CHN.
123. "中国艾滋病传播途径以性病传播为主" [Sex Becomes the Main Route of HIV/AIDS Transmission in China], *Docin.com.Inc.*, accessed February 20, 2012, http://www.docin.com/p-236465268.html.
124. "Grant Portfolio: India," *The Global Fund to Fight AIDS, Tuberculosis, and Malaria*, last modified December 23, 2011, http://portfolio.theglobalfund.org/en/Country/Index/IDA.
125. Interview with a Program Officer of an INGO [R2], Beijing, January 2011.
126. Interview with a National Director of an INGO [R7], Beijing, January 2011.
127. See "UN Security Council."

4 The Changing Face of Public Health Care Systems in China and India

1. King Lun Ngok, "Redefining Development in China: Towards a New Policy Paradigm for the New Century?" in *Changing Governance and Public Policy in East Asia*, ed. Ka Ho Mok and Ray Forrest (London: Routledge, 2009), 54.
2. "On Ten Major Relationships," *Selected Works of Mao Tse-tong*, accessed November 6. 2014, https://www.marxists.org/reference/archive/mao/selected-works/volume-5/mswv5_51.htm.
3. "On Ten Major Relationships."
4. Shao Guang Wang, "Uneven Economic Development," in *Critical Issues in Contemporary China*, ed. Czeslaw Tubilewicz (London: Routledge and Hong Kong: Open University of Hong Kong Press, 2006), 100.
5. Colin Mackerras, "Critical Social Issues" in *Critical Issues in Contemporary China*, ed. Czeslaw Tubilewicz (London: Routledge and Hong Kong: Open University of Hong Kong Press, 2006), 213.
6. Piya Mahtaney, *India, China and Globalization: The Emerging Superpower and the Future of Economic Development* (Great Britain: Palgrave Macmillan, 2007), 133.
7. Yuan Li Liu, "China's Public Health-Care System: Facing the Challenges," *Bulletin of the World Health Organization* 82, no. 7 (2004): 536.
8. Mahtaney, *Globalization*, 133.
9. Lei Yu Shi, "Health Care in China: A Rural–Urban Comparison after the Socioeconomic Reforms," *Bulletin of the World Health Organization* 71, no. 6 (1993): 724; Dong Zhe and Michael R. Phillips, "Evolution of China's Health-Care System," *The Lancet* 372, no. 9651 (2008): 1715.

10. Jean Drèze and Amartya Sen, *India: Development and Participation* (New York: Oxford University Press, 2002), 129.
11. Shi, "Health Care in China," 724; Zhe and Phillips, "Health-Care System," 1715.
12. Debabar Banerji, "Landmarks in the Development of Health Services in India," in *Public Health and the Poverty of Reforms: The South Asian Predicament*, ed. Imrana Qadeer, Kasturi Sen, and K. R. Nayar (New Delhi: Sage Publications, 2001), 43.
13. Meenakshi Gauthamk and M. Shyamprasad, "Needed: 'Basic' Doctors of Modern Medicine," *The Hindu*, November 9, 2009, accessed November 29, 2014, http://www.thehindu.com/opinion/lead/needed-basic-doctors-of-modern-medicine/article43383.ece.
14. "Report of The Health Survey and Development Committee," *Government of India*, accessed May 12, 2014, http://nihfw.org/NDC/DocumentationServices/Reports/bhore%20Committee%20Report%20VOL-1%20.pdf.
15. Ravi Duggal, "Bhore Committee (1946) and Its Relevance Today," *The Indian Journal of Paediatrics* 58, no. 4 (1991): 399.
16. Duggal, "Bhore Committee," 398.
17. Anwar Islam and M. Zaffar Tahir, "Health Sector Reform in South Asia: New Challenges and Constraints," *Health Policy* 60, no. 2 (2002): 159.
18. Ashok Vikhe Patil, K. V. Somasundaram, and R. C. Coyal, "Current Health Scenario in Rural India," *Australian Journal of Rural Health* 10, no. 2 (2002):133.
19. Nicholas C. Hope et al., "Introduction," in *Economic Reform in India: Challenges, Prospects, and Lessons*, ed. Nicholas C. Hope et al. (Cambridge: Cambridge University Press, 2013), 1.
20. Hope et al., "Introduction," 1.
21. Jagdish Bhagwati, "The Design of Indian Development," in *India's Economic Reform and Development: Essay for Manmohan Singh*, ed. Isher Judge Ahluwalia and I. M. D. Little (New Delhi: Oxford University Press, 1998), 27.
22. Hope et al., "Introduction," 2.
23. "Report of the Working Group on Medical Education," *National Knowledge Commission*, accessed May 12, 2010, http://www.knowledgecommission.gov.in/downloads/documents/wg_med.pdf.
24. Trevor J. B. Dummer and Ian G. Cook, "Health in China and India: A Cross-Country Comparison in a Context of Rapid Globalization," *Social Science & Medicine* 67, no. 4 (2008): 599.
25. "Rural Health Care System in India," *Bulletin on Rural Health Statistics in India*, last modified March 2008, http://www.mohfw.nic.in/Bulletin%20on%20RHS%20-%20March,%202008%20-%20PDF%20Version/Rural%20Health%20Care%20System%20in%20India.pdf.
26. Arvind Panagariya, "India: The Crisis in Rural Health Care," *Brookings*, last modified January 24, 2008, http://www.brookings.edu/opinions/2008/0124_health_care_panagariya.aspx.

27. "Rural Health Care."
28. Panagariya, "India: The Crisis."
29. Panagariya, "India: The Crisis."
30. Mahtaney, *Globalization*, 133.
31. Drèze and Sen, *Development and Participation*, 129.
32. Howard W. French, "Wealth Grows, but Health Care Withers in China," *New York Times*, January 14, 2006, accessed November 29, 2014, http://www.nytimes.com/2006/01/14/international/asia/14health.html?page wanted=all&_r=0.
33. Banerji, "Landmarks," 44.
34. David H. Peters, K. Sujatha Rao, and Robert Fryatt, "Lumping and Splitting: The Health Policy Agenda in India," *Health Policy and Planning* 18, no. 3 (2003): 250.
35. Ashok Vikhe Patil, K. V. Somasundaram, and R. C. Coyal, "Current Health Scenario in Rural India," *Australian Journal of Rural Health* 10, no. 2 (2002): 130.
36. Mahtaney, *Globalization*, 174.
37. Mahtaney, *Globalization*, 173–174.
38. Atul Kohli, "Politics of Economic Growth in India, 1980–2005. Part II: The 1990s and Beyond," *Economic and Political Weekly*, last modified April 8, 2006, http://www.newschool.edu/uploadedFiles/TCDS/Democracy_and_Diversity_Institutes/Kohli_PEGI_PartII.pdf.
39. Kohli, "Politics of Economic Growth."
40. Montek S. Ahluwalia, "India's Economic Reforms: An Appraisal," in *India in the Era of Economic Reforms*, ed. Jeffrey D. Sachs, Ashutosh Varshney, and Nirupam Bajpai (New Delhi: Oxford University Press, 1999), 28.
41. Uma Kapila, *Indian Economy: Performance and Policies* (New Delhi: Academic Foundation, 2008), 93.
42. Ahluwalia, "India's Economic Reforms," 28.
43. Azizur Rahman Khan and Carl Riskin, *Inequality and Poverty in China in the Age of Globalization* (New York: Oxford University Press, 2001), 4.
44. Related economic policies included Special Economic Zones (SEZ), Coastal Open Cities (COC), Economic and Technological Development Zones (ETDZ), Coastal Economic Open Zones (CEOZ), and Custom-Free Zones (CFZ).
45. van Stuijvenberg, "Structural Adjustment," 59.
46. van Stuijvenberg, "Structural Adjustment," 44.
47. Gregory C. Chow, "Economic Reform and Growth in China," *Annals of Economics and Finance* 5, no. 1 (2004): 127.
48. "Indian GDP Annual Growth Rate," *Trading Economic*, accessed November 21, 2014, http://www.tradingeconomics.com/india/gdp-growth-annual.
49. Wang, "Uneven Economic," 100.
50. Wang, "Uneven Economic," 100.
51. Wang, "Uneven Economic," 102.
52. Friedemann Wenzel, Fouad Bendimerad, and Ravi Sinha, "Megacities—Megarisks," *Natural Hazards* 42, no. 3 (2007): 482.

NOTES

53. "Preventing HIV/AIDS in India," *The World Bank*, last modified June 2005, http://siteresources.worldbank.org/INTINDIA/Resources/HIV-AIDS-brief-June2005-IN.pdf.
54. Gui Xien and Zhuang Ke, "AIDS in China," in *Emerging Infections in Asia*, ed. Yi-chen Lu, M. Essex, and Bryan Roberts (New York: Springer, 2008), 154.
55. Drèze and Sen, *Development and Participation*, 333.
56. Tony Saich, *Governance and Politics of China* (China: Palgrave Macmillan, 2004), 75–76; Ngok, "Redefining Development in China," 49.
57. Yip and Mahal, "The Health Care Systems," 927.
58. Yip and Mahal, "The Health Care Systems," 926.
59. van Stuijvenberg, "Structural Adjustment," 42. The slogan "Adjustment with a Human Face" was first advocated by The United Nations Children's Fund (UNICEF) and several bilateral donors from the Nordic countries, calling for protection of the poor and vulnerable populations affected by the Structural Adjustment Programs.
60. Yip and Mahal, "The Health Care Systems," 926.
61. Drèze and Sen, *Development and Participation*, 201.
62. "Project Performance Assessment Report," *The World Bank*, last modified July 2, 2003, http://lnweb90.worldbank.org/OED/oeddoclib.nsf/DocUNIDViewForJavaSearch/CF5907844F56853D85256D900073CB1D/$file/India_PPAR_26224.pdf; "UNGASS Country Progress Report 2010: India," *National AIDS Control Organization*, last modified March 31, 2010, http://data.unaids.org/pub/Report/2010/india_2010_country_progress_report_en.pdf.
63. "Fight Will Go on Despite Grant Cut," *NCAIDS, China CDC*, last modified November 10, 2011, http://www.chinaaids.cn/n1971/n2091/721831.html.
64. Drèze and Sen, *Development and Participation*, 313.
65. I. Qadeer, "Impact of Structural Adjustment Programs on Concept in Public Health," in *Public Health and the Poverty of Reforms: The South Asian Predicament*, ed. I. Qadeer, K. Sen, and K. R. Nayar (New Delhi: Sage Publications, 2001), 129.
66. Banerji, "Landmarks," 45–46.
67. Qadeer, "Impact of Structural Adjustment Programs," 129.
68. Liu, "China's Public Health-Care System," 533.
69. Khan and Riskin, *Inequality and Poverty*, 96; Joan Kaufman, "China: The Intersections between Poverty, Health Inequity, Reproductive Health and HIV/AIDS," *Development* 48, no. 4 (2005): 115.
70. Drèze and Sen, *Development and Participation*, 130.
71. Saich, *Governance and Politics*, 293.
72. van Stuijvenberg, "Structural Adjustment in India," 68; M. Govinda Rao and Choudhury Mita, "Health Care Financing Reforms in India," *National Institute of Public Finance and Policy*, accessed March 2012, http://www.nipfp.org.in/media/medialibrary/2013/04/wp_2012_100.pdf.
73. K. Seeta Prabhu, "The Impact of Structural Adjustment on Social Sector Expenditure: Evidence from Indian States," in *Economic Reforms and Poverty*

Alleviation in India, ed. C. H. Hanumantha Rao and Hans Linnemann (New Delhi: Sage Publications, 1996), 229.
74. Prabhu, "Structural Adjustment," 237.
75. S. P. Gupta, "Recent Economic Reforms in India and Their Impact on the Poor and Vulnerable Sections of Society," in *Economic Reforms and Poverty Alleviation in India*, ed. C. H. Hanumantha Rao and Hans Linnemann (New Delhi: Sage Publications, 1996), 147.
76. Gupta, "Recent Economic Reforms," 142.
77. Prabhu, "Structural Adjustment," 248.
78. Drèze and Sen, *Development and Participation*, 218.
79. Saich, *Governance and Politics*, 171.
80. Banerji, "Landmarks," 47.
81. Drèze and Sen, *Development and Participation*, 130.
82. Khan and Riskin, *Inequality and Poverty*, 158.
83. Saich, *Governance and Politics*, 293.
84. Liu, "China's Public Health-Care System," 536.
85. Mackerras, "Critical Social Issues," 214.
86. Yip and Mahal, "The Health Care Systems," 928.
87. Yip and Mahal, "The Health Care Systems," 928.
88. Drèze and Sen, *Development and Participation*, 206.
89. Drèze and Sen, *Development and Participation*, 206.
90. Yip and Mahal, "The Health Care Systems," 928.
91. "State Council Notice on Strengthening HIV/AIDS Prevention and Control." *NCAIDS, China CDC*. Last modified March 16, 2004. http://www.chinaaids.cn/n1971/n2301/n8034/32205.html.
92. "PM's address at the National Students and Youth Parliament Special Session on HIV/AIDS," *Government of India*, last modified November 7, 2004, http://pmindia.nic.in/speech/content.asp?id=44.
93. However, the negative aspect of "AIDS exceptionalism" may occur if there is an overwhelmingly policy preference toward a single disease. See Julia H. Smith, and Alan Whiteside, "The History of AIDS Exceptionalism," *Journal of the International AIDS Society* 13, no. 47 (2010): 1–8.
94. Madison Park, "The Price of Blood: China Faces HIV/AIDS Epidemic," *CNN*, December 10, 2012, accessed November 29, 2014, http://edition.cnn.com/2012/11/30/health/hiv-china-li/.
95. John Gittings, "The AIDS Scandal China Could Not Hush Up," *The Guardian*, June 11, 2001, accessed November 29, 2014, http://www.theguardian.com/world/2001/jun/11/china.internationaleducationnews.
96. French, "Wealth Grows."
97. Park, "The Price of Blood."

5 Securitizing HIV/AIDS in China

1. "Around the World; China Says Argentine Died of AIDS," *New York Times*, July 30, 1985, accessed November 10, 2014, http://www.nytimes.

com/1985/07/30/world/around-the-world-china-says-argentine-died-of-aids.html; Elena S. H. Yu et al., "HIV Infection and AIDS in China, 1985 through 1994," *American Journal of Public Health* 86, no. 8 (1996): 1116; Heather Xiao-quan Zhang, "The Gathering Storm: AIDS Policy in China." *Journal of International Development* 16, no. 8 (2004): 1156; Zun-you Wu et al., "Evolution of China's Response to HIV/AIDS," *The Lancet* 369, no. 9562 (2007): 679.
2. "China Epidemic: HIV and AIDS Estimate," *China AIDS Survey*, last modified August 7, 2007, http://www.aidsdatahub.org/files/documents/China_epidemic_HIV_and_AIDS_estimates.pdf.
3. "China Playing Its Part in World Anti-AIDS Battle," *Xinhua*, December 1, 1988, LexisNexis Newspapers.
4. "China Has No Sources for AIDS, Studies Show," *Xinhua*, January 22, 1988, LexisNexis Newspapers.
5. Jim Abrams, "China Discovers First AIDS Virus Carrier," *The Associated Press*, November 1, 1989, LexisNexis Newspapers.
6. "China Has No Sources."
7. Jon Cohen, "Changing Course to Break the HIV-Heroin Connection," *Science* 304, no. 5676 (2004): 1434; Zhang, "The Gathering Storm," 1156; Wu et al., "Evolution of China's Response," 679.
8. Zhi-min Liu, Zhi Lian, and Cheng-zheng Zhao, "Drug Use and HIV/AIDS in China," *Drug and Alcohol Review* 25, no. 2 (2006): 174; Yan Xiao et al., "Expansion of HIV/AIDS in China: Lessons from Yunnan Province," *Social Science & Medicine* 64, no. 3 (2007): 665.
9. Zhang, "The Gathering Storm," 1156; Wu et al., "Evolution of China's Response," 679.
10. Rajiv Chandra, "China: No Sex Please, We're Chinese!" *Inter Press Service*, September 17, 1993, LexisNexis Newspapers; "Ming Pao: Lack of Funds and Inadequate Publicity Hinder Control of AIDS," *BBC Summary of World Broadcasts*, June 11, 1994, LexisNexis Newspapers.
11. "China Reports 194 Infected by AIDS Virus," *Xinhua*, February 7, 1990, LexisNexis Newspapers.
12. Tian-xin Chu and Judith A. Levy, "Injection Drug Use and HIV/AIDS Transmission in China," *Cell Research* 15, nos. 11–12 (2005): 866.
13. Chris Beyrer, "An Epidemic of Denial: Stalled Responses to HIV/AIDS," *Harvard International Review* 25, no. 2 (2003): 64; Zhang, "The Gathering Storm," 1156; Kathleen Erwin, "The Circulatory System: Blood Procurement, AIDS, and the Social Body in China," *Medical Anthropology Quarterly* 20, no. 2 (2006): 140; Wu et al., "Evolution of China's Response," 679.
14. "2005 Update on the HIV/AIDS Epidemic and Response in China," *Ministry of Health, People's Republic of China & Joint United Nations Program on HIV/AIDS, World Health Organization*, last modified January 24, 2006, http://data.unaids.org/publications/External-Documents/rp_2005chinaestimation_25jan06_en.pdf.
15. Lei Sheng and Wu-kui Cao, "HIV/AIDS Epidemiology and Prevention in China," *Chinese Medical Journal* 121, no. 13 (2008): 1231.

16. Elisabeth Rosenthal, "In Rural China, a Steep Price of Poverty: Dying of AIDS," *New York Times*, October 28, 2000, accessed November 10, 2014, http://www.nytimes.com/2000/10/28/world/in-rural-china-a-steep-price-of-poverty-dying-of-aids.html; "Silent Plague: A Special Report; Deadly Shadow Darkens Remote Chinese Village," *New York Times*, May 28, 2001; accessed November 10, 2014, http://www.nytimes.com/2001/05/28/world/silent-plague-a-special-report-deadly-shadow-darkens-remote-chinese-village.html; "Silent Plague: AIDS Patients in China Lack Effective Treatment," *New York Times*, November 12, 2001, accessed November 10, 2014, http://www.nytimes.com/2001/11/12/international/asia/12AIDS.html; "AIDS Scourge in Rural China Leaves Villages of Orphans," *New York Times*, August 25, 2002, accessed November 10, 2014, http://www.nytimes.com/2002/08/25/world/aids-scourge-in-rural-china-leaves-villages-of-orphans.html.
17. 李宁, 王哲, 孙定勇 [Ning Li, Zhe Wang, and Ding-yong Sun,] 河南省艾滋病流行现状分析 ["Analysis of HIV/AIDS Epidemic in Henan Province,"] 医药论坛杂志 [*Journal of Medical Forum*] (2007年第28卷第19期) [28, no. 19 (2007)]: 23.
18. 张可 [Ke Zhang,] 既往有偿献血人员 HIV 感染者自然史分析 ["The Natural History of HIV Infection among Paid Blood Donors in Henan Province,"] 中国艾滋病性病 [*China Journal of AIDS and STD*] (2006年第12 卷第4 期) [12, no. 4 (2006)]: 292.
19. 李宁, 王哲, 孙定勇 [Li, Wang, and Sun,] 艾滋病分析 ["Analysis of HIV/AIDS,"] 23.
20. Calum MacLeod, "Bad Blood behind China's Crisis," *The Independent*, June 25, 2001, accessed November 10, 2014, http://www.independent.co.uk/life-style/health-and-families/health-news/bad-blood-behind-chinas-crisis-752731.html; "China Closes Blood Agencies to Curb AIDS," *China Daily*, March 28, 2005, accessed November 10, 2014, http://www.chinadaily.com.cn/english/doc/2005-03/28/content_428618.htm.
21. "China's HIV/AIDS-Infected Population Estimated at 780,000," *Xinhua*, November 29, 2011, accessed November 10, 2014, http://news.xinhuanet.com/english2010/china/2011-11/29/c_131277694.htm.
22. "Progress Made in HIV/AIDS Campaign," *NCAIDS, China CDC*, last modified November 25, 2011, http://www.chinaaids.cn/n1971/n2091/727369.html.
23. Shan Juan, "Gay Men Hit Hard by HIV/AIDS," *China Daily*, July 11, 2011, accessed November 10, 2014, http://www.chinadaily.com.cn/cndy/2011-07/11/content_12872203.htm.
24. "80-year-old Found with HIV by 'Unprotected Sex,'" *China Daily*, August 6, 2011, accessed November 10, 2014, http://www.chinadaily.com.cn/china/2011-08/06/content_13063132.htm.
25. "HIV/AIDS Cases Soar on College Campuses," *China Daily*, November 30, 2011, accessed November 10, 2014, http://www.chinadaily.com.cn/china/2011-11/30/content_14191608.htm.

26. Michael Martina, "China Says HIV/AIDS Cases Are Soaring," *Reuters*, November 30, 2011, accessed November 10, 2014, http://www.reuters.com/article/2011/11/30/us-china-aids-idUSTRE7AT1KC20111130.
27. "HIV/AIDS Cases Soar."
28. "Global Report—UNAIDS Report on the Global AIDS Epidemic 2013," *UNAID*, last modified September 2013, http://www.unaids.org/en/media/unaids/contentassets/documents/epidemiology/2013/gr2013/UNAIDS_Global_Report_2013_en.pdf.
29. "New HIV Rate in China Climbs Over 10% in First 10 Months of 2012," *International AIDS Society*, December 3, 2012, accessed January 31, 2015, https://www.iasociety.org/Default.aspx?pageId=5&elementId=14868.
30. "2014 China AIDS Response Progress Report," *National Health and Family Commission of the People's Republic of China*, June 2014, accessed January 31, 2015, http://www.unaids.org/sites/default/files/documents/CHN_narrative_report_2014.pdf.
31. "2014 China AIDS Response Progress Report."
32. "China Bars Import of Blood in an Effort to Prevent AIDS," *New York Times*, September 4, 1985, accessed November 10, 2014, http://www.nytimes.com/1985/09/04/world/china-bars-import-of-blood-in-an-effort-to-prevent-aids.html.
33. Donna Anderson, "Peking Daily Cautions against Western Threats of AIDS, Drugs," *The Associated Press*, February 4, 1987, LexisNexis Newspapers.
34. "China Makes Efforts to Prevent AIDS," *Xinhua*, September 27, 1987, LexisNexis Newspapers.
35. "AIDS Can Be Checked in China—Experts," *Xinhua*, July 22, 1987, LexisNexis Newspapers.
36. "Correction China Focuses on Women, Again Ignores Gays in AIDS Fight," *Deutsche Presse-Agentur*, July 12, 1996, LexisNexis Newspapers.
37. Han-zhu Qian et al., "Injection Drug Use and HIV/AIDS in China: Review of Current Situation, Prevention and Policy Implications," *Harm Reduction Journal* 3, no. 4 (2006): 4.
38. Qian et al., "Injection Drug Use," 4.
39. Qian et al., "Injection Drug Use," 4.
40. "China Epidemic: HIV and AIDS Estimate."
41. "China Bars Import of Blood."
42. "China Set Up National AIDS Committee," *Xinhua*, March 1, 1990, LexisNexis Newspapers.
43. "Frontier Health and Quarantine Law of the People's Republic of China," *China.org.cn*, accessed February 23, 2010, http://lanzhou.china.com.cn/english/travel/40418.htm.
44. Zhang, "The Gathering Storm," 1161.
45. Jie Shen and Dong-bao Yu, "Governmental Policies on HIV Infection in China," *Cell Research* 15, nos. 11–12 (2005): 903.
46. "China Issues Regulations on AIDS," *Xinhua*, January 14, 1988, LexisNexis Newspapers.

47. Shen and Yu, "Governmental Policies," 903.
48. Shen and Yu, "Governmental Policies," 903.
49. Wen-yuan Yin and Zun-you Wu, "Challenges and Opportunities: The Expanded Government-Led HIV/AIDS Programs in China," *Virologica Sinica* 22, no. 6 (2007): 495.
50. "HIV/AIDS: China's Titanic Peril," *UNAIDS/WHO*, last modified June 2002, http://www.hivpolicy.org/Library/HPP000056.pdf.
51. "China's Titanic Peril."
52. "The Paris Declaration," *Paris AIDS Summit*, last modified December 1, 1994. http://data.unaids.org/pub/externaldocument/2007/theparisdeclaration_en.pdf.
53. Yan Cui, Adrian Liau, and Zun-you Wu, "An Overview of the History of Epidemic of and Response to HIV/AIDS in China: Achievements and Challenges," *Chinese Medical Journal* 122, no. 19 (2009): 2253.
54. Exchange rate: 1 CNY equals to 0.156 USD, on September 15, 2011.
55. Cui, Liau, and Wu, "An Overview of the History," 2253.
56. Patricia K. Wajda, "AIDS," in *A Comparative Perspective on Major Social Problems*, ed. Rita J. Simon (Lanham, MD: Lexington Books, 2001), 228.
57. "China's Titanic Peril."
58. "China's Titanic Peril."
59. "China's Titanic Peril."
60. Zun-you Wu, Ke-ming Rou, and Hai-xia Cui, "The HIV/AIDS Epidemic in China: History, Current Strategies and Future Challenges," *AIDS Education and Prevention* 16, Supplementary A (2004): 13.
61. Shen and Yu, "Governmental Policies," 904.
62. Shen and Yu, "Governmental Policies," 904; Yin and Yu, "Challenges and Opportunities," 495.
63. "National Center for AIDS/STD Control and Prevention," *China Center for Disease Control*, accessed February 24, 2010, http://www.chinaids.org.cn/n443289/n443290/n447111/index.html.
64. "China—China's Once-Hidden HIV Fears Now Out in the Open," *ChinaOnline*, February 24, 2010, LexisNexis Newspapers.
65. J. Stephen Morrison, and Bates Gill, "Averting a Full-Blown HIV/AIDS Epidemic in China," *Center for Strategic and International Studies*, last modified February 2003, http://csis.org/files/media/csis/pubs/0302_avertepidemicchina.pdf.
66. "China's Titanic Peril."
67. Elisabeth Rosenthal, "Scientists Warn of Inaction as AIDS Spreads in China," *New York Times*, August 2, 2000, accessed November 10, 2014, http://www.nytimes.com/2000/08/02/world/scientists-warn-of-inaction-as-aids-spreads-in-china.html.
68. Ilavenil Ramiah, "Securitizing the AIDS Issue in Asia," in *Non-Traditional Security in Asia: Dilemmas in Securitization*, ed. Mely Caballero-Anthony, Ralf Emmers, and Amitav Acharya (England: Ashgate Publishing Limited, 2006a), 161.

69. China's President Jiang Zemin on January 7, 2000, in his reply to the President of the World Bank James Wolfensohn's call for action of Asian Government to halting the spread of HIV/AIDS. See "China's Titanic Peril."
70. Elisabeth Rosenthal, "Suddenly, AIDS Makes the News in China," *New York Times*, December 5, 2001, accessed November 10, 2014, http://www.nytimes.com/2001/12/05/world/suddenly-aids-makes-the-news-in-china.html.
71. "China to Act Sternly against Illegal Blood Deals," *People's Daily Online*, August 23, 2001, http://www.english.peopledaily.com.cn/english/200108/23/eng20010823_78118.html.
72. "A Joint Assessment of HIV/AIDS Prevention, Treatment and Care in China (2003)," *Ministry of Health & UN Theme Group on HIV/AIDS in China*, last modified December 1, 2003, http://data.unaids.org/UNA-docs/china_joint_assessment_2003_en.pdf.
73. "A Joint Assessment of HIV/AIDS Prevention, Treatment and Care in China (2004)," *State Council AIDS Working Committee Office & UN Theme Group on HIV/AIDS in China*, last modified December 1, 2004, http://www.chinaids.org.cn/worknet/download/2004/report2004en.pdf.
74. Bin Xue, "HIV/AIDS Policy and Policy Evolution in China," *International Journal of STD & AIDS* 16, no. 7 (2005): 460.
75. Xiu-lan Zhang, Pierre Miège, and Yu-rong Zhang, "Decentralization of the Provision of Health Services to People Living with HIV/AIDS in Rural China: The Case of Three Counties," *Health Research Policy and Systems* 9, no. 9 (2011): 2.
76. "Speech by Executive Vice Minister of Health, Mr. Gao Qiang, at the HIV/AIDS High-Level Meeting of the UN General Assembly," *Permanent Mission of the People's Republic of China to the UN*, last modified September 22, 2003, http://www.china-un.org/eng/lhghyywj/ldhy/previousga/58/t28511.htm.
77. "Speech by Executive Vice Minister of Health."
78. "Speech by Executive Vice Minister of Health."
79. "A Joint Assessment (2004)."
80. Meng-jie Han et al., "Design and Implementation of a China Comprehensive AIDS Response Program (China CARES), 2003–08," *International Journal of Epidemiology* 39, Supplementary 2 (2010): 48; Feng Zhou et al., "Expenditure for the Care of HIV-Infected Patients in Rural Areas in China's Antiretroviral Therapy Programs," *BMC Medicine* 9, no. 6 (2011): 1. The main activities of China CARES include: (1) strengthening HIV/AIDS surveillance; (2) distributing comprehensive HIV/AIDS prevention activities such IEC; free VCT; condom use promotion, STD diagnosis and treatment; needle exchange and MMT; PMTCT; (3) providing HIV care and treatment such as ARV treatment, care, and support to people living with HIV/AIDS and free schooling for children orphaned by HIV/AIDS; and also (4) ensuring the safety of the blood supply.
81. Han et al., "Design and Implementation," 47.
82. Han et al., "Design and Implementation," 54.

83. "A Joint Assessment (2004)" ; Han et al., "Design and Implementation," 51.
84. Yun-zhen Cao and Hong-zhou Lu, "Care of HIV-Infected Patients in China," *Cell Research* 15, nos. 11–12 (2005): 885.
85. Fu-jie Zhang et al., "The Chinese Free Antiretroviral Treatment Program: Challenges and Responses," *AIDS* 21, Supplementary 8 (2007): 143.
86. 张福杰 [Fu-jie Zhang et al.,] 艾滋病的抗病毒治疗 与我国的免费 治 疗现状 ["Antiretroviral Therapy for HIV/AIDS and Current Situation of China Free ARV Program,"] 科技1717 [*Science & Technology Review*] (2005年第23卷第7期) [23, no. 7 (2005)]: 25.
87. "State Council Notice on Strengthening HIV/AIDS Prevention and Control," NCAIDS, China CDC, last modified March 16, 2004, http://www.chinaaids.cn/n1971/n2301/n8034/32205.html.
88. 国务院关于进一步加强艾滋病防治工作的通知 ["State Council Notice on Further Strengthening HIV/AIDS Prevention and Control,"] 国发48号 *[State Council Document No. 48,]* (二〇一〇年十二月三十一日) [last modified December 31, 2010,] http://www.gov.cn/zwgk/2011-02/16/content_1804536.htm.
89. "2012 China AIDS Response Progress Report," *Ministry of Health of the People's Republic of China*, last modified March 31, 2012, http://www.unaids.org/en/dataanalysis/monitoringcountryprogress/progressreports/2012countries/ce_CN_Narrative_Report[1].pdf.
90. "Progress Made in HIV/AIDS Campaign."
91. "A Joint Assessment of HIV/AIDS Prevention, Treatment and Care in China (2007)," *State Council AIDS Working Committee Office & UN Theme Group on AIDS in China*, last modified December 1, 2007, http://www.undp.org.cn/downloads/otherlocal/HIV/20080104.pdf; "2011 Estimate for the HIV/AIDS Epidemic in China," *Ministry of Health, Joint United Nations Program on HIV/AIDS, World Health Organization*, last modified November 2010, http://www.chinaids.org.cn/n1971/n2151/n777994.files/n777993.pdf.
92. Yin and Yu, "Challenges and Opportunities," 494.
93. "A Joint Assessment (2004)."
94. "Four Free" refers to (1) free ARV drugs to HIV/AIDS patients who are rural residents or people with financial difficulties living in urban areas; (2) free voluntary counseling and HIV/AIDS screening testing; (3) free drugs to HIV-infected pregnant women to prevent mother-to-child transmission, and HIV/AIDS testing of newborn babies; and (4) free schooling for children orphaned by HIV/AIDS; meanwhile, "One Care" refers to care and financial assistance to the households of people living with HIV/AIDS.
95. Harm reduction includes: (1) information and education, including safe sex education and condom distribution; (2) treatment and substitution programs; (3) outreach and peer-education; (4) increasing access to sterile injecting equipment and safe disposal; and (5) voluntary counseling and testing for HIV.
96. Sheena G. Sullivan and Zun-you Wu, "Rapid Scale Up of Harm Reduction in China," *International Journal of Drug Policy* 18, no. 2 (2007): 121.
97. "China Amends Disease Law, Bans Blood Trade," *People's Daily Online*, August 30, 2004, accessed May 5, 2012, http://english.peopledaily.com.cn/200408/30/eng20040830_155306.html.

98. "China Beefs Up Prevention and Control of Contagious Disease," *People's Daily Online*, August 28, 2004, accessed January 4, 2010, http://www.nytimes.com/1985/09/04/world/china-bars-import-of-blood-in-an-effort-to-prevent-aids.html.
99. "China's Lawmakers Mull Enacting Law for AIDS Prevention, Control," *People's Daily Online*, June 22, 2004, accessed February 25, 2010, http://english.peopledaily.com.cn/200406/22/eng20040622_147216.html.
100. "China's Lawmakers."
101. "Law Spreads the Load in AIDS Battle; NPC Hands Local Governments Responsibility for Fighting Disease, Including Policing Blood Sales, *South China Morning Post*, August 29, 2004, LexisNexis Newspapers.
102. "China Puts Independent Clause of AIDS Prevention into Law," *People's Daily Online*, August 25, 2004, accessed February 25, 2010, http://english.peopledaily.com.cn/200408/25/eng20040825_154760.html.
103. "Independent Clause."
104. "China Lifts Travel Restrictions for HIV Carriers," *BBC News*, April 28, 2010, accessed June 24, 2011, http://news.bbc.co.uk/2/hi/8647592.stm.
105. "Premier Wen Vows More Aid to AIDS Patients," *NCAIDS, China CDC*, last modified December 1, 2011, http://www.chinaaids.cn/n1971/n2091/729286.html.
106. "Progress Made in HIV/AIDS Campaign."
107. 国务院通知 ["State Council Notice."]
108. Interview with a government official of the Ministry of Health [R37], Beijing, May 2011.
109. "President Hu Tells HIV Carriers, Communities Not to Be Daunted by Disease," *People's Daily Online*, December 1, 2007, accessed March 12, 2012, http://english.peopledaily.com.cn/90001/90782/90880/6312983.html.
110. "President Hu."
111. Interview with a project manager of an INGO [R8], Beijing, January 2011.
112. Interview with a national director of an INGO [R7], Beijing, January 2011.
113. Philip P. Pan, "China Meets AIDS Crisis with Force; Police, Not Physicians, Answer Villagers' Pleas," *The Washington Post*, August 18, 2003, LexisNexis Newspapers.
114. Pan, "China Meets AIDS."
115. Lai-ha Chan, Pak K. Lee, and Gerald Chan, "China Engages Global Health Governance: Processes and Dilemmas," *Global Public Health* 4, no. 1 (2009): 8.
116. Pan, "China Meets AIDS."
117. Interview with the chairperson of a local NGO [R31], Shanghai, May 2011.
118. Interview with Dr. Qao Qi, the Chinese University of Hong Kong, Hong Kong, January 2011.
119. Maureen Fan, "Provinces Undermines Beijing's Goals on AIDS," *The Washington Post*, September 19, 2007, accessed January 8, 2010, http://www.washingtonpost.com/wp-dyn/content/article/2007/09/18/AR2007091802083.html; "AIDS Blood Scandals: What China Can Learn from the World's Mistakes," *Asia Catalyst*, last modified September 2007, http://www.asiacatalyst.org/news/AIDS_blood_scandals_rpt_0907.pdf.

120. "An Alleyway in Hell: China's Abusive Black Jails," *Human Rights Watch*, last modified November 2009, http://www.hrw.org/sites/default/files/reports/china1109web_1.pdf.
121. "An Alleyway in Hell."
122. "China: House Arrests Stifle HIV/AIDS Petitions," *Human Rights Watch*, last modified March 12, 2006, http://www.hrw.org/en/news/2006/03/10/china-house-arrests-stifle-hivaids-petitions.
123. "China: Secret 'Black Jails' Hide Severe Rights Abuses," *Human Rights Watch*, last modified November 11, 2009, http://www.hrw.org/en/news/2009/11/02/china-secret-black-jails-hide-severe-rights-abuses.
124. Chris Buckley, "Exclusive—Secret Chinese Jail Makes Silencing Protest a Business," *Reuters*, September 11, 2007, accessed January 8, 2010, http://in.reuters.com/article/worldNews/idINIndia-29454320070911?pageNumber=2&virtualBrandChannel=0.
125. Keith Alcorn, "Chinese HIV Prevention with Drug Users Undermined by Police," *Aidsmap*, last modified December 11, 2008, http://www.aidsmap.com/Chinese-HIV-prevention-with-drug-users-undermined-by-police/page/1432754/.
126. "Restrictions on AIDS NGOs in Asia," *Asia Catalysts*, last modified December 1, 2009, http://www.asiacatalyst.org/news/restrictionsAIDSngos1209.pdf.
127. Chris Hogg, "State Media Praises Shanghai Gays," *BBC News*, June 10, 2009, accessed November 10, 2014, http://news.bbc.co.uk/2/hi/asia-pacific/8092516.stm.
128. Yan-feng Qian and Hong-yi Wang, "Gay Party Starts to Lose Its Sparkle," *China Daily*, June 12, 2009, accessed January 26, 2012, http://www.chinadaily.com.cn/china/2009-06/12/content_8275477.htm.
129. Christine Laskowski, "Inaugural Gay Pageant Order to Shut Down," *China Daily*, January 16, 2010, accessed November 10, 2014, http://www.chinadaily.com.cn/china/2010-01/16/content_9330189.htm.
130. Andrew Jacobs, "Police Raid Shanghai Gay Bar and Detain More than 60," *New York Times*, April 4, 2011, accessed November 10, 2014, http://www.nytimes.com/2011/04/05/world/asia/05shanghai.html?_r=0.
131. Melissa G. Curley, "Levels of Analysis Issues in the Migration—Security Nexus," in *Security and Migration: The Dynamics of Securitization*, ed. Melissa G. Curley and Siu-lun Wong (London: Routledge, 2008), 28–29.
132. Curley, "Levels of Analysis," 29.
133. John Balzano and Ping Jia, "Coming Out of Denial: An Analysis of AIDS Law and Policy in China (1987–2006)," *Loyola University Chicago International Law Review* 3, no. 2 (2005–2006): 194.
134. Kenneth Lieberthal and Michel Oksenberg, *Policy Making in China: Leaders, Structures, and Processes* (Princeton: Princeton University Press, 1988), 401.
135. "State Council Notice."

6 Audience Acceptance in China: Case Studies in Beijing, Shanghai, and Kunming

1. 国务院关于进一步加强艾滋病防治工作的通知 ["State Council Notice on Further Strengthening HIV/AIDS Prevention and Control,"] 国发48号 [*State Council Document No. 48,*] (二〇一〇年十二月三十一日) [last modified December 31, 2010,] http://www.gov.cn/zwgk/2011-02/16/content_1804536.htm.
2. Fieldworks in China were conducted in January and May 2011.
3. Michael C. Williams, "The Continuing Evolution of Securitization Theory," in *Securitization Theory: How Security Problems Emerge and Dissolve*, ed. Thierry Balzacq (London: Routledge, 2011), 215.
4. "Around the World; China Says Argentine Died of AIDS," *New York Times*, July 30, 1985, accessed November 10, 2014, http://www.nytimes.com/1985/07/30/world/around-the-world-china-says-argentine-died-of-aids.html.
5. "Over 70% of the HIV Infected in Beijing are Immigrants; Lower Criteria for Eligibility to MMT to be Piloted," *NCAIDS, China CDC*, last modified June 22, 2010, http://www.chinaids.org.cn/n1971/n2091/439308.html.
6. "Over 70%."
7. "New HIV/AIDS Cases Rise Over 50% in Beijing," *China Daily*, November 21, 2007, accessed November 10, 2014, http://www.chinadaily.com.cn/china/2012-11/29/content_15973852.htm.
8. "New HIV/AIDS Cases Surge in Beijing," *China Daily*, July 10, 2009, accessed November 10, 2014, http://www.chinadaily.com.cn/cndy/2009-07/10/content_8405065.htm.
9. Interview with a program officer of an NGO [R3], Beijing, January 2011.
10. Interview with an officer of the UNAIDS China Office [R1], Beijing, January 2011; Interview with an officer of a grassroots NGO [R6], Beijing, January 2011; Interview with a Program Coordinator of an INGO [R12], Beijing, January 2011.
11. 12 out of 16 participants in Beijing who have answered this question believed that HIV/AIDS is the most serious public health problem in the eyes of the government.
12. Interview with a country program manager of an INGO [R5], Beijing, January 2011.
13. Interview with a program officer of an NGO [R3], Beijing, January 2011.
14. Interview with a program development director of an INGO [R9], Beijing, January 2011.
15. 11 out of 16 interviewees believed that HIV/AIDS is a top/high priority issue on the government agenda.
16. Interview with a project manager of an INGO [R8], Beijing, January 2011.
17. Interview with a program development director of an INGO [R9], Beijing, January 2011.

18. "Shanghai Brings AIDS Prevention Under Legal Framework," *Xinhua*, March 1, 1999, LexisNexis Newspapers.
19. Edmund Settle, "AIDS in China: An Annotated Chronology 1985–2003," *China AIDS Survey*, last modified November 14, 2003, http://portal.unesco.org/education/en/file_download.php/82b973698fcdf215528d63d2b6796087AIDSchron_111603.pdf.
20. Fei-ran Lu, "AIDS on Increase in Shanghai," *People's Daily Online*, November 29, 2010, accessed November 10, 2014, http://english.people.com.cn/90882/7659183.html.
21. Wen-jun Cai, "Free Condoms Join AIDS Fight," *Shanghai Daily*, July 28, 2010, accessed November 8, 2011, http://www.shanghaidaily.com/sp/article/2010/201007/20100728/article_444527.htm.
22. "Gay Men HIV Cases Quintuple in Shanghai," *China Daily*, June 20, 2009, accessed November 10, 2014, http://www.chinadaily.com.cn/world/samesex/2009-06/20/content_8323083.htm.
23. "Shanghai Sees More HIV/AIDS Cases among Men Who Have Sex with Men," *Xinhua*, June 19, 2009, accessed November 10, 2014, http://news.xinhuanet.com/english/2009-06/19/content_11566218.htm.
24. Cai, "Free Condoms."
25. "Growing Tolerance Towards Homosexuals in China," *People's Daily Online*, December 10, 2004, accessed November 10, 2014, http://english.peopledaily.com.cn/200412/10/eng20041210_166876.html.
26. Yu-ji Feng, Zun-you Wu, and Roger Detels, "Evolution of Men Who Have Sex with Men Community and Experienced Stigma among Men Who Have Sex with Men in Chengdu, China," *Journal of Acquired Immune Deficiency Syndromes* 53, Supplementary 1 (2010): 98.
27. Peter Ellingsen, "Shanghai's Gays Slowly Make Their Way Out of the Closet; China," *Sydney Morning Herald*, March 10, 1989, LexisNexis Newspapers.
28. Seth Faison, "China's Gays Venture Out of the Closet at Last," *The Guardian*, September 6, 1997, LexisNexis Newspapers.
29. Kyung-hee Choi et al., "The Influence of Social and Sexual Networks in the Spread of HIV and Syphilis among Men Who Have Sex with Men in Shanghai, China," *Journal of Acquired Immune Deficiency Syndromes* 45, no. 1 (2007): 84; T. S. K. Kong, "Risk Factors Affecting Condom Use among Male Sex Workers Who Serve Men in China: A Qualitative Study," *Sexually Transmitted Infections* 84, no. 6 (2008): 444.
30. Jenny X. Liu and Kyung Choi, "Experiences of Social Discrimination among Men Who Have Sex with Men in Shanghai, China," *AIDS and Behavior* 10, Supplementary 1 (2006): 26.
31. Five out of five respondents have stated that HIV/AIDS prevalence among MSM will be increased in Shanghai in the future.
32. Two out of four respondents in Shanghai believed that HIV/AIDS is the most serious problem in the eyes of the Chinese government.
33. Interview with a leader of a local NGO [R31], Shanghai, May 2011.
34. Interview with Tony Zheng, Chairperson of Shanghai CSW & MSM Center, Shanghai, May 2011.

35. Interview with a leader of a local NGO [R31], Shanghai, May 2011.
36. Zhi-min Liu, Zhi Lian, and Cheng-zheng Zhao, "Drug Use and HIV/AIDS in China," *Drug and Alcohol Review* 25, no. 2 (2006): 174; Yan Xiao et al., "Expansion of HIV/AIDS in China: Lessons from Yunnan Province," *Social Science & Medicine* 64, no. 3 (2007): 665.
37. Xiao et al., "Expansion of HIV/AIDS," 666.
38. Xi-wen Zheng et al., "Injecting Drug Use and HIV Infection in Southwest China," *AIDS* 8, no. 8 (1994): 1141.
39. Xiao et al., "Expansion of HIV/AIDS," 666.
40. Man-hong Jia et al., "The HIV Epidemic in Yunnan Province, China, 1989–2007," *Journal of Acquired Immune Deficiency Syndromes* 53, Supplementary 1 (2010): 34.
41. Theodore M. Hammett et al., "Patterns of HIV Prevalence and HIV Risk Behaviors among Injection Drug Users Prior to and 24 Months Following Implementation of Cross-Border HIV Prevention Interventions in Northern Vietnam and Southern China," *AIDS Education and Prevention* 18, no. 2 (2006): 98; Zhi Hu et al., "Epidemiological Characteristics of HIV/AIDS in West China," *International Journal of STD & AIDS* 17, no. 5 (2006): 326; Liu et al., "Drug Use and HIV/AIDS in China," 174.
42. "HIV Infections Exceed 90,000 in SW China's Yunnan," *People's Daily Online*, November 30, 2011, accessed November 13, 2014, http://english.peopledaily.com.cn/90882/7662239.html.
43. Jia et al., "The HIV Epidemic," 38.
44. Chris Beyrer et al., "Overland Heroin Trafficking Routes and HIV-1 Spread in South and South-East Asia," *AIDS* 14, no. 1 (2000): 78; Tian-xin Chu and Judith A. Levy, "Injection Drug Use and HIV/AIDS Transmission in China," *Cell Research* 15, nos. 11–12 (2005): 865.
45. Beyrer et al., "Overland Heroin," 80.
46. "Heroin Movement Worldwide—Southeast Asia," *Central Intelligence Agency*, last modified December 12, 2008, https://www.cia.gov/library/publications/additional-publications/heroin-movement-worldwide/southeast-asia.html.
47. Nicolas Bacaër, Xamxinur Abdurahman, and Jian-li Ye, "Modeling the HIV/AIDS Epidemic among Injecting Drug Users and Sex Workers in Kunming, China," *Bulletin of Mathematical Biology* 68, no. 3 (2006): 527.
48. 昆明累计报告艾滋病1.5万余例 ["The Cumulative Reported Number of HIV/AIDS in Kunming is above 15,000,"] 云南网 [*Yunnan Wang,*] [last modified December 2, 2010,] http://special.yunnan.cn/feature3/html/2010-12/02/content_1427519.htm.
49. "Kunming HIV/AIDS Prevention and Control Working Report," *Kunming CDC*, last modified October 2010, http://www.info.gov.hk/aids/rrc/english/lions_rep/ppt10_08.pdf.
50. Interview with a HIV/AIDS consultant [R26], Kunming, May 2011.
51. Interview with a program officer of an INGO [R28], Kunming, May 2011.
52. Interview with an officer of an INGO [R20], Kunming, May 2011.

53. Six out of ten participants in Kunming who have responded to this question believed that HIV/AIDS is the most serious public health problem in the eyes of the government.
54. Interview with an officer working in an INGO [R24], Kunming, May 2011.
55. Interview with an officer of an INGO [R20], Kunming, May 2011.
56. Interview with Dr. Zhang Kai-ning, director of Yunnan Health and Development Research Association, Kunming, May 2011.
57. Six out of ten interviewees believed that HIV/AIDS is a top/high priority issue on the government agenda.
58. Interview with Dr. Zhang Kai-ning, director of Yunnan Health and Development Research Association, Kunming, May 2011.
59. Interview with the vice director of a drug treatment center [R22], Kunming, May 2011.
60. Arni S. R. Srinivasa Rao et al., "HIV/AIDS Epidemic in India and Predicting the Impact of the National Response: Mathematical Modeling and Analysis," *Mathematical Biosciences and Engineering* 6, no. 4 (2009): 781.
61. Nine out of 16 respondents in Beijing and three out of four respondents in Shanghai stated that HIV/AIDS is the most serious public health problem in China
62. Interview with a program coordinator of a grassroots NGO [R6], Beijing, January 2011.
63. Interview with a country program manager of an INGO [R5], Beijing, January 2011.
64. One out of 16 respondents in Beijing and one out of four respondents in Shanghai stated that HIV/AIDS is not a serious problem in China.
65. Six out of 16 respondents in Beijing and 0 out of four respondents in Shanghai stated that HIV/AIDS is only one of the most serious public health problems in China.
66. Interview with the director of a national NGO [R35], Beijing, May 2011.
67. Interview with a leader of a local NGO [R31], Shanghai, May 2011.
68. Interview with an HIV/AIDS consultant [R26], Kunming, May 2011.
69. Three out of ten respondents in Kunming stated that HIV/AIDS is the most serious public health problem in China.
70. Interview with the vice director of a drug treatment center [R22], Kunming, May 2011.
71. Interview with an officer of an INGO [R24], Kunming, May 2011.
72. Interview with a project officer of a national NGO [R25], Kunming, May 2011.
73. Interview with an officer of an INGO [R24], Kunming, May 2011.
74. Nine out of 16 respondents in Beijing recognized the NGOs' involvement in national HIV/AIDS programs.
75. Three out of four respondents in Shanghai recognized the NGOs' involvement in national HIV/AIDS programs.
76. Six out of ten respondents in Kunming mentioned that NGOs' involvement in national HIV/AIDS programs.

NOTES 215

77. Interview with the founder of an HIV/AIDS-related self-help group [R29], Shanghai, May 2011.
78. Interview with an officer of an INGO [R24], Kunming, May 2011.
79. Interview with an HIV/AIDS consultant [R26], Kunming, May 2011.
80. Interview with an officer of an INGO [R20], Kunming, May 2011.
81. Interview with an officer of a grassroots NGO [R21], Kunming, May 2011.
82. Interview with a program officer of an NGO [R3], Beijing, January 2011.
83. Interview with a project manager of an INGO [R8], Beijing, January 2011.
84. Interview with a chairperson of a grassroots NGO [R13], Beijing, January 2011.
85. Interview with a country program manager of an INGO [R5], Beijing, January 2011.
86. Interview with a program coordinator of a grassroots NGO [R6], Beijing, January 2011.
87. "500 Million Suspected to Carry Tuberculosis Virus," *People's Daily Online*, March 23, 2011, accessed November 10, 2014, http://english.people.com.cn/90001/90776/90882/7329035.html?amp.
88. "China's HIV/AIDS-Infected Population Estimated at 780,000," *Xinhua*, November 29, 2011, accessed November 10, 2014, http://news.xinhuanet.com/english2010/china/2011-11/29/c_131277694.htm.
89. "500 Million."
90. Three out of 16 respondents in Beijing and 1 out of 10 respondents in Kunming believed that TB is more serious than HIV/AIDS.
91. Interview with a country program manager of an INGO [R5], Beijing, January 2011.
92. Interview with an officer of an INGO [R20], Kunming, May 2011.
93. Three out of 16 respondents in Beijing and three out of four respondents in Shanghai believed that HIV/AIDS is the most serious problem among three.
94. Interview with a project manager of an INGO [R8], Beijing, January 2011.
95. Interview with an HIV/AIDS consultant [R26], Kunming, May 2011.
96. Interview with the director of a national NGO [R35], Beijing, May 2011.
97. Interview with an officer of the UNAIDS China Office [R1], Beijing, January 2011.
98. Interview with the department head of an INGO [R19], Kunming, May 2011.
99. Interview with a project manager of an INGO [R8], Beijing, January 2011.
100. Interview with Tony Zheng, chairperson of Shanghai CSW & MSM Center, Shanghai, May 2011.
101. Interview with a program coordinator of an INGO [R12], Beijing, January 2011.
102. Five out of 16 respondents in Beijing believed that HIV/AIDS-TB coinfection is the most serious problem in China.
103. Interview with Lin Oi-chu, chief executive of Hong Kong AIDS Foundation, Hong Kong, February 2011.

104. Lei Gao et al., "HIV/TB Co-infection in Mainland China: A Meta-Analysis," *PLoS ONE* 5, no. 5 (2010): 3–4.
105. Interview with a program coordinator of a grassroots NGO [R6], Beijing, January 2011; interview with a country program manager of an INGO [R5], Beijing, January 2011.
106. 18 out of 30 of the respondents in this study believe that HIV/AIDS-related NGOs have been involved by the national government.
107. Drew Thompson, and Xiao-qing Lu, "China's Evolving Civil Society: From Environment to Health," *Woodrow Wilson International Center for Scholars*, accessed February 15, 2012, http://208elmp02.blackmesh.com/sites/default/files/CEF_Feature.2.pdf.
108. Thompson and Lu, "China's Evolving."
109. "A Joint Assessment of HIV/AIDS Prevention, Treatment and Care in China (2004)," *State Council AIDS Working Committee Office & UN Theme Group on HIV/AIDS in China*, last modified December 1, 2004, http://www.chinaids.org.cn/worknet/download/2004/report2004en.pdf.
110. "NGOs Play 'Outstanding' Role in Fighting against HIV/AIDS: Vice Health Minister," *People's Daily Online*, September 1, 2005, accessed November 10, 2014, http://english.people.com.cn/200509/01/eng20050901_205717.html.
111. "China Encourages NGO's Participation in Fighting against AIDS," *China.org.cn*, March 23, 2006, accessed November 10, 2014, http://www.china.org.cn/english/2006/Mar/162981.htm.
112. Gui-ying Wang, "Gao Qiang Set Requirements for Future Response to HIV/AIDS in China," *NCAIDS/China CDC*, accessed February 22, 2012, http://www.chinaaids.cn/n1971/n2091/111203.html.
113. Wang, "Gao Qiang."
114. Shan Juan, "Red Ribbon Forum Redoubles AIDS Fighting Bid," *China Daily*, July 6, 2010, accessed November 10, 2014, http://www.chinadaily.com.cn/china/2010-07/06/content_10067737.htm.
115. Bin Xue, "HIV/AIDS Policy and Policy Evolution in China," *International Journal of STD & AIDS* 16, no. 7 (2005): 462.
116. "Fight Will Go on Despite Grant Cut," *NCAIDS, China CDC*, last modified November 10, 2011, http://www.chinaaids.cn/n1971/n2091/721831.html.
117. "Grant Portfolio: China," *The Global Fund to Fight AIDS, Tuberculosis and Malaria*, last modified January 25, 2012, http://portfolio.theglobalfund.org/en/Country/Index/CHN.
118. "NGO Perspectives on the Global Fund," *International Council of AIDS Service Organizations*, last modified June 2004, http://www.hivpolicy.org/Library/HPP000321.pdf.
119. "China: 'At a Critical Stage,'" *International Federation for Human Rights*, last modified April 2005, http://www.fidh.org/IMG/pdf/cn413a.pdf.
120. "NGO Perspectives."
121. "Grant Portfolio: China."
122. Thompson and Lu, "China's Evolving."

123. 中国艾滋病传播途径以性病传播为主 ["Sex Becomes the Main Route of HIV/AIDS Transmission in China,"] *Docin.com.Inc,* accessed February 20, 2012, http://www.docin.com/p-236465268.html.
124. 中国艾滋病传播途径 ["HIV/AIDS Transmission in China."]
125. 2007 年国家艾滋病防治社会动员经费支持<目一览表 ["A Table Shows the Budget of HIV/AIDS Prevention and Treatment Supported through Social Mobilization Program in 2007,"] *Docin.com.Inc.,* accessed February 20, 2012, http://www.docin.com/p-262618485.html.
126. 2008 年国家艾滋病防治社会动员经费支持<目一览表 ["A Table Shows the Budget of HIV/AIDS Prevention and Treatment Supported through Social Mobilization Program in 2008,"] *Docin.com.Inc.,* accessed February 20, 2012, http://www.docin.com/p-31402759.html.
127. "China Global Fund Program Principle Recipient," *Chinese Center for Disease Control and Prevention,* accessed February 18, 2012, http://www.chinaglobalfund.org/en/090720/ff808081221b6499012296034cf900f1.html.
128. "National Program Office of China Global Fund AIDS Program (Round 6)," *National Center for AIDS/STD Control and Prevention, China CDC,* accessed December 19, 2011, http://www.chinaaids.cn/n443289/n443290/n447113/n447525/n457450/index.html.
129. "National Program (Round 6)."
130. Interview with Lin Oi-chu, chief executive of Hong Kong AIDS Foundation, Hong Kong, February 2011.
131. Interview with an officer of a national NGO [R25], Kunming, May 2011.
132. Yan-zhong Huang, "Asia Unbound: The Global Fund, China, and Civil Society," *Councils on Foreign Relations,* last modified June 1, 2011, http://blogs.cfr.org/asia/2011/06/01/the-global-fund-china-and-civil-society/.
133. "Global Fund Lifts China Grant Freeze," *The Body,* last modified August 24, 2011, http://www.thebody.com/content/63640/global-fund-lifts-china-grant-freeze.html.
134. "Fight Will Go on Despite Grant Cut."
135. Based on the Chinese official data, 304 out of 352 NGOs working on HIV/AIDS issues are grassroots NGOs.
136. Interview with an officer of a grassroots NGO [R21], Kunming, May 2011.
137. Interview with Tony Zheng, chairperson of Shanghai CSW & MSM Center, Shanghai, May 2011.
138. Interview with a program coordinator of a grassroots NGO [R6], Beijing, January 2011.
139. Interview with a program officer of an INGO [R2], Beijing, January 2011.
140. Ying Xu and Li-tao Zhao, "China's Rapidly Growing Non-Governmental Organizations," *EAI Background Brief No. 514,* last modified March 25, 2010, http://www.eai.nus.edu.sg/BB514.pdf.
141. Carolyn Hsu, "Beyond Civil Society: An Organizational Perspective on State-NGO Relations in the People's Republic of China," *Journal of Civil Society* 6, no. 3 (2010): 261-262; Hui Li et al., "From Spectators to Implementers: Civil Society Organizations Involved in AIDS Programs in China," *International Journal of Epidemiology* 39, Supplementary 2 (2010): 66.

142. Li et al., "From Spectators," 67.
143. Xu and Zhao, "China's Rapidly."
144. Thompson and Lu, "China's Evolving."
145. Interview with a program coordinator of a grassroots NGO [R6], Beijing, January 2011.
146. Tian-ran Xu, "Restructuring to Result in Less Red Tape for NGO's," *Global Times*, October 14, 2010, accessed October 9, 2011, http://china.globaltimes.cn/society/2010-10/581806.html.
147. Interview with a program coordinator of a grassroots NGO [R6], Beijing, January 2011.
148. Li et al., "From Spectators," 67.
149. Interview with the vice director of a drug treatment center [R22], Kunming, May 2011.
150. Xiao-hua Liu, "NGOs in China: An Overview," *International Community Foundation*, last modified September 2002, www.icfdn.org/publications/NGOsinChina-ICFWhitePaper.doc.
151. Juan, "Red Ribbon Forum."
152. J. T. F. Lau et al., "Public Health Challenges of the Emerging HIV Epidemic among Men Who Have Sex with Men in China," *Public Health* 125, no. 5 (2011): 263.
153. Thompson and Lu, "China's Evolving."
154. Sharon LaFraniere, "AIDS Funds Frozen for China in Grant Dispute," *New York Times*, May 20, 2011, accessed November 10, 2014, http://www.nytimes.com/2011/05/21/world/asia/21china.html?pagewanted=all&_r=0.
155. Li et al., "From Spectators," 67.
156. Li et al., "From Spectators," 68.
157. Melissa G. Curley, "The Role of Civil Society in East Asian Region Building," in *Advancing East Asian Regionalism*, ed. Melissa G. Curley and Nicholas Thomas (London: Routledge, 2007), 190.
158. Interview with a program coordinator of a grassroots NGO [R6], Beijing, January 2011.
159. LaFraniere, "AIDS Funds."
160. LaFraniere, "AIDS Funds."
161. Interview with a program officer of an INGO [R2], Beijing, January 2011.
162. Interview with a high-ranked government official [R33], Shanghai, May 2011.
163. "Global Fund."
164. Catherine Boone and Jake Batsell, "Politics and AIDS in Africa: Research Agendas in Political Science and International Relations," in *HIV/AIDS and the Threat to National and International Security*, ed. R. L. Ostergard (London: Palgrave Macmillan, 2007), 15.
165. Boone and Batsell, "Politics and AIDS," 14.
166. "China: Country Summary," *Human Rights Watch*, last modified January 2007, http://www.hrw.org/sites/default/files/related_material/china_0.pdf.
167. "China Bans AIDS Right Meeting, Group Says," *Reuters*, July 29, 2007, accessed February 29, 2012, http://www.reuters.com/article/2007/07/29/us-china-aids-idUSPEK26767220070729.

168. Pinar Bilgin, "Making Turkey's Transformation Possible: Claiming 'Security-Speak'—Not Desecuritization!," *Southeast European and Black Sea Studies* 7, no. 4 (2007): 560.
169. Tania Branigan, "HIV/AIDS Activist Fled China for US," *The Guardian*, May 10, 2010, accessed December 13, 2011, http://www.guardian.co.uk/world/2010/may/10/aids-activist-flees-china-america; Juliana Liu, "Exiled China AIDS Activist Mourns Her Former Life," *BBC News*, October 20, 2010, accessed December 13, 2011, http://www.bbc.co.uk/news/world-11446636.
170. Melissa G. Curley and Jonathan Herington, "The Securitization of Avian Influenza: International Discourses and Domestic Politics in Asia," *Review of International Studies* 37, no. 1 (2011): 164.
171. Thompson and Lu, "China's Evolving."
172. Bilgin, "Making Turkey's," 559.
173. Qiu-sha Ma, "Defining Chinese Nongovernmental Organizations," *Voluntas: International Journal of Voluntary and Nonprofit Organizations* 13, no. 2 (2002): 125.
174. Hsu, "Civil Society," 267.
175. Hsu, "Civil Society," 267.

7 Securitizing HIV/AIDS in India

1. Arvind Pandey et al., "Improved Estimates of India's HIV Burden in 2006," *Indian Journal of Medical Research* 129, no. 1 (2009): 52.
2. K. S. Jayaraman, "Pool of Infected Women?" *Nature* 321, no. 6066 (1986): 103.
3. "India Has Most HIV Cases, 20 Per Cent of Men Have Sexually Transmitted Diseases," *BBC Monitoring South Asia—Political*, September 3, 1999, LexisNexis Newspapers.
4. Jayati Ghosh, "A Geographical Perspective on HIV/AIDS in India," *Geographical Review* 92, no. 1 (2002): 115.
5. Andre Picard, "India 'Sitting on Top of Volcano' 100 Million at Risk, Health Experts Say," *The Globe and Mail*, July 1, 1998, LexisNexis Newspapers.
6. Sheena Asthana, "AIDS-Related Policies, Legislation and Program Implementation in India," *Health Policy and Planning* 11, no. 2 (1996): 185.
7. "Monitoring the UNGASS Goals of Sexual and Reproductive Health in the Context of HIV/AIDS: India Country Report," *The Cell for AIDS Research Action and Training, Tata Institute of Social Sciences, Mumbai, India*, last modified February 2008, http://ungassforum.files.wordpress.com/2008/02/ungass-india-report.pdf.
8. Akram A. Khan and Nazli Bano, "HIV/AIDS Epidemic in India: A Critical Health and Development Issue," in *Economics of Education and Health in India*, ed. Anil Kumar Thakur and Abdus Salam (New Delhi: The Indian Economic Association, 2008), 478.

9. "HIV Epidemic Reaches Advanced Stage in India," *Xinhua*, July 9, 1997, LexisNexis Newspapers; "AIDS Ballooning in India; Maharashtra Tops," *The Press Trust of India*, July 15, 2000, LexisNexis Newspapers.
10. Ghosh, "A Geographical Perspective," 116.
11. "Annual Report 2008–2009," *National AIDS Control Organization*, accessed February 8, 2010, https://www.nacoonline.org/upload/Publication/Annual_Report_NACO_2008–09.pdf.
12. Pandey et al., "Improved Estimates," 52.
13. Samir Lakhashe et al., "HIV Infection in India: Epidemiology, Molecular Epidemiology and Pathogenesis," *Journal of Biosciences* 33, no. 4 (2008): 516.
14. Lakhashe et al., "HIV Infection in India," 516.
15. "Monitoring the UNGASS Goals."
16. Shankar Raghuraman, "India to Lose 16m to AIDS by '26,'" *Times of India*, August 9, 2006, accessed April 26, 2012, http://articles.timesofindia.indiatimes.com/2006-08-09/india/27810016_1_aids-population-projections-death-rate.
17. "HIV & AIDS in India," *AVERT*, last modified October 1, 2014, http://www.avert.org/hiv-aids-india.htm.
18. "Annual Report 2010–2011," *National AIDS Control Organization*, last modified March 15, 2011, http"//aidsdatahub.org/dmdocuments/NACO_Annual_Report_2010_11.pdf.
19. "UNGASS Country Progress Report 2010: India," *National AIDS Control Organization*, last modified March 31, 2010, http://data.unaids.org/pub/Report/2010/india_2010_country_progress_report_en.pdf.
20. Thomas E. Rotnem and Tinaz Pavri, "The HIV/AIDS Pandemic in Comparative Perspective: The Cases of India and Russia" (paper presented at the Georgia Political Science Association, Conference Proceedings, 2006); William Stones and Saseendran Pallikadavath, "HIV and AIDS in India: Will the Next 20 Years Be Different?," *Harvard Health Policy Review* 7, no. 2 (2006): 115; Sonal R. Doshi and Bindi Gandhi, "Women in India: The Context and Impact of HIV/AIDS," *Journal of Human Behavior in the Social Environment* 17, nos. 3–4 (2008): 423; Arni S. R. Srinivasa Rao et al., "HIV/AIDS Epidemic in India and Predicting the Impact of the National Response: Mathematical Modeling and Analysis," *Mathematical Biosciences and Engineering* 6, no. 4 (2009): 781; "UNAIDS Outlook Report 2010," *UNAIDS*, last modified July 2010, http://data.unaids.org/pub/Outlook/2010/20100713_outlook_report_web_en.pdf.
21. Interview with S. Samraj, executive director of Christian AIDS National Alliance, New Delhi, March 2011.
22. Interview with Gopal Mukherjee, program manager of Family Health International, March 2011.
23. Arvind Singhal, and Everett M. Rogers, *Combating AIDS: Communication Strategies in Action* (India: Sage Publications, 2003), 115; Doshi and Gandhi, "Women in India," 425; Khan and Bano, "HIV/AIDS Epidemic in India," 478.

24. M. Llewellyn, "India's Denial of Death; The Cutting Edge: AIDS in India—The New Untouchables on SBS at 8.30 pm," *Sydney Morning Herald*, October 10, 1994, LexisNexis Newspapers.
25. Mark Fineman, "Superstition, Poverty May Bring AIDS Crisis in India," *Los Angeles Times*, May 28, 1990, accessed November 10, 2014, http://articles.latimes.com/1990-05-28/news/mn-51_1_aids-crisis.
26. "India: AIDS Spreading in Kerala, Punjab," *Inter-Press Service*, March 20, 1992, LexisNexis Newspapers.
27. Daniel Malini, "AIDS in India: Denial and Disaster," *Harvard International Review* 25, no. 2 (2003): 9; Pramit Mitra, "India at the Crossroads: Battling the HIV/AIDS Pandemic," *The Washington Quarterly* 27, no. 4 (2004): 98.
28. "AIDS Screen for All Foreigners, Almost," *The Statement*, May 17, 2002, LexisNexis Newspapers.
29. "Foreigners in India to Undergo AIDS Test," *Xinhua*, April 28, 1988, LexisNexis Newspapers.
30. Philippa Hawker, "Time Running Out for India's AIDS Response," *The Age*, October 11, 1994, LexisNexis Newspapers.
31. Asthana, "AIDS-Related Policies," 187.
32. Khan and Bano, "HIV/AIDS Epidemic in India," 485.
33. Stones and Pallikadavath, "HIV and AIDS in India," 117.
34. "Indians Urged to Be Involved in AIDS Awareness Activities," *Xinhua*, December 1, 1997, LexisNexis Newspapers.
35. "Annual Report 2010–2011."
36. "Annual Report 2010–2011."
37. Interview with S. Samraj, executive director of Christian AIDS National Alliance, New Delhi, March 2011.
38. Jayaraman, "Pool of Infected Women?," 103.
39. Sanjay A. Pai, "Agencies Disagree on AIDS Deaths Rates for India," *The Lancet Infectious Diseases* 2, no. 4 (2002): 199.
40. Padma Chandrasekaran et al., "Containing HIV/AIDS in India: The Unfinished Agenda," *The Lancet Infectious Diseases* 6, no. 8 (2006): 513.
41. Interview with a government official working in an HIV/AIDS-related department [R47], New Delhi, March 2011.
42. At the conversion rate of Rs. 45.6 to US$ 1.
43. "Project Performance Assessment Report," *The World Bank*, last modified July 2, 2003, http://lnweb90.worldbank.org/OED/oeddoclib.nsf/DocUNIDViewForJavaSearch/CF5907844F56853D85256D900073CB1D/$file/India_PPAR_26224.pdf.
44. "The National AIDS Control Program."
45. "The National AIDS Control Program."
46. "'Controversial' Bill on Disclosure of AIDS Sufferers Withdrawn," *BBC Summary of World Broadcasts*, December 7, 1991, LexisNexis Newspapers.
47. Khan and Bano, "HIV/AIDS Epidemic in India," 478.
48. G. P. Kumar, "New Plan to Check Spread of HIV in Manipur," *The Hindu*, November 16, 1998), LexisNexis Newspapers.

49. "India: 250 AIDS Patients Detected in a Single District," *Inter Press Service*, January 9, 1992, LexisNexis Newspapers.
50. "Address by the Prime Minister Stri Atal Bihari Vajpayee at the Meeting on National Program for Prevention and Control of HIV/AIDS New Delhi," *Embassy of India*, last modified December 12, 1998, http://www.indianembassy.org/policy/AIDS/prime_minister_AIDS.html.
51. "Indian Premier Seeks Cooperation of Industrial Houses to Contain AIDS," *BBC Monitoring South Asia—Political*, December 1, 2000, LexisNexis Newspapers.
52. "National AIDS Prevention and Control Policy," *National AIDS Control Organization*, last modified April 15, 2003, http://www.hsph.harvard.edu/population/aids/india.aids.02.pdf.
53. "Prime Minister's Speech at the 58th UN General Assembly," *Embassy of India*, last modified September 25, 2003, http://www.indianembassy.org/pic/pm/vajpayee/pm_sept_25_03.htm.
54. Mead Over et al., *HIV/AIDS Treatment and Prevention in India: Modeling the Cost and Consequences* (Washington, DC: The World Bank, 2004), 17.
55. "World Bank to Give India 191M US Dollars for AIDS Control," *BBC Monitoring South Asia—Political*, September 15, 1999, LexisNexis Newspapers.
56. "Government Fears Slowdown in Anti-HIV Drive," *The Statement*, September 2, 1999, LexisNexis Newspapers.
57. "Swaraj," *The Press Trust of India*, December 1, 2003, LexisNexis Newspapers.
58. "India to Provide AIDS Medicines in Government Hospitals," *BBC Summary of World Broadcasts*, November 30, 2003, LexisNexis Newspapers.
59. "Indian Government to Give HIV-Positive Children Free Drugs," *Deutsche Presse-Agentur*, October 5, 2003, LexisNexis Newspapers.
60. Dinesh C. Sharma, "India's Free Antiretroviral Program Gets Off to Slow Start," *The Lancet* 363, no. 9416 (2004): 1205.
61. "Project Performance Assessment Report."
62. "Indian Minister: Put Health on Agenda," *Associated Press Online*, July 27, 2003, LexisNexis Newspapers.
63. Rajesh Mahapatra, "India Rejects U.S. Government Warning on Spread of HIV/AIDS," *Associated Press Worldstream*, November 8, 2002, LexisNexis Newspapers.
64. Luke Harding, "India Rebuffs Bill Gates in AIDS Row," *The Guardian*, November 11, 2002, accessed May 5, 2012, http://www.guardian.co.uk/world/2002/nov/11/india.microsoft.
65. Donald G. McNeil, "India, Said to Play Down AIDS, Has Many Fewer with Virus than Thought, Study Finds," *New York Times*, June 8, 2007, accessed November 10, 2014, http://www.nytimes.com/2007/06/08/world/asia/08aids.html?gwh=D539307E1112BA4D5221D0B8FBC62C77&gwt=pay.
66. Harding, "India Rebuffs Bill Gates."
67. Vir Sanghvi, "The ABC of Sex Education," *Hindustan Times*, July 22, 2007, accessed May 5, 2012, http://www.hindustantimes.com/News-Feed/ViewsVirSanghvi/The-ABC-of-sex-education/Article1-237966.aspx.

68. Deepa A. Tnn, "Holistic Approach Needed for Prevention of AIDS," *Times of India*, June 1, 2003, accessed June 5, 2012, http://articles.timesof india.indiatimes.com/2003-06-01/mumbai/27174652_1_aids-prevention-programmes-health-budget-health-activists.
69. Sanghvi, "The ABC of Sex Education."
70. Ranjit Devraj, "Health-India: Anti-AIDS Group Assailed for 'Misuse of Funds,'" *Inter Press Service*, August 21, 2004, LexisNexis Newspapers.
71. Khan and Bano, "HIV/AIDS Epidemic in India," 478.
72. "PM's Address at the National Students and Youth Parliament Special Session on HIV/AIDS," *Government of India*, last modified November 7, 2004, http://pmindia.nic.in/speech/content.asp?id=44.
73. "XV International AIDS Conference Ends with Leaders Calling for Increased Commitment to Fight HIV/AIDS Worldwide," *Kaiser Family Foundation*, last modified July 16, 2004, http://dailyreports.kff.org/Daily-Reports/2004/July/16/dr00024798.aspx.
74. "National Common Minimum Program," *Government of India*, last modified May 2004, http://pmindia.nic.in/cmp.pdf.
75. "Prime Minister Addresses Media Leaders Summit on HIV/AIDS," *Hindustan Times,* January 6, 2005, LexisNexis Newspapers.
76. "Bollywood Film on HIV/AIDS Opens to Mixed Review, Could Represent Ideological Shift on HIV/AIDS in India," *The Body*, last modified August 30, 2004, http://www.thebody.com/content/art11067.html.
77. Steve Sternberg, "In India, Sex Trade Fuels HIV's Spread," *USA Today*, last modified February 24, 2005, http://www.usatoday.com/news/health/2005-02-23-aids-india-cover_x.htm.
78. "DD to Air Soap to Increase AIDS Awareness," *The Hindu Business Line*, April 5, 2005, accessed May 5, 2012, http://www.thehindubusinessline.in/2005/04/06/stories/2005040601250900.htm.
79. "Condom Ads May Make a Comeback on DD," *The Hindu Business Line*, July 27, 2004, accessed March 4, 2010, http://www.thehindubusinessline.com/bline/2004/07/27/stories/2004072701060400.htm.
80. "National AIDS Control Organization," *National AIDS Control Organization*, accessed March 4, 2010, http://www.nacoonline.org/About_NACO/.
81. "UNGASS Country Progress Report 2010: India." Twenty-five states include Andhra Pradesh, Arunachal Pradesh, Assam, Andaman and Nicobar Islands, Bihar, Daman and Diu, Delhi, Gujarat, Haryana, Himachal Pradesh, Jammu and Kashmir, Karnataka, Maharashtra, Manipur, Mizoram, Nagaland, Orissa, Punjab, Sikkim, Tamil Nadu, Tripura, Uttar Pradesh, and West Bengal.
82. "Meeting of State Project Directors on National AIDS Control Program," *Hindustan Times*, July 12, 2005, LexisNexis Newspapers.
83. "Department of AIDS Control: Outcome Budget 2011–12," *Ministry of Health & Family Welfare, Government of India*, accessed October 29, 2011, http://nacoonline.org/upload/Finance/OutcomeBudget%202011-12%20final.pdf.
84. Jyoti Thottam, "India's Historic Ruling on Gay Rights," *Time*, July 2, 2009, accessed November 10, 2014, http://www.time.com/time/world/article/0,8599,1908406,00.html.

85. "Decriminalize Homosexuality Says Delhi High Court," *Thaindian News*, July 2, 2009, accessed May 5, 2012, http://www.thaindian.com/newsportal/india-news/decriminalise-homosexuality-says-delhi-high-court_100212245.html.
86. "Decriminalize Homosexuality."
87. "Letter to Indian Prime Minister Singh," *Human Rights Watch*, last modified January 11, 2006, http://www.hrw.org/news/2006/01/09/letter-indian-prime-minister-singh.
88. Jim Lobe, "Health-India: Police Tactics Spread AIDS—Report," *Inter Press Service*, July 9, 2002, accessed May 5, 2012, http://ipsnews.net/news.asp?idnews=91762.
89. Matt Wade, "India's Gays Happy to Remain in the Closet," *The Age*, March 20, 2010, accessed April 23, 2012, http://www.theage.com.au/world/indias-gays-happy-to-remain-in-the-closet-20100319-qm69.html.
90. Interview with Dr. Nabeel M. K., research associate of UNAIDS, New Delhi, March 2011.
91. "Restrictions on People Living with HIV Lifted," *The Hindu*, November 27, 2010, accessed November 2, 2011, http://www.hindu.com/2010/11/27/stories/2010112754671600.htm.
92. "Community Feedback Must in India's AIDS Program," *Thaindian News*, May 5, 2011, accessed November 7, 2011, http://www.thaindian.com/newsportal/uncategorized/community-feedback-must-in-indias-aids-programme_100533912.html.
93. "Introduce HIV/AIDS Bill in Parliament, Demand Affected People," *Thaindian News*, July 4, 2011, accessed November 7, 2011, http://www.thaindian.com/newsportal/uncategorized/introduce-hivaids-bill-in-parliament-demand-affected-people_100547301.html.
94. "HIV/AIDS Bill Still Pending: Azad," *Thaindian News*, August 19, 2011, accessed November 7, 2011, http://www.thaindian.com/newsportal/health1/hivaids-bill-still-pending-azad_100557697.html.
95. Interview with a government official of the National AIDS Research Institute [R39], Pune, November 2010.
96. "Government to Drop Treatment Clause from HIV/AIDS Bill," *Thaindian News*, July 4, 2011, accessed November 7, 2011, http://www.thaindian.com/newsportal/uncategorized/government-to-drop-treatment-clause-from-hivaids-bill-lead_100547362.html.
97. "Government to Drop Treatment Clause."
98. "National Rural Health Mission (2005–2012) Document," *Ministry of Health & Family Welfare, Government of India*, accessed May 17, 2010, http://www.mohfw.nic.in/NRHM/Documents/Mission_Document.pdf.
99. Arvind Panagariya, "India: The Crisis in Rural Health Care," *Brookings*, last modified January 24, 2008, http://www.brookings.edu/opinions/2008/0124_health_care_panagariya.aspx; Ravi Duggal, "Sinking Flagships and Health Budgets in India," *Economic & Political Weekly* 14, no. 33 (2009): 15.
100. "National Rural Health Mission Framework for Implementation (2005–2012)," *Ministry of Health & Family Welfare, Government of India*, accessed May

11, 2010, http://mohfw.nic.in/NRHM/Documents/NRHM_Framework_Latest.pdf.
101. "Resolution on NRHM," *National Rural Health Mission*, last modified February 29, 2008, http://mohfw.nic.in/NRHM/RESOLUTIONon%20NRHM.htm.
102. "Health Mission Likely to Get Extension till 2020," *Thaindian News*, April 13, 2010, accessed November 7, 2011, http://www.thaindian.com/newsportal/health1/health-mission-likely-to-get-extension-till-2020_100347290.html.
103. Robert Compton, "Dynamics of HIV/AIDS in China and India: Assessing Governmental Response," in *HIV/AIDS and the Threat to National and International Security*, ed. Robert L. Ostergard (London: Palgrave Macmillan, 2007), 234.
104. "India: Country Situation 2009," *UNAIDS*, accessed December 5, 2011, http://www.unaids.org/ctrysa/ASIIND_en.pdf.
105. "UNGASS Country Progress Report 2010: India."
106. "UNGASS Country Progress Report 2010: India."
107. "NACO Newsletter," *National AIDS Control Organization*, last modified October-December 2009, http://www.nacoonline.org/upload/IEC%20Division/NACO_Newsletter%20(%20Oct-Dec)%202009%20English.pdf.
108. "Annual Report 2010–2011."
109. "UNGASS Country Progress Report 2010: India."
110. Interview with a government official of a HIV/AIDS-related department [R48], New Delhi, March 2011.
111. Interview with Amita Chebbi, country director of Clinton Health Access Initiative, New Delhi, March 2011.
112. Interview with S. Samraj, executive director of Christian AIDS National Alliance, New Delhi, March 2011.
113. Interview with Padma Buggineni, program manager of International HIV/AIDS Alliance, New Delhi, March 2011.
114. Interview with Dr. I. S. Gilada, managing director and consultant in Skin, STDs & HIV/AIDS of Unison Medicare & Research Care Pvt Ltd, Mumbai, November 2010.
115. Interview with Loon Gangte, executive director of Delhi Network for People Living with HIV/AIDS, New Delhi, March 2011.
116. Interview with Sujit Kumar Sahu, program coordinator HIV & AIDS of The Evangelical Fellowship of India Commission Relief, New Delhi, March 2011.
117. Interview with Vinod Bhanu, executive director of Centre for Legislative Research and Advocacy, New Delhi, March 2011.
118. Interview with a government official of a HIV/AIDS-related department [R46], New Delhi, March 2011.
119. Interview with Dr. Thokchom Meinya, Member of Parliament (Lok Sabha), New Delhi, March 2011.
120. Interview with a government official of a HIV/AIDS-related department [R47], New Delhi, March 2011.

121. Interview with Gopal Mukherjee, program manager of Family Health International, New Delhi, March 2011.
122. Interview with Gopal Mukherjee, program manager of Family Health International, New Delhi, March 2011.

8 Audience Acceptance in India: Case Studies in New Delhi, Mumbai, and Imphal

1. Fieldworks in India were conducted in November 2010 and March 2011.
2. Michael C. Williams, "The Continuing Evolution of Securitization Theory," in *Securitization Theory: How Security Problems Emerge and Dissolve*, ed. Thierry Balzacq (London: Routledge, 2011), 215.
3. "HIV/AIDS Scenario in Delhi," *Delhi State AIDS Control Society*, last modified May 21, 2010, http://delhi.gov.in/wps/wcm/connect/doit_dsacs/DSACS/Home/HIV+-+AIDS+Scenario/HIV+or+AIDS+Scenario+in+Delhi.
4. "HIV/AIDS Scenario."
5. "HIV/AIDS Scenario."
6. "Delhi Home to Over 32,000 HIV/AIDS Patients," *Thaindian News*, July 10, 2008, accessed November 10, 2014, http://www.thaindian.com/newsportal/health/delhi-home-to-over-32000-hivaids-patients_10070096.html.
7. "Delhi Home."
8. Pareena G. Lawrence and Maria C. Brun, "NGOs and HIV/AIDS Advocacy in India: Identifying the Challenges," *South Asia: Journal of South Asian Studies* 34, no. 1 (2011): 72.
9. "Delhi Home."
10. Six out of 15 respondents in New Delhi stated that HIV/AIDS is the most serious public health problem in the eyes of the Indian government.
11. Interview with Amita Chebbi, country director of Clinton Health Access Initiative, New Delhi, March 2011.
12. Interview with Dr. Nabeel M. K., research associate, Solution Exchange AIDS Community, UNAIDS India Office, New Delhi, March 2011.
13. Interview with Sujit Kumar Sahu, program coordinator HIV & AIDS of The Evangelical Fellowship of India Commission Relief, New Delhi, March 2011.
14. Four out of 15 respondents stated that HIV/AIDS has occupied a high priority on the government agenda.
15. Interview with Pallavi Upadhyaya, prevention programs coordinator of AIDS Healthcare Foundation India Cares, New Delhi, March 2011.
16. Interview with Vinod Bhanu, executive director of Centre for Legislative Research and Advocacy, New Delhi, March 2011.
17. Eight out of 15 respondents stated that HIV/AIDS is not the top priority issue in the Indian government.

18. Interview with Dr. Nabeel M. K., research associate, Solution Exchange AIDS Community, UNAIDS India Office, New Delhi, March 2011.
19. Interview with Siddhartha Vatsyayan, director of AIDS Awareness Group, New Delhi, March 2011.
20. Interview with Gopal Mukherjee, program manager of Family Health International, New Delhi, March 2011.
21. "Will Balbir Pasha Get AIDS? Case Study: An Innovative Approach to Reduce HIV/AIDS Prevalence through Targeted Mass Media Communications in Mumbai, India," *Population Services International*, last modified May 2003, http://pdf.usaid.gov/pdf_docs/PNADE789.pdf.
22. Mark Fineman, "Superstition, Poverty May Bring AIDS Crisis in India," *Los Angeles Times*, May 28, 1990, accessed November 10, 2014, http://articles.latimes.com/1990-05-28/news/mn-51_1_aids-crisis; Sanjoy Hazarika, "In an Unaware India, AIDS Threat is Growing," *New York Times*, August 9, 1990, accessed November 10, 2014, http://www.nytimes.com/1990/08/09/world/in-an-unaware-india-aids-threat-is-growing.html.
23. "Rape for Profit: Trafficking of Nepali Girls and Women to India's Brothels," *Human Rights Watch*, last modified October 1995, http://www.hrw.org/reports/1995/India.htm.
24. John Ward Anderson and Molly Moore, "AIDS Nears Epidemic Rate in India; Prostitution, Blood Supply, Drug Use Blamed for Spread of Disease," *The Washington Post*, September 14, 1992, LexisNexis Newspapers.
25. Haima Deshpande, "Using Minors in Prostitution Is a Billion Dollar Industry in the City," *Daily News & Analysis*, March 9, 2007, accessed November 10, 2014, http://www.dnaindia.com/mumbai/report-using-minors-in-prostitution-is-a-billion-dollar-industry-in-the-city-1083952.
26. Kausalya Mohan Babu, "Nepal's Sex Trade Victims; Corrupt Police Allow Trafficking of Girls, Women into Bombay Brothels," *The Washington Times*, September 28, 2002, LexisNexis Newspapers.
27. "India Has Most HIV Cases, 20 Per Cent of Men Have Sexually Transmitted Diseases," *BBC Monitoring South Asia—Political*, September 3, 1999, LexisNexis Newspapers.
28. Anderson and Moore, "AIDS Nears."
29. Fineman, "Superstition."
30. "AIDS Ballooning in India; Maharashtra Tops," *The Press Trust of India*, July 15, 2000, LexisNexis Newspapers.
31. Anuradha Mascarenhas, "HIV Prevalence Rate among MSM in City a Big Worry," *Indian Express*, March 21, 2008, accessed April 8, 2010, http://www.expressindia.com/story_print.php?storyId=286955.
32. Matt Wade, "India's Gays Happy to Remain in the Closet," *The Age*, March 20, 2010, accessed November 10, 2014, http://www.theage.com.au/world/indias-gays-happy-to-remain-in-the-closet-20100319-qm69.html.
33. Kounteya Sinha, "India's Fight against AIDS to Focus on Gays," *Times of India*, August 7, 2008, accessed November 10, 2014, http://timesofindia.indiatimes.com/world/rest-of-world/Indias-fight-against-AIDS-to-focus-on-gays/articleshow/3335285.cms.

34. Sarah Hawkes and K. G. Santhya, "Diverse Realities: Sexually Transmitted Infections and HIV in India," *Sexually Transmitted Infections* 78, Supplementary 1 (2002): 32.
35. Wade, "India's Gays."
36. Wade, "India's Gays."
37. Niranjan S. Karnik, "Locating HIV/AIDS and India: Cautionary Notes on the Globalization of Categories," *Science, Technology, & Human Values* 26, no. 3 (2001): 327.
38. Sinha, "India's Fight."
39. "A Baseline Understanding of MSM Commercial Sex Activity at Mumbai Truck Terminal," *The Humsafar Trust*, accessed April 8, 2010, http://www.humsafar.org/rc/MSW%20truckers%20baseline%20report.pdf.
40. Alexandra L. Hernandez et al., "Sexual Behavior among Men Who Have Sex with Women, Men, and *Hijras* in Mumbai, India—Multiple Sexual Risks," *AIDS and Behavior* 10, Supplementary 1 (2006): 8.
41. "Annual HIV Sentinel Surveillance Country Report 2006," *National AIDS Control Organization*, accessed May 10, 2010, http://www.nacoonline.org/upload/NACO%20PDF/HIV%20Sentinel%20Surveillance%202006_India%20Country%20Report.pdf.
42. Sameer Kumta et al., "Bisexuality, Sexual Risk Taking, and HIV Prevalence among Men Who Have Sex with Men Accessing Voluntary Counseling and Testing Services in Mumbai, India," *Journal of Acquired Immune Deficiency Syndromes* 53, no. 2 (2010): 227–233.
43. Sumitra Deb Roy, "HIV Prevalence in City Has Dipped: AIDS Body," *Times of India*, March 7, 2011.
44. 3 out 7 respondents in Mumbai stated that HIV/AIDS is the most serious public health problem in the eyes of the Indian government.
45. Interview with Umesh Tandel, project manager of Mukti Sadan Foundation, Mumbai, November 2010.
46. Five out of seven respondents stated that HIV/AIDS is not a top priority on the government agenda.
47. Interview with a program director of an INGO [R43], Mumbai, November 2010.
48. Interview with Yuvraj Shirde, administration officer of Network of Maharashtra by People Living with HIV/AIDS, Pune, November 2010.
49. Interview with Vinay Vasta, president of Social Activities Integration, Mumbai, November 2010.
50. Happymon Jacob, "Impact of HIV/AIDS on Governance in Manipur and Nagaland," *AIDS, Security, and Conflict Initiative Research Report*, last modified April 2008, http://asci.researchhub.ssrc.org/impact-of-hiv-aids-on-governance-in-manipur-and-nagaland/attachment.
51. Amarjeet M. Singh, "Combating Drug Abuse and HIV/AIDS in Manipur," *Manipur Online*, October 19, 2003, accessed January 15, 2010, http://www.manipuronline.com/Features/October2003/combatingdrugs19_4.htm.
52. Rasheeda Bhagat, "Manipur: A Heady Cocktail of Alcohol, AIDS & Drugs," *The Hindu Business Line*, August 8, 2002, accessed November 10, 2014, http://

www.thehindubusinessline.com/2002/08/08/stories/2002080800580200.htm.
53. "HIV-AIDS Situation in North Eastern States," *International Studies of HIV/AIDS*, accessed April 29, 2012, http://medind.nic.in/haa/t04/i1/haa t04i1p147.pdf.
54. Rasheeda Bhagat, "HIV/AIDS in Manipur: In the 'State' of Despair," *The Hindu Business Online*, July 10, 2002, accessed November 10, 2014, http://www.thehindubusinessline.com/2002/07/10/stories/2002071001300900.htm; Thiyam Bharlat, "Dilemma of HIV/AIDS in Northeast India Particularly Manipur," *Asian Harm Reduction Network*, last modified October 18, 2004, http://www.ahrn.net/index2.php?option=content&do_pdf=1&id=1060; "Hindustan Times: AIDS Infection Rate among Women Rising Alarmingly in Manipur," *Burmanet*, last modified December 5, 2005, http://www.burmanet.org/news/2005/12/05/hindustan-times-aids-infection-rate-among-women-rising-alarmingly-in-manipur/.
55. See S. Sarkar et al., "Rapid Spread of HIV among Injecting Drug Users in North-Eastern States of India," *Bulletin on Narcotics* 45, no. 1 (1993): 91–105.
56. "AIDS Cases on the Rise in N-E," *The Statement*, April 19, 1998, LexisNexis Newspapers.
57. "Epidemiological Analysis of HIV/AIDS in Manipur 2011," *Manipur State AIDS Control Society*, accessed April 25, 2012, http://manipursacs.nic.in/assets/docs/epidem_jan_2011.pdf.
58. "AIDS Scene Remains Grim in Manipur," *The Tribune*, November 30, 2009, accessed April 23, 2012, http://www.tribuneindia.com/2009/20091130/nation.htm#18.
59. "ADB Project to Help Check AIDS in NE," *The Assam Tribune*, February 1, 2010, accessed November 10, 2014, http://www.assamtribune.com/scripts/detailsnew.asp?id=feb0210/oth06.
60. "Epidemiological Analysis of HIV/AIDS in Manipur 2009," *Manipur State AIDS Control Society*, accessed March 30, 2010, http://manipursacs.nic.in/assets/docs/epidem%202009.pdf.
61. "Epidemiological Analysis."
62. "UNGASS Country Progress Report 2010: India," *National AIDS Control Organization*, last modified March 31, 2010, http://data.unaids.org/pub/Report/2010/india_2010_country_progress_report_en.pdf.
63. "629 AIDS Cases Found in Manipur," *Xinhua*, July 7, 1990, LexisNexis Newspapers.
64. Mukta Sharma et al., "Five Years of Needle Syringe Exchange in Manipur, India: Program and Contextual Issues," *International Journal of Drug Policy* 14, nos. 5–6 (2003): 408.
65. Sarlima Laishram, "Epidemiological Analysis of HIV/AIDS in Manipur," *E-PAO*, last modified May 30, 2008, http://www.e-pao.net/epSubPageExtractor.asp?src=education.Health_Issue.Drug_Awareness_Education.Epidemiological_Analysis_of_HIVAIDS.
66. Interview with a high-ranked government official in Manipur State AIDS Control Society [R64], Imphal, March 2011.

67. Interview with Dr. K. Priyokumar Singh, physician, Nodal Officer of Jawaharlal Nehru Hospital, Imphal, March 2011.
68. "On the Frontline of Northeast India," *Transnational Institute*, last modified March 2011, http://www.tni.org/sites/www.tni.org/files/download/On%20 the%20Frontline%20of%20Northeast%20India.pdf.
69. Interview with Dr. K. Priyokumar Singh, physician, Nodal Officer of Jawaharlal Nehru Hospital, Imphal, March 2011.
70. "AIDS Scene."
71. "On the Frontline."
72. Jacob, "Impact of HIV/AIDS."
73. Interview with R. K. Gyanandra Singh, program officer of Catholic Relief Services, Guwahati, March 2011.
74. Interview with R. K. Gyanandra Singh, program officer of Catholic Relief Services, Guwahati, March 2011.
75. Three out of six respondents stated that HIV/AIDS is the most serious public health problem in India.
76. Interview with Amun Leivon, director of Calvary Counseling Centre, Imphal, March 2011.
77. Interview with a government official of National AIDS Control Organization-North East Regional Office [R63], Guwahati, March 2011.
78. Three out of six respondents stated that HIV/AIDS is a top priority on the government agenda.
79. Interview with R. K. Gyanandra Singh, program officer of Catholic Relief Services, Guwahati, March 2011.
80. Interview with Amun Leivon, director of Calvary Counseling Centre, Imphal, March 2011.
81. Four out of seven respondents in Mumbai and four out of six respondents in Imphal believed that HIV/AIDS is the most serious public health problem in India.
82. Interview with Amun Leivon, director of Calvary Counseling Centre, Imphal, March 2011.
83. Interview with a program director of an INGO [R43], Mumbai, November 2010.
84. Five out of 15 respondents in New Delhi believed that HIV/AIDS is the most serious public health problem in India.
85. Interview with Anuradha Mukherjee, programs manager of The Naz Foundation (India) Trust, New Delhi, March 2011.
86. Interview with Gopal Mukherjee, program manager of Family Health International, New Delhi, March 2011.
87. Interview with a project director of a national NGO [R54], New Delhi, March 2011.
88. Interview with Kajal Bhardwaj, an independent legal researcher, New Delhi, March 2011.
89. Interview with Akhila Sivadas, executive director of Centre for Advocacy and Research, New Delhi, March 2011.

90. Interview with a campaign coordinator of an INGO [R69], New Delhi, March 2011.
91. Interview with Sujit Kumar Sahu, program coordinator HIV&AIDS of The Evangelical Fellowship of India Commission Relief, New Delhi, March 2011.
92. Four out of seven respondents in Mumbai have recognized the NGOs' involvement in national HIV/AIDS programs.
93. 13 out of 15 respondents in New Delhi have recognized the NGOs' involvement in national HIV/AIDS programs.
94. Four out of six respondents in Imphal have recognized the NGOs' involvement in national HIV/AIDS programs.
95. Interview with Sujit Kumar Sahu, program coordinator HIV & AIDS of The Evangelical Fellowship of India Commission Relief, New Delhi, March 2011.
96. Interview with Padma Buggineni, program manager: Policy of International HIV/AIDS Alliance, New Delhi, March 2011.
97. Interview with Akhila Sivadas, executive director of Centre for Advocacy and Research, New Delhi, March 2011.
98. Interview with Umesh Tandel, project manager of Mukti Sadan Foundation, Mumbai, November 2010.
99. Interview with Vinay Vasta, president of Social Activities Integration, Mumbai, November 2010.
100. Interview with Amun Leivon, director of Calvary Counseling Centre, Imphal, March 2011.
101. Interview with Loon Gangte, executive director of Delhi Network for People Living with HIV/AIDS, New Delhi, March 2011.
102. Interview with Padma Buggineni, program manager: Policy of International HIV/AIDS Alliance, New Delhi, March 2011.
103. Interview with a project director of a national NGO [R54], New Delhi, March 2011.
104. Interview with Vinod Bhanu, executive director of Centre for Legislative Research and Advocacy, New Delhi, March 2011.
105. Aarti Dhar, "Half of Patients in Asia Live in India," *The Hindu*, December 1, 2011, accessed November 10, 2014, http://www.thehindu.com/todays-paper/tp-national/half-of-hiv-patients-in-asia-live-in-india/article2676106.ece.
106. Pradeep Seth, "The Situation of HIV/M. Tuberculosis Co-infection in India," *The Open Infectious Disease Journal* 5, Supplementary 1-M5 (2011): 51.
107. Aarti Dhar, "Say WHO: India Has the Highest Number of Multidrug Resistant TB in South East Asia," *The Hindu*, March 23, 2012, accessed November 10, 2014, http://www.thehindu.com/news/national/says-who-india-has-highest-number-of-multidrugresistant-tb-in-south-east-asia/article3156259.ece.
108. Dhar, "Say WHO."

109. "World Malaria Report 2011," *World Health Organization*, accessed April 24, 2011, http://www.who.int/malaria/world_malaria_report_2011/9789241564403_eng.pdf.
110. "70% Indians Are Prone to Malaria Infection," *Times of India*, December 15, 2011, accessed November 10, 2014, http://timesofindia.indiatimes.com/india/70-Indians-are-prone-to-malaria-infection/articleshow/11114459.cms.
111. Kounteya Sinha, "India to Raise Malaria Toll Figure 40-Fold," *Times of India*, February 4, 2012, accessed November 10, 2014, http://timesofindia.indiatimes.com/india/India-to-raise-malaria-toll-figure-40-fold/articleshow/11747962.cms.
112. Interview with Lincoln Choudhury, UNAIDS representative, Guwahati, March 2011.
113. Interview with Dr. Nabeel M. K., research associate, Solution Exchange AIDS Community, UNAIDS India Office, New Delhi, March 2011.
114. Timothy Gaikwad, "Living with HIV in Mumbai," *The Guardian*, June 8, 2011.
115. Uma Kapila, *Indian Economy: Performance and Policies* (New Delhi: Academic Foundation, 2008–2009), 260.
116. Interview with a campaign coordinator of an INGO [R69], New Delhi, March 2011.
117. "Table 6: Command Over Resources, The Rise of the South: Human Progress in a Diverse World," *United Nations Development Program*, last modified March 14, 2013, http://www.undp.org/content/dam/undp/library/corporate/HDR/2013GlobalHDR/English/HDR2013%20Report%20English.pdf.
118. "INTERVIEW—India not Treating AIDS Patients Early—Global Fund," *Reuters Africa*, September 9, 2010, accessed March 21, 2012, http://af.reuters.com/article/southAfricaNews/idAFSGE6880AA20100909?pageNumber=2&virtualBrandChannel=0.
119. N. J. Kurian, "Financing Healthcare in India," *The Hindu*, January 15, 2010, accessed November 10, 2014, http://www.thehindu.com/opinion/lead/financing-healthcare-in-india/article80956.ece?css=print.
120. Interview with Siddhartha Vatsysyan, director of AIDS Awareness Group, New Delhi, March 2011.
121. Two out of 15 respondents believed that HIV/AIDS is the most serious problem among all.
122. Interview with Loon Gangte, executive director of Delhi Network for People Living with HIV/AIDS, New Delhi, March 2011.
123. Interview with Padma Buggineni, program manager of Policy of International HIV/AIDS Alliance, New Delhi, March 2011.
124. One out of 15 respondents in New Delhi stated that maternal and child health is more serious than HIV/AIDS in India.
125. Interview with Sujit Kumar Sahu, program coordinator HIV&AIDS of The Evangelical Fellowship of India Commission Relief, New Delhi, March 2011.

126. Five out of 15 respondents believed that TB is the most serious problem among all.
127. Interview with Pallavi Upadhyaya, prevention program coordinator of AIDS Healthcare Foundation—India Cares, New Delhi, March 2011.
128. Interview with Amita Chebbi, country director of Clinton Health Access Initiative, New Delhi, March 2011.
129. Four out of 15 respondents believed that HIV/AIDS, TB and malaria are all the most serious problems in India.
130. Interview with Gopal Mukherjee, program manager of Family Health International, New Delhi, March 2011.
131. Interview with a campaign coordinator of an INGO [R69], New Delhi, March 2011.
132. Interview with Anuradha Mukherjee, programs manager of The Naz Foundation (India) Trust, New Delhi, March 2011.
133. Kurian, "Financing Healthcare in India."
134. Seven out of 15 respondents in New Delhi believed that NACP should be incorporated into NRHM.
135. Interview with a project director of a national NGO [R54], New Delhi, March 2011.
136. Interview with Akhila Sivadas, executive director of Centre for Advocacy and Research, New Delhi, March 2011.
137. Six out of 15 of the respondents in New Delhi believed that NACP should not be incorporated into NRHM program.
138. Interview with Dr. Nabeel M. K., research associate, Solution Exchange AIDS Community of UNAIDS India Office, New Delhi, March 2011.
139. Interview with a campaign coordinator of an INGO [R69], New Delhi, March 2011.
140. Interview with Sujit Kumar Sahu, program coordinator HIV&AIDS of The Evangelical Fellowship of India Commission Relief, New Delhi, March 2011.
141. Four out of six respondents in Imphal believed that NACP should not be incorporated into NRHM.
142. Interview with R. K. Gyanandra Singh, program officer of Catholic Relief Services, Guwahati, March 2011.
143. Interview with Dr. K. Priyokumar Singh, physician, Nodal Officer of Jawaharlal Nehru Hospital, Imphal, March 2011.
144. Qiu-sha Ma, "Defining Chinese Nongovernmental Organizations," *Voluntas: International Journal of Voluntary and Nonprofit Organizations* 13, no. 2 (2002): 118.
145. Thierry Balzacq, "The Three Faces of Securitization: Political Agency, Audience and Context," *European Journal of International Relations* 11, no. 2 (2005): 185.
146. Catherine Boone and Jake Batsell, "Politics and AIDS in Africa: Research Agendas in Political Science and International Relations," in *HIV/AIDS and the Threat to National and International Security*, ed. R. L. Ostergard (London: Palgrave Macmillan, 2007), 14.

147. Interview with Kajal Bhardwaj, an independent legal research, New Delhi, March 2011.
148. "NGO/CBO Operational Guidelines—Section," *National AIDS Control Organization*, last modified April 10, 2007, http://upsacs.nic.in/ti%20documents/NGO%20CBO%20Operational%20Guidelines.pdf.
149. Interview with a government official in HIV/AIDS-related department [R47], New Delhi, March 2011.
150. "UNGASS Country."
151. "Targeted Interventions Under NACP-III: Core High Risk Groups," *National AIDS Control Organization*, last modified October 2007, http://www.nacoonline.org/upload/Policies%20&%20Guidelines/27,%20NACP-III.pdf.
152. Ilavenil Ramiah, "Securitizing the AIDS Issue in Asia," in *Non-Traditional Security in Asia: Dilemmas in Securitization*, ed. Mely Caballero-Anthony, Ralf Emmers, and Amitav Acharya (England: Ashgate Publishing Limited, 2006a), 151.
153. Interview with a government official of an HIV/AIDS-related department [R47], New Delhi, March 2011.
154. Interview with a project director of national NGO [R54], New Delhi, March 2011.
155. Interview with Akhila Sivadas, executive director of Centre for Advocacy and Research, New Delhi, March 2011.
156. Interview with a campaign coordinator of an INGO [R69], New Delhi, March 2011.
157. Interview with Dr. Nabeel M. K., research associate, Solution Exchange AIDS Community of UNAIDS India Office, New Delhi, March 2011.
158. Interview with Akhila Sivadas, executive director of Centre for Advocacy and Research, New Delhi, March 2011.
159. Interview with Sujit Kumar Sahu, program coordinator, HIV&AIDS of The Evangelical Fellowship of India Commission Relief, New Delhi, March 2011.
160. Interview with Vinod Bhanu, executive director of Centre for Legislative Research and Advocacy, New Delhi, March 2011.
161. Interview with Padma Buggineni, program manager: Policy of International HIV/AIDS Alliance, New Delhi, March 2011.
162. Interview with R. K. Gyanandra Singh, program officer of Catholic Relief Services, Guwahati, Mach 2011.
163. "Grant Portfolio: India," *The Global Fund to Fight AIDS, Tuberculosis, and Malaria*, last modified December 23, 2011, http://portfolio.theglobalfund.org/en/Country/Index/IDA.
164. *Barriers to Sustainable Access of Children and Families to ART Centers in Rural India* (New Delhi: India HIV/AIDS Alliance, 2009).
165. "Applicant—Disease Profile," *India Country Coordinating Mechanism—HIV/AIDS*, last modified August 11, 2011, http://www.india-ccm.org/global-fund-grant-india-HIV.php.
166. *Policy Brief* (New Delhi: Indian HIV/AIDS Alliance, Undated).

167. *Learning from Our Role in the HIV Response in India: Annual Report 2009–10* (New Delhi: India HIV/AIDS Alliance, Undated).
168. *Learning from Our Role.*
169. *Learning from Our Role.*
170. *Learning from Our Role.*
171. "$25M for MSM and TG Communities in India," *International HIV/AIDS Alliance*, last modified September 13, 2010, http://www.aidsalliance.org/NewsDetails.aspx?Id=687.

9 Conclusion: Reconsidering HIV/AIDS Securitization

1. See Ole Wæver, "Securitization: Taking Stock of a Research Program in Security Studies," unpublished draft, 2003, 27–28.
2. Simon Rushton, "The Development of the HIV/AIDS and Security Discourse: The Role of CSOs" (paper presented at Peter Wall Institute's London Workshop on Civil Society Organizations and Global Health Governance, October 2007).
3. Lene Hansen, "The Little Mermaid's Silent Security Dilemma and the Absence of Gender in the Copenhagen School," *Millennium Journal of International Studies* 29, no. 2 (2000): 296.
4. Barry Buzan and Lene Hansen, *The Evolution of International Studies* (Cambridge: Cambridge University Press, 2009), 216.
5. Rita Floyd, "Can Securitization Theory Be Used in Normative Analysis? Towards a Just Securitization Theory," *Security Dialogue* 42, nos. 4–5 (2011): 429.
6. Floyd, "Can Securitization Theory," 429.
7. Colin McInnes and Simon Rushton, "HIV, AIDS and Security: Where Are We Now?" *International Affairs* 86, no. 1 (2010): 244.
8. Wæver, "Securitization," 23.
9. Barry Buzan, Ole Wæver, and Jaap de Wilde, *Security: A New Framework for Analysis* (Boulder, CO: Lynne Rienner Publishers, 1998), 29.
10. Juha A. Vuori, "Illocutionary Logic and Strands of Securitization: Applying the Theory of Securitization to the Study of Non-Democratic Political Orders," *European Journal of International Relations* 14, no. 1 (2008): 72; McInnes and Rushton, "HIV, AIDS and Security," 244.
11. "National Program Office of China Global Fund AIDS Program (Round 6)," *NCAIDS, China CDC*, accessed December 19, 2011, http://www.chinaaids.cn/n443289/n443290/n447113/n447525/n457450/index.html.
12. J. T. F. Lau et al., "Public Health Challenges of the Emerging HIV Epidemic among Men Who Have Sex with Men in China," *Public Health* 125, no. 5 (2011): 263.
13. Drew Thompson and Xiao-qing Lu, "China's Evolving Civil Society: From Environment to Health," *Woodrow Wilson International Center for Scholars*,

accessed February 15, 2012, http://208elmp02.blackmesh.com/sites/default/files/CEF_Feature.2.pdf.
14. Pinar Bilgin, "Making Turkey's Transformation Possible: Claiming 'Security-Speak'—not Desecuritization!" *Southeast European and Black Sea Studies* 7, no. 4 (2007): 560.
15. Park Madison, "As HIV Epidemic Grows, Florida City Grapples with Fear and Denial," *CNN*, November 29, 2011, accessed November 2014, http://edition.cnn.com/2011/11/29/health/jacksonville-hiv-florida/index.html; Julia Medew, "Warning as HIV Cases Increase," *Sydney Morning Herald*, October 19, 2010, accessed November 10, 2014, http://www.smh.com.au/lifestyle/diet-and-fitness/warning-as-hiv-cases-increase-20091108-i3kc.html.
16. "HIV and AIDS in the UK," *AVERT*, accessed May 28, 2012, http://www.avert.org/aids-uk.htm#contentTable0.
17. "After Years of Decline, HIV Rate Starts to Increase in Many US Cities," *Voice of America*, last modified October 29, 2009, http://www.voanews.com/content/a-13-a-2002-11-29-16-after-67253707/379188.html.
18. Kate Benson Health, "HIV Rate Rising but Other Infection Less Common," *Sydney Morning Herald*, October 19, 2010, http://www.smh.com.au/lifestyle/diet-and-fitness/hiv-rate-rising-but-other-infections-less-common-20101018-16qxf.html.

Bibliography

"A Baseline Understanding of MSM Commercial Sex Activity at Mumbai Truck Terminal." *The Humsafar Trust.* Accessed April 8, 2010. http://www.humsafar.org/rc/MSW%20truckers%20baseline%20report.pdf.

"A Joint Assessment of HIV/AIDS Prevention, Treatment and Care in China (2003)." *Ministry of Health and UN Theme Group on HIV/AIDS in China.* Last modified December 1, 2003. http://data.unaids.org/UNA-docs/china_joint_assessment_2003_en.pdf.

"A Joint Assessment of HIV/AIDS Prevention, Treatment and Care in China (2004)." *State Council AIDS Working Committee Office and UN Theme Group on HIV/AIDS in China.* Last modified December 1, 2004. http://www.chinaids.org.cn/worknet/download/2004/report2004en.pdf.

"A Joint Assessment of HIV/AIDS Prevention, Treatment and Care in China (2007)." *State Council AIDS Working Committee Office and UN Theme Group on AIDS in China.* Last modified December 1, 2007. http://www.undp.org.cn/downloads/otherlocal/HIV/20080104.pdf.

"About AIDS Vaccines: Why a Vaccine." *International AIDS Vaccine Initiative.* Accessed September 10, 2009. http://www.iavi.org/why-a-vaccine/Pages/about-AIDS-vaccine.aspx.

"Act Now: Asia Pacific Leaders Respond to HIV/AIDS." *UNAIDS/Asia Pacific Leadership Forum on HIV/AIDS and Development.* Accessed April 14, 2012. http://data.unaids.org/publications/External-Documents/apfl_actnow_en.pdf.

"Address by the Prime Minister Sri Atal Bihari Vajpayee at the meeting on National Program for Prevention and Control of HIV/AIDS New Delhi." *Embassy of India.* Last modified December 12, 1998. http://www.indianembassy.org/policy/AIDS/prime_minister_AIDS.html.

"After Years of Decline, HIV Rate Starts to Increase in Many US Cities." *Voice of America.* Last modified October 29, 2009. http://www.voanews.com/content/a-13-a-2002-11-29-16-after-67253707/379188.html.

Ahluwalia, Montek S. "India's Economic Reforms: An Appraisal." In *India in the Era of Economic Reforms*, edited by Jeffrey D. Sachs, Ashutosh Varshney, and Nirupam Bajpai, 26–80. New Delhi: Oxford University Press, 1999.

"AIDS Blood Scandals: What China Can Learn from the World's Mistakes." *Asia Catalyst.* Last modified September 2007. http://www.asiacatalyst.org/news/AIDS_blood_scandals_rpt_0907.pdf.

"AIDS Prevention and Care in the Workplace: Enhancing the Role of the Private Sector." *World Health Organization.* Last modified January 12–13, 1995. http://whqlibdoc.who.int/searo/1994-99/SEA_AIDS_90.pdf.
Alcorn, Keith. "Chinese HIV Prevention with Drug Users Undermined by Police." *Aidsmap.* Last modified December 11, 2008. http://www.aidsmap.com/Chinese-HIV-prevention-with-drug-users-undermined-by-police/page/1432754/.
Alder, Emanuel. "Seizing the Middle Ground: Constructivism in World Politics." *European Journal of International Relations* 3, no. 3 (1997): 319–363.
Altman, Dennis. "AIDS and Security." *International Relations* 17, no. 4 (2003): 417–427.
"An Alleyway in Hell: China's Abusive Black Jails." *Human Rights Watch.* Last modified November 2009. http://www.hrw.org/sites/default/files/reports/china1109web_1.pdf.
"Annual HIV Sentinel Surveillance Country Report 2006." *National AIDS Control Organization.* Accessed May 10, 2010. http://www.nacoonline.org/upload/NACO%20PDF/HIV%20Sentinel%20Surveillance%202006_India%20Country%20Report.pdf.
"Annual Report 2008–2009." *National AIDS Control Organization.* Accessed February 8, 2010. https://www.nacoonline.org/upload/Publication/Annual_Report_NACO_2008-09.pdf.
"Annual Report 2010–2011." *National AIDS Control Organization, Department of AIDS Control.* Last modified March 15, 2011. http://aidsdatahub.org/dmdocuments/NACO_Annual_Report_2010_11.pdf.
"Applicant—Disease Profile." *India Country Coordinating Mechanism—HIV/AIDS.* Last modified August 11, 2011. http://www.india-ccm.org/global-fund-grant-india-HIV.php.
Asthana, Sheena. "AIDS-Related Policies, Legislation and Program Implementation in India." *Health Policy and Planning* 11, no. 2 (1996): 184–197.
Austin, John Langshaw. *How to Do Things with Words.* Oxford: Oxford University Press, 1962.
Bacaër, Nicolas, Xamxinur Abdurahman, and Jian-li Ye. "Modeling the HIV/AIDS Epidemic among Injecting Drug Users and Sex Workers in Kunming, China." *Bulletin of Mathematical Biology* 68, no. 3 (2006): 525–550.
Balzacq, Thierry. "The Three Faces of Securitization: Political Agency, Audience and Context." *European Journal of International Relations* 11, no. 2 (2005): 171–201.
Balzano, John and Ping Jia. "Coming Out of Denial: An Analysis of AIDS Law and Policy in China (1987– 2006)." *Loyola University Chicago International Law Review* 3, no. 2 (2005–2006): 187–212.
Barnett, Tony. "A Long-Wave Event. HIV/AIDS, Politics, Governance and 'Security': Sundering the Intergenerational Bond?" *International Affairs* 82, no. 2 (2006): 297–313.
Barnett, Tony. "HIV/AIDS, a Long Wave Event: Sundering the Intergenerational Bond." In *AIDS and Governance*, edited by Nana K. Poku, Alan Whiteside, and Bjorn Sandkjaer, 29–47. England: Ashgate Publishing Limited, 2007.

Barnett, Tony and Gwyn Prins. "HIV/AIDS and Security: Fact, Fiction, Evidences—A Report to UNAIDS." *International Affairs* 82, no. 2 (2006): 359–368.

Banerji, Debabar. "Landmarks in the Development of Health Services in India." In *Public Health and the Poverty of Reforms: The South Asian Predicament*, edited by Imrana Qadeer, Kasturi Sen, and K. R. Nayar, 109–114. New Delhi: Sage Publications, 2001.

Barriers to Sustainable Access of Children and Families to ART Centres in Rural India. New Delhi: India HIV/AIDS Alliance, 2009.

Beyrer, Chris. "An Epidemic of Denial: Stalled Responses to HIV/AIDS." *Harvard International Review* 25, no. 2 (2003): 64–68.

Beyrer, Chris, Myat Htoo Razak, Khomdon Lisam, Jie Chen, Wei Lui, and Xiao Fang Yu. "Overland Heroin Trafficking Routes and HIV-1 Spread in South and South-East Asia." *AIDS* 14, no. 1 (2000): 75–83.

Bhagwati, Jagdish. "The Design of Indian Development." In *India's Economic Reform and Development: Essay for Manmohan Singh*, edited by Isher Judge Ahluwalia and I. M. D. Little, 25–42. New Delhi: Oxford University Press, 1998.

Bharlat, Thiyam. "Dilemma of HIV/AIDS in Northeast India Particularly Manipur." *Asian Harm Reduction Network*. Last modified October 18, 2004. http://www.ahrn.net/index2.php?option=content&do_pdf=1&id=1060.

Bilgin, Pinar. "Making Turkey's Transformation Possible: Claiming 'Security-Speak'—not Desecuritization!" *Southeast European and Black Sea Studies* 7, no. 4 (2007): 555–571.

"Bollywood Film on HIV/AIDS Opens to Mixed Review, Could Represent Ideological Shift on HIV/AIDS in India." *The Body*. Last modified August 30, 2004. http://www.thebody.com/content/art11067.html.

Boone, Catherine and Jake Batsell. "Politics and AIDS in Africa: Research Agendas in Political Science and International Relations." In *HIV/AIDS and the Threat to National and International Security*, edited by R. L. Ostergard, 3–35. London: Palgrave Macmillan, 2007.

Brown, Garrett W. and Ronald Labonté. "Globalization and Its Methodological Discontents: Contextualizing Globalization through the Study of HIV/AIDS." *Globalization and Health* 7, no. 29 (2011): 1–12.

Brown, Lisanne, Kate Macintyre, and Lea Trujillo. "Interventions to Reduce HIV/AIDS Stigma: What Have We Learned?" *AIDS Education and Prevention* 15, no. 1 (2003): 49–69.

Brugha, Ruairí, Martine Donoghue, Mary Starling, Phillimon Ndubani, Freddie Ssengooba, Benedita Fernandes, and Gill Walt. "The Global Fund: Managing Great Expectations." *The Lancet* 364, no. 9428 (2004): 95–100.

Buruma, Ian. "After America." *The New Yorker*. Last modified April 21, 2008. http://www.newyorker.com/arts/critics/atlarge/2008/04/21/080421crat_atlarge_buruma.

Buzan, Barry. *People, States and Fear: An Agenda for International Security Studies in the Post-Cold War Era*. Great Britain: Hartnolls Limited, 1991.

Buzan, Barry and Lene Hansen. *The Evolution of International Studies.* Cambridge: Cambridge University Press, 2009.

Buzan, Barry, Ole Wæver, and Jaap de Wilde. *Security: A New Framework for Analysis.* Boulder, CO: Lynne Rienner Publishers, 1998.

Caballero-Anthony, Mely. "Combating Infectious Diseases in East Asia: Securitization and Global Public Goods for Health and Human Security." *Journal of International Affairs* 59, no. 2 (2006): 105–127.

Caballero-Anthony, Mely. "Human Security and Primary Health Care in Asia: Realities and Challenges." In *Global Health Challenges for Human Security*, edited by Lincoln C. Chen, Jennifer Leaning, and Vasant Narasimhan, 233–255. Cambridge, MA: Global Equity Initiative, Asia Center, Harvard University, 2003.

Caballero-Anthony, Mely and Ralf Emmers. "Understanding the Dynamics of Securitizing Non-Traditional Security." In *Non-Traditional Security in Asia: Dilemmas in Securitization*, edited by Mely Caballero-Anthony, Ralf Emmers, and Amitav Acharya, 1–12. Singapore: Ashgate Publishing Limited, 2006a.

Caballero-Anthony, Mely and Ralf Emmers. "The Dynamics of Securitization in Asia." In *Studying Non-Traditional Security in Asia: Trends and Issues*, edited by Ralf Emmers, Mely Caballero-Anthony, and Amitav Acharya, 21–35. Singapore: Marshall Cavendish Academic, 2006b.

Cao, Yun-zhen and Hong-zhou Lu. "Care of HIV-Infected Patients in China." *Cell Research* 15, no. 11–12 (2005): 883–890.

Ceyhan, Ayse and Anastassia Tsoukala. "The Securitization of Migration in Western Societies: Ambivalent Discourses and Policies." *Alternatives* 27, no. 1 (2002): 21–39.

Chan, Lai-ha, Pak K. Lee, and Gerald Chan. "China Engages Global Health Governance: Processes and Dilemmas." *Global Public Health* 4, no. 1 (2009): 1–30.

Chandler, David. "Review Essay: Human Security: The Dog That Didn't Bark." *Security Dialogue* 39, no. 4 (2008): 427–438.

Chandrasekaran, Padma, Gina Dallabetta, Virginia Loo, Sujata Rao, Helene Gayle, and Ashok Alexander. "Containing HIV/AIDS in India: The Unfinished Agenda." *The Lancet Infectious Diseases* 6, no. 8 (2006): 508–521.

"Chapter 2: New Dimension of Human Security." *Human Development Report 1994, United Nations Development Program.* Accessed September 27, 2009. http://hdr.undp.org/en/media/hdr_1994_en_chap2.pdf.

Chen, Lincoln C., "Health as a Human Security Priority for the 21st Century." Paper for Human Security Track III, Helsinki Process, December 7, 2004.

Chin, James. *The AIDS Pandemic: The Collision of Epidemiology with Political Correctness.* Oxford: Radcliffe Publishing Limited, 2007.

"China: 'At a Critical Stage.'" *International Federation for Human Rights.* Last modified April 2005. http://www.fidh.org/IMG/pdf/cn413a.pdf.

"China: Country Summary." *Human Rights Watch.* Last modified January 2007. http://www.hrw.org/sites/default/files/related_material/china_0.pdf.

"China Epidemic: HIV and AIDS Estimate." *China AIDS Survey*. Last modified August 7, 2007. http://www.aidsdatahub.org/files/documents/China_epidemic_HIV_and_AIDS_estimates.pdf.

"China Global Fund Program Principle Recipient." *Chinese Center for Disease Control and Prevention*. Accessed February 18, 2012. http://www.chinaglobalfund.org/en/090720/ff808081221b6499012296034cf900f1.html.

"China: House Arrests Stifle HIV/AIDS Petitions." *Human Rights Watch*. Last modified March 12, 2006. http://www.hrw.org/en/news/2006/03/10/china-house-arrests-stifle-hivaids-petitions.

"China: Secret 'Black Jails' Hide Severe Rights Abuses." *Human Rights Watch*. Last modified November 11, 2009. http://www.hrw.org/en/news/2009/11/02/china-secret-black-jails-hide-severe-rights-abuses.

"China 2010 UNGASS Country Progress Report (2008–2009)." *Ministry of Health of the People's Republic of China*. Last modified April 2, 2010. http://data.unaids.org/pub/Report/2010/china_2010_country_progress_report_en.pdf.

Choi, Kyung-hee, Zhen Ning, Steven Gregorich, and Qi-chao Pan. "The Influence of Social and Sexual Networks in the Spread of HIV and Syphilis among Men Who Have Sex with Men in Shanghai, China." *Journal of Acquired Immune Deficiency Syndromes* 45, no. 1 (2007): 77–84.

Chow, Gregory C. "Economic Reform and Growth in China." *Annals of Economics and Finance* 5, no. 1(2004): 127–152.

Chu, Tian-xin and Judith A. Levy. "Injection Drug Use and HIV/AIDS Transmission in China." *Cell Research* 15, no. 11-12 (2005): 865–869.

Ciută, Felix. "Security and the Problem of Context: A Hermeneutical Critique of Securitization Theory." *Review of International Studies* 35, no. 2 (2009): 301–326.

Cohen, Jon. "Changing Course to Break the HIV-Heroin Connection." *Science* 304, no. 5676 (2004): 1434–1435.

Compton, Robert. "Dynamics of HIV/AIDS in China and India: Assessing Governmental Response." In *HIV/AIDS and the Threat to National and International Security*, edited by Robert L. Ostergard, 223–240. London: Palgrave Macmillan, 2007.

"Constitution of the World Health Organization." *World Health Organization*. Accessed September 18, 2009. http://www.who.int/governance/eb/who_constitution_en.pdf.

"Core Structures." *The Global Fund to Fight AIDS, Tuberculosis and Malaria*. Accessed April 28, 2012. http://www.theglobalfund.org/en/about/structures/.

Cui, Yan, Adrian Liau, and Zun-you Wu. "An Overview of the History of Epidemic of and Response to HIV/AIDS in China: Achievements and Challenges." *Chinese Medical Journal* 122, no. 19 (2009): 2251–2257.

Curley, Melissa G. "Levels of Analysis Issues in the Migration—Security Nexus." In *Security and Migration: The Dynamics of Securitization*, edited by Melissa G. Curley and Siu-lun Wong, 19–34. London: Routledge, 2008.

Curley, Melissa G. "The Role of Civil Society in East Asian Region Building." In *Advancing East Asian Regionalism*, edited by Melissa G. Curley and Nicholas Thomas, 179–201. London: Routledge, 2007.

Curley, Melissa G. and Jonathan Herington. "The Securitization of Avian Influenza: International Discourses and Domestic Politics in Asia." *Review of International Studies* 37, no. 1 (2011): 141–166.
Curley, Melissa G. and Nicholas Thomas. "Human Security and Public Health in Southeast Asia: The SARS Outbreak." *Australian Journal of International Affairs* 58, no. 1 (2004): 17–32.
Curley, Melissa G. and Siu-lun Wong. *Security and Migration in Asia: The Dynamics of Securitization*. London: Routledge, 2008.
Datta, Rekha. *Beyond Realism: Human Security in India and Pakistan in the Twenty-First Century*. Lanham: Lexington Books, 2008.
Davies, Sara E. "Securitizing Infectious Disease." *International Affairs* 84, no. 2 (2008): 295–313.
de Waal, Alex. "HIV/AIDS: The Security Issue of a Lifetime." In *Global Health Challenges for Human Security*, edited by Lincoln C. Chen, Jennifer Leaning, and Vasant Narasimhan, 125–137. Cambridge, MA: Global Equity Initiative, Asia Center, Harvard University, 2003.
"Declaration on Commitment of HIV/AIDS." *United Nations General Assembly*. Last modified August 2, 2011. http://www.un.org/ga/aids/docs/aress262.pdf.
"Declaration of Commitment on HIV/AIDS Interventions." *Centers of Disease Control, Republic of China*. Last modified December 19, 2001. http://www.cdc.gov.tw/ct.asp?xItem=595&ctNode=1069&mp=220.
"Department of AIDS Control: Outcome Budget 2011–2012." *Ministry of Health and Family Welfare, Government of India*. Accessed October 29, 2011. http://nacoonline.org/upload/Finance/OutcomeBudget%202011-12%20final.pdf.
Deudney, Daniel. "The Case against Linking Environmental Degradation and National Security." *Millennium Journal of International Studies* 19, no. 3 (1990): 461–476.
Doshi, Sonal R. and Bindi Gandhi. "Women in India: The Context and Impact of HIV/AIDS." *Journal of Human Behavior in the Social Environment* 17, no. 3–4 (2008): 413–442.
Drexler, Madeline. *Secret Agents: The Menace of Emerging Infections*. Washington, DC: Joseph Henry Press, 2002.
Drèze, Jean and Amartya Sen. *India: Development and Participation*. New York: Oxford University Press, 2002.
Duggal, Ravi. "Bhore Committee (1946) and Its Relevance Today." *The Indian Journal of Paediatrics* 58, no. 4 (1991): 395–406.
Duggal, Ravi. "Sinking Flagships and Health Budgets in India." *Economic and Political Weekly* 14, no. 33 (2009): 14–17.
Dummer, Trevor J. B. and Ian G. Cook. "Health in China and India: A Cross-Country Comparison in a Context of Rapid Globalization." *Social Science and Medicine* 67, no. 4 (2008): 590–605.
Easton, David. *A Framework for Political Analysis*. Englewood Cliffs: Prentice-Hall, 1965.
Elbe, Stefan. "Pandemics on the Radar Screen: Health Security, Infectious Disease and the Medicalization of Insecurity." *Political Studies* 59, no. 4 (2011): 848–866.

Elbe, Stefan. "Should HIV/AIDS Be Securitized? The Ethical Dilemmas of Linking HIV/AIDS and Security." *International Studies Quarterly* 50, no. 1 (2006): 119–144.

"Emerging and Re-Emerging Infectious Diseases: Introduction and Goals." *National Institute of Allergy and Infectious Diseases, National Institutes of Health*. Last modified March 10, 2010. http://www.niaid.nih.gov/topics/emerging/pages/introduction.aspx.

Emmers, Ralf. "ASEAN and the Securitization of Transnational Crime in Southeast Asia." *The Pacific Review* 16, no. 3 (2003): 419–438.

Emmers, Ralf, Greener B. Barcham, and Nicholas Thomas. "Securitizing Human Trafficking in the Asia-Pacific: Regional Organizations and Response Strategies." In *Security and Migration in Asia: The Dynamics of Securitization*, edited by Melissa G. Curley and Siu-lun Wong, 59–82. London: Routledge, 2008.

"Epidemiological Analysis of HIV/AIDS in Manipur 2009." *Manipur State AIDS Control Society*. Accessed March 30, 2010. http://manipursacs.nic.in/assets/docs/epidem%202009.pdf.

"Epidemiological Analysis of HIV/AIDS in Manipur 2011." *Manipur State AIDS Control Society*. Accessed April 25, 2012. http://manipursacs.nic.in/assets/docs/epidem_jan_2011.pdf.

Eriksson, Johan. "Agendas, Threats and Politics: Securitization in Sweden." Paper presented at the ECPR Joint Sessions, workshop "Redefining Security," Mannheim, March 26–31, 1999.

Erwin, Kathleen. "The Circulatory System: Blood Procurement, AIDS, and the Social Body in China." *Medical Anthropology Quarterly* 20, no. 2 (2006): 139–159.

"Exploring the Waste Land." Last modified September 29, 2002. http://world.std.com/~raparker/exploring/thewasteland/explore.html.

Fauci, Anthony. "Fauci: Why There Is No AIDS Vaccine." *msnbc.com*. Last modified March 31, 2009. http://www.msnbc.msn.com/id/29898087/.

Feng, Yu-ji, Zun-you Wu, and Roger Detels. "Evolution of Men Who Have Sex with Men Community and Experienced Stigma among Men Who Have Sex with Men in Chengdu, China." *Journal of Acquired Immune Deficiency Syndromes* 53, Supplementary 1 (2010): 98–103.

Fidler, David P. "A Pathology of Public Health Securitism: Approaching Pandemics as Security Threats." In *Governing Global Health: Challenge, Response, Innovation*, edited by Andrew F. Cooper, John J. Kirton, and Ted Schrecker, 41–66. England: Ashgate Publishing Limited, 2007.

"Fight Will Go on Despite Grant Cut." *NCAIDS, China CDC*. Last modified November 10, 2011. http://www.chinaaids.cn/n1971/n2091/721831.html.

"Finance Minister P. Chidambaram's Budget Speech." *Rediff*. Last modified February 28, 2007. http://www.rediff.com/money/2007/feb/28bud26.htm.

Floyd, Rita. "Can Securitization Theory Be Used in Normative Analysis? Towards a Just Securitization Theory." *Security Dialogue* 42, no. 4–5 (2011): 427–439.

Floyd, Rita. "Human Security and the Copenhagen School's Securitization Approach: Conceptualizing Human Security as a Securitizing Move." *Human Security Journal* 5, (2007a): 38–49.

Floyd, Rita. "Towards a Consequentialist Evaluation of Security: Bringing Together the Copenhagen and the Welsh Schools of Security Studies." *Review of International Studies* 33, no. 2 (2007b): 327–350.

Fourie, Pieter. "The Relationship between the AIDS Pandemic and State Fragility." *Global Change, Peace and Security* 19, no. 3 (2007): 281–300.

Friedlander, Mark P. *Outbreak: Disease Detectives at Work*. New York: Lerner Publications Company, 2000.

"Frontier Health and Quarantine Law of the People's Republic of China." *China.org.cn*. Accessed February 23, 2010. http://lanzhou.china.com.cn/english/travel/40418.htm.

Gao, Lei, Feng Zhou, Xiang-wei Li, and Qi Jin. "HIV/TB Co-Infection in Mainland China: A Meta-Analysis." *PLoS ONE* 5, no. 5 (2010): 1–6.

Garrett, Laurie. "HIV and National Security: Where Are the Links?" *Council on Foreign Relations*. Accessed January 4, 2010. http://www.cfr.org/content/publications/attachments/HIV_National_Security.pdf.

Garrett, Laurie. *The Coming Plague: Newly Emerging Diseases in a World Out of Balance*. New York: Penguin Group, 1994.

Garrett, Laurie. "The Return of Infectious Diseases." In *Plagues and Politics*, edited by Andrew T. Price-Smith, 183–194. London: Palgrave Macmillan, 2001.

Gauri, Varun and Evan S. Lieberman. "AIDS and the State: The Politics of Government Responses to the Epidemic in Brazil and South Africa." Paper presented at the annual meetings for the American Political Science Association, Chicago, IL, September 2–5, 2004.

Gauri, Varun and Evan S. Lieberman. "Boundary Institutions and HIV/AIDS Policy in Brazil and South Africa." *Studies in Comparative International Development* 41, no. 3 (2006): 47–73.

Ghosh, Jayati. "A Geographical Perspective on HIV/AIDS in India." *Geographical Review* 92, no. 1 (2002): 115–116.

Giblin, James Cross. *When Plague Strikes: The Black Death, Smallpox, AIDS*. New York: HarperCollins Publishers, 1995.

Girshick, Rachel. "Adopting Institutional Changes: HIV/AIDS and the Changing Institution of Security." Paper presented in the Annual Conference for the International Studies Association, Montreal, Quebec, March 18, 2004.

"Global AIDS Overview." *AIDS.gov*. Last modified December 18, 2013. http://www.aids.gov/federal-resources/arounglobal-aidsd-the-world/-overview/.

"Global Fund Lifts China Grant Freeze." *The Body*. Last modified August 24, 2011. http://www.thebody.com/content/63640/global-fund-lifts-china-grant-freeze.html.

"Global Report—UNAIDS Report on the Global AIDS Epidemic 2013." *UNAID*. Last modified September 2013. http://www.unaids.org/en/media/unaids/contentassets/documents/epidemiology/2013/gr2013/UNAIDS_Global_Report_2013_en.pdf.

"Global Risks 2009: A Global Risk Network Report." *World Economic Forum*. Last modified January 2009. https://members.weforum.org/pdf/globalrisk/2009.pdf.

Godbole, Sheela and Sanjay Mehendale. "HIV/AIDS Epidemic in India: Risk Factors, Risk Behavior and Strategies for Prevention and Control." *Indian Journal of Medical Research* 121, no. 4 (2005): 356–368.
Gómez, Eduardo J. "The Politics of Government Response to HIV/AIDS in Brazil: Democratization, International Pressures, and the Civic Sources of Institutional Change." Rough draft, July 1, 2008: 1–55.
"Grant Portfolio: China." *The Global Fund to Fight AIDS, Tuberculosis and Malaria.* Last modified January 25, 2012. http://portfolio.theglobalfund.org /en/Country/Index/CHN.
"Grant Portfolio: India." *The Global Fund to Fight AIDS, Tuberculosis, and Malaria.* Last modified December 23, 2011. http://portfolio.theglobalfund .org/en/Country/Index/IDA.
Grmek, Mirko D. *History of AIDS: Emergence and Origin of a Modern Pandemic.* Princeton: Princeton University Press, 1990.
Grusky, Oscar, Hong-jie Liu, and Michael Johnston. "HIV/AIDS in China: 1990–2001." *AIDS and Behavior* 6, no. 4 (2002): 381–393.
Gupta, S. P. "Recent Economic Reforms in India and Their Impact on the Poor and Vulnerable Sections of Society." In *Economic Reforms and Poverty Alleviation in India*, edited by C. H. Hanumantha Rao and Hans Linnemann, 126–170. New Delhi: Sage Publications, 1996.
Gupte, Mirko D., Vidya Ramachandran, and R. K. Mutatkar. "Epidemiological Profile of India: Historical and Contemporary Perspectives." *Journal of Biosciences* 26, no. 4 (2001): 437–464.
Hammett, Theodore M., Ryan Kling, Patrick Johnston, Wei Liu, Doan Ngu, Patricia Friedmann, Kieu Thanh Binh, Ha Viet Dong, Van Ly Kieu, Donghua Meng, Yi Chen, and Jarlais Don C. Des. "Patterns of HIV Prevalence and HIV Risk Behaviors among Injection Drug Users Prior to and 24 Months Following Implementation of Cross-Border HIV Prevention Interventions in Northern Vietnam and Southern China." *AIDS Education and Prevention* 18, no. 2 (2006): 97–115.
Han, Meng-jie, Qing-feng Chen, Yang Hao, Yi-fei Hu, Dong-mei Wang, Yan Gao, and Marc Bulterys. "Design and Implementation of a China Comprehensive AIDS Response Program (China CARES), 2003–2008." *International Journal of Epidemiology* 39, Supplementary 2 (2010): 47–55.
Hansen, Lene. "The Little Mermaid's Silent Security Dilemma and the Absence of Gender in the Copenhagen School." *Millennium Journal of International Studies* 29, no. 2 (2000): 285–306.
Hansen, Lene. "The Politics of Securitization and the Muhammad Cartoon Crisis: A Post-Structuralist Perspective." *Security Dialogue* 42, no. 4–5 (2011): 357–369.
Hawkes, Sarah and K. G. Santhya. "Diverse Realities: Sexually Transmitted Infections and HIV in India." *Sexually Transmitted Infections* 78, Supplementary 1 (2002): 31–39.
Hays, J. N. *Epidemics and Pandemics: Their Impacts on Human History.* Santa Barbara, CA: ABC-CLIO, 2005.

Heinecken, Lindy. "Facing a Merciless Enemy: HIV/AIDS and the South African Armed Forces." *Armed Forces and Society* 29, no. 2 (2003): 281–300.
Hernandez, Alexandra L., Christina P. Lindan, Meenakshi Mathur, Maria Ekstrand, Purnima Madhivanan, Ellen S. Stein, Steven Gregorich, Sanjukta Kundu, Alka Gogate, and Hema R. Jerajani. "Sexual Behavior among Men Who Have Sex with Women, Men, and *Hijras* in Mumbai, India—Multiple Sexual Risks." *AIDS and Behavior* 10, Supplementary 1 (2006): 5–16.
"Heroin Movement Worldwide—Southeast Asia." *Central Intelligence Agency*. Last modified December 12, 2008. https://www.cia.gov/library/publications/additional-publications/heroin-movement-worldwide/southeast-asia.html.
Heymann, David L. "Evolving Infectious Disease Threats to National and Global Security." In *Global Health Challenges for Human Security*, edited by Lincoln C. Chen, Jennifer Leaning and Vasant Narasimhan, 105–123. Cambridge, MA: Global Equity Initiative, Asia Center, Harvard University, 2003.
"Hindustan Times: AIDS Infection Rate among Women Rising Alarmingly in Manipur." *Burmanet*. Last modified December 5, 2005. http://www.burmanet.org/news/2005/12/05/hindustan-times-aids-infection-rate-among-women-rising-alarmingly-in-manipur/.
"HIV Estimates in India, 1981–2004." *UNAIDS*. Last modified March 11, 2010. http://www.unaids.org.in/displaymore.asp?page=17&pagenav=title&subitemkey=439&subchkey=0&itemid=322&chname=HIV%20Epidemic%20in%20India&subchnm=.
"HIV/AIDS: China's Titanic Peril." *UNAIDS/WHO*. Last modified June 2002. http://www.hivpolicy.org/Library/HPP000056.pdf.
"HIV and AIDS in Russia, Eastern Europe and Central Asia." *AVERT*. Last modified July 23, 2010. http://www.avert.org/aids-russia.htm.
"HIV and AIDS in the UK." *AVERT*. Accessed May 28, 2012. http://www.avert.org/aids-uk.htm#contentTable0.
"HIV/AIDS in India: An Epidemic of Abuse." *Human Rights Watch*. Last modified July 11, 2002. http://www.hrw.org/en/news/2002/07/09/hivaids-india-epidemic-abuse.
"HIV/AIDS Laws of the World." *Harvard School of Public Health*. Last modified February 2, 2010. http://www.hsph.harvard.edu/population/aids/aids.htm.
"HIV/AIDS Scenario in Delhi." *Delhi State AIDS Control Society*. Last modified May 21, 2010. http://delhi.gov.in/wps/wcm/connect/doit_dsacs/DSACS/Home/HIV+-+AIDS+Scenario/HIV+or+AIDS+Scenario+in+Delhi.
"HIV-AIDS Situation in North Eastern States." *International Studies of HIV/AIDS*. Accessed April 29, 2012. http://medind.nic.in/haa/t04/i1/haat04i1p147.pdf.
Hope, Nicholas C., Anjini Kochar, Roger Noll, and T. N. Srinivasan. "Introduction." In *Economic Reform in India: Challenges, Prospects, and Lessons*, edited by Nicholas C. Hope, Anjini Kochar, Roger Noll, and T. N. Srinivasan, 1–30. Cambridge: Cambridge University Press, 2013.
Howlett, Michael, M. Ramesh, and Anthony Perl. *Studying Public Policy: Policy Cycles and Policy Subsystems*. Toronto: Oxford University Press, 2009.
Hsu, Carolyn. "Beyond Civil Society: An Organizational Perspective on State-NGO Relations in the People's Republic of China." *Journal of Civil Society* 6, no. 3 (2010): 259–277.

Hu, Zhi, Xia Qin, Min-zhen Zhu, Sen Yang, and Xue-jun Zhang. "Epidemiological Characteristics of HIV/AIDS in West China." *International Journal of STD and AIDS* 17, no. 5 (2006): 324–328.

Huang, Yan-zhong. "Asia Unbound: The Global Fund, China, and Civil Society." *Councils on Foreign Relations*. Last modified June 1, 2011. http://blogs.cfr.org/asia/2011/06/01/the-global-fund-china-and-civil-society/.

Huysmans, Jef. "Revisiting Copenhagen: Or, on the Creative Development of a Security Studies Agenda in Europe." *European Journal of International Relations* 4, no. 4 (1998): 479–505.

Hyun, In-taek, Sung-han Kim, and Geun Lee. "Bringing Politics Back in: Globalization, Pluralism, and Securitization in East Asia." In *Studying Non-Traditional Security in Asia: Trends and Issues*, edited by Ralf Emmers, Mely Caballero-Anthony, and Amitav Acharya, 108–128. Singapore: Marshall Cavendish Academic, 2006b.

"India: Country Situation 2009." *UNAIDS*. Accessed December 5, 2011. http://www.unaids.org/ctrysa/ASIIND_en.pdf.

"Indian GDP Annual Growth Rate." *Trading Economic*. Accessed November 21, 2014. http://www.tradingeconomics.com/india/gdp-growth-annual.

Iqbal, Javed Mohammad. "AIDS and the State: A Comparison of Brazil, India and South Africa." *South Asian Survey* 16, no. 1 (2009): 119–135.

Irengbam, Rajeev. "HIV/AIDS in Manipur: Some Issues and Concerns." *Journal of Health and Development* 1, no. 1 (2005): 15–23.

Islam, Anwar and M. Zaffar Tahir. "Health Sector Reform in South Asia: New Challenges and Constraints." *Health Policy* 60, no. 2 (2002): 151–169.

Jackson, Nicole J. "International Organizations, Security Dichotomies and the Trafficking of Persons and Narcotics in Post-Soviet Central Asia: A Critique of the Securitization Framework." *Security Dialogue* 37, no. 3 (2006): 299–317.

Jacob, Happymon. "Impact of HIV/AIDS on Governance in Manipur and Nagaland." *AIDS, Security, and Conflict Initiative Research Report*. Last modified April 2008. http://asci.researchhub.ssrc.org/impact-of-hiv-aids-on-governance-in-manipur-and-nagaland/attachment.

Jayaraman, K. S. "Pool of Infected Women?" *Nature* 321, no. 6066 (1986): 103.

Jia, Man-hong, Hong-bing Luo, Yan-ling Ma, Ning Wang, Kumi Smith, Jiang-yuan Mei, Ran Lu, Ji-yun Lu, Li-ru Fu, Qiang Zhang, Zun-you Wu, and Lin Lu. "The HIV Epidemic in Yunnan Province, China, 1989-2007." *Journal of Acquired Immune Deficiency Syndromes* 53, Supplementary 1 (2010): 34–40.

Jönsson, Kristina. "Issue without Boundaries: HIV/AIDS in Southeast Asia." *Centre for East and South-East Asian Studies, Lund University, Sweden, Working Paper No. 19*. Accessed August 30, 2010. http://www.lu.se/images/Syd_och_sydostasienstudier/working_papers/Jonsson.pdf.

Karnik, Niranjan S. "Locating HIV/AIDS and India: Cautionary Notes on the Globalization of Categories." *Science, Technology, and Human Values* 26, no. 3 (2001): 322–348.

Kanki, Phyllis J. and Myron E. Essex. "Virology." In *The AIDS Pandemic: Impact on Science and Society*, edited by Kenneth H. Mayer and H. F. Pizer, 13–35. New York: Elsevier Academic Press, 2005.

Kapila, Uma. *Indian Economy: Performance and Policies.* New Delhi: Academic Foundation, 2008–2009.
Karlen, Arno. *Plague's Progress: A Social History of Man and Disease.* London: Gollancz, 1995.
Kaufman, Joan. "China: The Intersections between Poverty, Health Inequity, Reproductive Health and HIV/AIDS." *Development* 48, no. 4 (2005): 115–119.
Khan, Akram A. and Nazli Bano. "HIV/AIDS Epidemic in India: A Critical Health and Development Issue." In *Economics of Education and Health in India*, edited by Anil Kumar Thakur and Abdus Salam, 468–492. New Delhi: The Indian Economic Association, 2008.
Khan, Azizur Rahman and Carl Riskin. *Inequality and Poverty in China in the Age of Globalization.* New York: Oxford University Press, 2001.
Kohli, Atul. "Politics of Economic Growth in India, 1980–2005. Part II: The 1990s and beyond." *Economic and Political Weekly.* Last modified April 8, 2006. http://www.newschool.edu/uploadedFiles/TCDS/Democracy_and _Diversity_Institutes/Kohli_PEGI_PartII.pdf.
Kong, T. S. K. "Risk Factors Affecting Condom Use among Male Sex Workers Who Serve Men in China: A Qualitative Study." *Sexually Transmitted Infections* 84, no. 6 (2008): 444–448.
Krause, Keith and Michael C. Williams. "Broadening the Agenda of Security Studies: Politics and Methods." *Mershon International Studies Review* 40, no. 2 (1996): 229–254.
"Kunming HIV/AIDS Prevention and Control Working Report." *Kunming CDC.* Last modified October 2010. http://www.info.gov.hk/aids/rrc/english/lions_ rep/ppt10_08.pdf.
Kumta, Sameer, Mark Lurie, Sherry Weitzen, Hemangi Jerajani, Alka Gogate, Row-kavi Ashok, Vivek Anand, Harvey Makadon, and Kenneth H. Mayer. "Bisexuality, Sexual Risk Taking, and HIV Prevalence among Men Who Have Sex with Men Accessing Voluntary Counseling and Testing Services in Mumbai, India." *Journal of Acquired Immune Deficiency Syndromes* 53, no. 2 (2010): 227–233.
Kuo, Steve Hsu-sung, Su-fen Tsai, and Yen-fang Huang. "Taiwan." In *Fighting a Rising Tide: The Response to AIDS in East Asia*, edited by Tadashi Yamamoto and Satoko Itoh, 226–246. Tokyo: Japan Center for International Exchange, 2006.
Laishram, Sarlima. "Epidemiological Analysis of HIV/AIDS in Manipur." *E-PAO.* Last modified May 30, 2008. http://www.e-pao.net/epSubPage-Extractor.asp?src=education.Health_Issue.Drug_Awareness_Education. Epidemiological_Analysis_of_HIVAIDS.
Lakhashe, Samir, Madhuri Thakar, Sheela Godbole, Srikanth Tripathy, and Ramesh Paranjape. "HIV Infection in India: Epidemiology, Molecular Epidemiology and Pathogenesis." *Journal of Biosciences* 33, no. 4 (2008): 515–525.
Lan, Yu-ching, Tarek Elbeik, JoAnn Dileanis, Valerie Ng, Yen-ju Chen, Hsieh-shong Leu, Shu-hsing Cheng, Jen-chien Wong, Wing-wai Wong, and Yi-ming

A. Chen. "Molecular Epidemiology of HIV-1 Subtypes and Drug Resistant Strains in Taiwan." *Journal of Medical Virology* 80, no. 2 (2008): 183–191.
Lanegran, Kim and Goran Hyden. "Mapping the Politics of AIDS: Illustrations from East Africa." *Population and Environment* 14, no. 3 (1993): 245–263.
Lau, J. T. F., C. Lin, Chun Hao, X. Xu, and J. Gu. "Public Health Challenges of the Emerging HIV Epidemic among Men Who Have Sex with Men in China." *Public Health* 125, no. 5 (2011): 260–265.
Laustsen, Carsten Bagge, and Ole Wæver. "In Defense of Religion: Sacred Referent Objects for Securitization." *Millennium Journal of International Studies* 29, no. 3 (2000): 705–739.
Lawrence, Pareena G. and Maria C. Brun. "NGOs and HIV/AIDS Advocacy in India: Identifying the Challenges." *South Asia: Journal of South Asian Studies* 34, no. 1 (2011): 65–88.
Learning from Our Role in the HIV Response in India: Annual Report 2009–2010. New Delhi: India HIV/AIDS Alliance, Undated.
"Letter to Indian Prime Minister Singh." *Human Rights Watch*. Last modified January 11, 2006. http://www.hrw.org/news/2006/01/09/letter-indian-prime-minister-singh.
Li, Hui, Nana Taona Kuo, Hui Liu, Christine Korhonen, Ellenie Pond, Hao-yan Guo, Liz Smith, Hui Xue, and Jiang-ping Sun. "From Spectators to Implementers: Civil Society Organizations Involved in AIDS Programs in China." *International Journal of Epidemiology* 39, Supplementary 2 (2010): 65–71.
Lieberthal, Kenneth and Michel Oksenberg. *Policy Making in China: Leaders, Structures, and Processes*. Princeton: Princeton University Press, 1988.
"List of Emerging and Re-emerging Diseases." *National Institute of Allergy and Infectious Diseases, National Institutes of Health*. Last modified August 8, 2014 . http://www.niaid.nih.gov/topics/BiodefenseRelated/Biodefense/Pages/CatA.aspx.
Liu, Jenny X. and Kyung Choi. "Experiences of Social Discrimination among Men Who Have Sex with Men in Shanghai, China." *AIDS and Behavior* 10, Supplementary 1 (2006): 25–33.
Liu, Xiao-hua. "NGOs in China: An Overview." *International Community Foundation*. Last modified September 2002. www.icfdn.org/publications/NGOsinChina-ICFWhitePaper.doc.
Liu, Yuan Li. "China's Public Health-Care System: Facing the Challenges." *Bulletin of the World Health Organization* 82, no. 7 (2004): 532–538.
Liu, Zhi-min, Zhi Lian, and Cheng-zheng Zhao. "Drug Use and HIV/AIDS in China." *Drug and Alcohol Review* 25, no. 2 (2006): 173–175.
Lo, Catherine Yuk-ping and Nicholas Thomas. "How Is Health a Security Issue? Politics, Responses and Issues." *Health Policy and Planning* 25, no. 6 (2010): 447–453.
Lu, Yi-yi. "The Autonomy of Chinese NGOs: A New Perspective." *China: An International Journal* 5, no. 2 (2007): 173–203.
Lu, Yi-yi. "The Limitations of NGOs: A Preliminary Study of Non-Governmental Social Welfare Organizations in China." *CCS International Working Paper 13*.

Accessed February 6, 2012. http://eprints.lse.ac.uk/29218/1/IWP13LuYiyi.pdf.
Lu, Lin, Man-hong Jia, Yan-ling Ma, Li Yang, Zhiwei Chen, David D. Ho, Yan Jiang, and Lin-qi Zhang. "The Changing Face of HIV in China." *Nature* 455, no. 7213 (2008): 609–611.
Lu, Lin, Yu-xia Fang, and Xi Wang. "Drug Abuse in China: Past, Present and Future." *Cellular and Molecular Neurobiology* 28, no. 4 (2008): 479–490.
Ma, Qiu-sha. "Defining Chinese Nongovernmental Organizations." *Voluntas: International Journal of Voluntary and Nonprofit Organizations* 13, no. 2 (2002): 113–130.
Mackerras, Colin. "Critical Social Issues." In *Critical Issues in Contemporary China*, edited by Czeslaw Tubilewicz, 193–226. London: Routledge and Hong Kong: Open University of Hong Kong Press, 2006.
Maclean, Sandra J. "Microbes, Mad Cows and Militaries: Exploring the Links between Health and Security." *Security Dialogue* 39, no. 5 (2008): 475–494.
Mahtaney, Piya. *India, China and Globalization: The Emerging Superpower and the Future of Economic Development*. Great Britain: Palgrave Macmillan, 2007.
Malini, Daniel. "AIDS in India: Denial and Disaster." *Harvard International Review* 25, no. 2 (2003): 9–10.
"Mapping the Global Future: Report of the National Intelligence Council's 2020 Project." *National Intelligence Council*. Accessed May 28, 2012. http://www.dni.gov/nic/NIC_globaltrend2020_s2.html.
Marshall, Martin N. "Sampling for Qualitative Research." *Family Practice* 13, no. 6 (1996): 522–525.
Mathews, Jessica Tuchman. "Redefining Security." *Foreign Affairs* 68, no. 2 (1989): 162–177.
Matsumoto, David. *Cultural Influences on Research Methods and Statistics*. Pacific Grove, CA: Brooks/Cole Publishing Company, 1994.
Mbeki, Thabo. "Speech of the Opening of the 13th International AIDS Conference, Durban." *JournAIDS*. Last modified July 9, 2000. http://www.southafrica-newyork.net/consulate/aidsspeech.htm.
McDonald, Matt. "Securitization and the Construction of Security." *European Journal of International Relations* 14, no. 4 (2008): 563–587.
McInnes, Colin. "HIV/AIDS and Security." *International Affairs* 82, no. 2 (2006): 315–326.
McInnes, Colin and Kelley Lee. "Health, Security and Foreign Policy." *Review of International Studies* 32, no. 1 (2006): 5–23.
McInnes, Colin and Simon Rushton. "HIV/AIDS and Securitization Theory." *European Journal of International Relations* 19, no. 1 (2013): 115-138.
McInnes, Colin and Simon Rushton. "HIV, AIDS and Security: Where Are We Now?" *International Affairs* 86, no. 1 (2010): 225–245.
Mitra, Pramit. "India at the Crossroads: Battling the HIV/AIDS Pandemic." *The Washington Quarterly* 27, no. 4 (2004): 95–107.
Mitra, Pramit, Vibhuti Haté, and Teresita Schaffer. "India: Fitting HIV/AIDS into a Public Health Strategy." *Center for Strategic and International*

Studies. Last modified November 2007. http://csis.org/files/media/csis/pubs/071120_india__hivaids_public_health_strategy.pdf.

Möller, Frank. "Photographic Interventions in Post-9/11 Security Policy." *Security Dialogue* 38, no. 2 (2007): 179–196.

"Monitoring the UNGASS Goals of Sexual and Reproductive Health in the Context of HIV/AIDS: India Country Report." *The Cell for AIDS Research Action and Training, Tata Institute of Social Sciences, Mumbai, India*. Last modified February 2008. http://ungassforum.files.wordpress.com/2008/02/ungass-india-report.pdf.

Morrison, J. Stephen and Bates Gill. "Averting a Full-Blown HIV/AIDS Epidemic in China." *Center for Strategic and International Studies*. Last modified February 2003. http://csis.org/files/media/csis/pubs/0302_avertepidemicchina.pdf.

Morrison, J. Stephen and Todd Summers. "United to Fight HIV/AIDS?" *The Washington Quarterly*. Accessed January 30, 2012. http://www.twq.com/03autumn/docs/03autumn_morrison.pdf.

Murphy, Thérèse and Noel Whitty. "Is Human Rights Prepared? Risk, Rights and Public Health Emergencies." *Medical Law Review* 17, no. 2 (2009): 219–244.

"NACO Newsletter." *National AIDS Control Organization*. Last modified October-December 2009. http://www.nacoonline.org/upload/IEC%20Division/NACO_Newsletter%20(%20Oct-Dec)%202009%20English.pdf.

"National AIDS Control Organization." *National AIDS Control Organization*. Accessed March 4, 2010. http://www.nacoonline.org/About_NACO/.

"National AIDS Prevention and Control Policy." *National AIDS Control Organization*. Last modified April 15, 2003. http://www.hsph.harvard.edu/population/aids/india.aids.02.pdf.

"National Center for AIDS/STD Control and Prevention." *China Center for Disease Control*. Accessed February 24, 2010. http://www.chinaids.org.cn/n443289/n443290/n447111/index.html.

"National Common Minimum Program." *Government of India*. Last modified May 2004. http://pmindia.nic.in/cmp.pdf.

"National Program Office of China Global Fund AIDS Program (Round 6)." *NCAIDS, China CDC*. Accessed December 19, 2011. http://www.chinaaids.cn/n443289/n443290/n447113/n447525/n457450/index.html.

"National Rural Health Mission (2005–2012) Mission Document." *Ministry of Health and Family Welfare, Government of India*. Accessed May 17, 2010. http://www.mohfw.nic.in/NRHM/Documents/Mission_Document.pdf.

"National Rural Health Mission Framework for Implementation (2005–2012)." *Ministry of Health and Family Welfare, Government of India*. Accessed May 11, 2010. http://mohfw.nic.in/NRHM/Documents/NRHM_Framework_Latest.pdf.

Neack, Laura. *Elusive Security: States First, People Last*. Lanham, MD: Rowman and Littlefield Publishers Inc, 2007.

"New HIV Rate in China Climbs Over 10% in First 10 Months of 2012," *International AIDS Society*, December 3, 2012, accessed January 31, 2015, https://www.iasociety.org/Default.aspx?pageId=5&elementId=14868.

Newman, Edward. "Critical Human Security Studies." *Review of International Studies* 36, no. 1 (2010): 77–94.
Newman, Edward. "Human Security and Constructivism." *International Studies Perspectives* 2, no. 3 (2001): 239–251.
"NGO/CBO Operational Guidelines—Section." *National AIDS Control Organization.* Last modified April 10, 2007. http://upsacs.nic.in/ti%20documents/NGO%20CBO%20Operational%20Guidelines.pdf.
"NGO Perspectives on the Global Fund." *International Council of AIDS Service Organizations.* Last modified June 2004. http://www.hivpolicy.org/Library/HPP000321.pdf.
Ngok, King Lun. "Redefining Development in China: Towards a New Policy Paradigm for the New Century?" In *Changing Governance and Public Policy in East Asia*, edited by Ka Ho Mok and Ray Forrest, 49–66. London: Routledge, 2009.
O'Manique, Colleen. "The 'Securitization' of HIV/AIDS in Sub-Saharan Africa: A Critical Feminist Lens." *Policy and Society* 24, no. 1 (2005): 24–47.
"On Ten Major Relationships." *Selected Works of Mao Tse-tong.* Accessed November 6. 2014. https://www.marxists.org/reference/archive/mao/selected-works/volume-5/mswv5_51.htm.
"On the Frontline of Northeast India." *Transnational Institute.* Last modified March 2011. http://www.tni.org/sites/www.tni.org/files/download/On%20the%20Frontline%20of%20Northeast%20India.pdf.
Orbinski, James. "Global Health, Social Movements, and Governance." In *Governing Global Health: Challenge, Response, Innovation*, edited by Andrew F. Cooper, John J. Kirton, and Ted Schrecker, 29–40. England: Ashgate Publishing Limited, 2007.
Ostergard, Robert L. "HIV/AIDS, State Capacity, and the Threat to National and International Security: A Theoretical Overview." In *HIV/AIDS and the Threat to National and International Security*, edited by Robert L. Ostergard, 65–76. London: Palgrave Macmillan, 2007.
Over, Mead, Peter Heywood, Julian Gold, Indrani Gupta, Subhash Hira, and Elliot Marseille. *HIV/AIDS Treatment and Prevention in India: Modeling the Cost and Consequences.* Washington, DC: The World Bank, 2004.
"Over 70% of the HIV Infected in Beijing Are Immigrants; Lower Criteria for Eligibility to MMT to Be Piloted." *NCAIDS, China CDC.* Last modified June 22, 2010. http://www.chinaids.org.cn/n1971/n2091/439308.html.
"Overview: An Agenda for the Social Summit." *Human Development Report 1994, United Nations Development Program.* Accessed September 24, 2009. http://hdr.undp.org/en/media/hdr_1994_en_overview.pdf.
"Overview of Civil Society Organizations: India." *Asian Development Bank.* Last modified June 1, 2009. http://www.adb.org/sites/default/files/pub/2009/CSB-IND.pdf.
"Overview of HIV and AIDS in India." *AVERT.* Last modified October 29, 2009. http://www.avert.org/aidsindia.htm.
Pai, Sanjay A. "Agencies Disagree on AIDS Deaths Rates for India." *The Lancet Infectious Diseases* 2, no. 4 (2002): 199.

Panagariya, Arvind. "India: The Crisis in Rural Health Care." *Brookings*. Last modified January 24, 2008. http://www.brookings.edu/opinions/2008/0124 _health_care_panagariya.aspx.
Pandey, Arvind, Dandu C. S. Reddy, Peter D. Ghys, Mariamma Thomas, Damodar Sahu, Madhulekha Bhattacharya, Kanchan D. Maiti, Fred Arnold, Shashi Kant, Ajay Khera, and Renu Garg. "Improved Estimates of India's HIV Burden in 2006." *Indian Journal of Medical Research* 129, no. 1 (2009): 50–58.
Patil, Ashok Vikhe, K. V. Somasundaram, and R. C. Coyal. "Current Health Scenario in Rural India." *Australian Journal of Rural Health* 10, no. 2 (2002):129–135.
Peters, David H., K. Sujatha Rao, and Robert Fryatt. "Lumping and Splitting: The Health Policy Agenda in India." *Health Policy and Planning* 18, no. 3 (2003): 249–260.
Piot, Peter, Richard G. A. Feachem, Jong-wook Lee, and James D. Wolfensohn. "A Global Response to AIDS: Lessons Learned, Next Steps." *Science* 304, no. 5679 (2004): 1909–1910.
"PM's Address at the National Students and Youth Parliament Special Session on HIV/AIDS." *Government of India*. Last modified November 7, 2004. http:// pmindia.nic.in/speech/content.asp?id=44.
Policy Brief. New Delhi: Indian HIV/AIDS Alliance, Undated.
"Political Declaration on HIV/AIDS." *United Nations General Assembly*. Last modified June 15, 2006. http://data.unaids.org/pub/Report/2006 /20060615_hlm_politicaldeclaration_ares60262_en.pdf.
"Political Declaration on HIV/AIDS: Intensifying Our Efforts to Eliminate HIV/ AIDS." *United Nations General Assembly*. Last modified June 8, 2011. http:// daccess-dds-ny.un.org/doc/UNDOC/LTD/N11/367/84/PDF/N1136784 .pdf?OpenElement.
Porapakkham, Yaowarat, Somjai Pramarnpol, Supatra Athibhoddhi, and Richard Bernhard. "The Evolution of HIV/AIDS Policy in Thailand: 1984–1994." *United States Agency for International Development*. Accessed August 2, 2010. http://pdf.usaid.gov/pdf_docs/PNACG546.pdf.
Prabhu, K. Seeta, "The Impact of Structural Adjustment on Social Sector Expenditure: Evidence from Indian States." In *Economic Reforms and Poverty Alleviation in India*, edited by C. H. Hanumantha Rao and Hans Linnemann, 228–254. New Delhi: Sage Publications, 1996.
"Premier Wen Vows More Aid to AIDS Patients." *NCAIDS, China CDC*. Last modified December 1, 2011. http://www.chinaaids.cn/n1971/n2091/729286 .html.
"Preventing HIV/AIDS in India." *The World Bank*. Last modified June 2005. http://siteresources.worldbank.org/INTINDIA/Resources/HIV-AIDS-brief -June2005-IN.pdf.
"Prime Minister's Speech at the 58th UN General Assembly." *Embassy of India*. Last modified September 25, 2003. http://www.indianembassy.org/pic/pm /vajpayee/pm_sept_25_03.htm.

Prins, Gwyn. "AIDS and Global Security." *International Affairs* 80, no. 5 (2004): 931–952.
"Progress Made in HIV/AIDS Campaign." *NCAIDS, China CDC*. Last modified November 25, 2011. http://www.chinaaids.cn/n1971/n2091/727369.html.
"Progress on Global Access to HIV Antiretroviral Therapy: A Report on '3 by 5' and Beyond." *WHO/UNAIDS*. Last modified March 2006. http://www.who.int/hiv/fullreport_en_highres.pdf.
"Project Performance Assessment Report." *The World Bank*. Last modified July 2, 2003. http://lnweb90.worldbank.org/OED/oeddoclib.nsf/Doc UNIDViewForJavaSearch/CF5907844F56853D85256D900073CB1D/$file /India_PPAR_26224.pdf.
Putin, Vladimir. "Opening Remarks at State Council Presidium Meeting on Urgent Measures to Combat the Spread of HIV-AIDS in the Russian Federation." *Official Web Portal: President of Russia*. Last modified April 21, 2006. http://archive.kremlin.ru/eng/text/speeches/2006/04/21/2148_type 82912type82913_104797.shtml#.
Qian, Han-zhu, Joseph E. Schumacher, Huey T. Chen, and Yu-hua Ruan. "Injection Drug Use and HIV/AIDS in China: Review of Current Situation, Prevention and Policy Implications." *Harm Reduction Journal* 3, no. 4 (2006): 1–8.
Qian, Z. H., Sten H. Vermund, and N. Wang. "Risk of HIV/AIDS in China: Subpopulations of Special Importance." *Sexually Transmitted Infections* 81, no. 6 (2005): 442–447.
"Race for HIV Cure Overshadows Prevention, Says Expert." *Aids Cure*. Last modified February 19, 2009. http://aidscure-top.blogspot.com/2009/02/race-for -hiv-cure-overshadows.html.
Rai, Mohammad A., Haider J. Warraich, Syed H. Ali, and Vivek R. Nerurkar. "HIV/AIDS in Pakistan: The Battle Begins." *Retrovirology* 4, no. 22 (2007): 1–3.
Raman, Jaishankar. "A Comparison of the Economic Reform Experiences in China and India." In *Economic Development in India and China: New Perspectives on Progress and Change*, edited by Penelope B. Prime and Kishore G. Kulkarni, 97–113. New Delhi: Serials Publications, 2007.
Ramiah, Ilavenil. "Securitizing the AIDS Issue in Asia." In *Non-Traditional Security in Asia: Dilemmas in Securitization*, edited by Mely Caballero-Anthony, Ralf Emmers, and Amitav Acharya, 136–167. England: Ashgate Publishing Limited, 2006a.
Rao, Arni S. R. Srinivasa, Kurien Thomas, Kurapati Sudhakar, and Philip K. Maini. "HIV/AIDS Epidemic in India and Predicting the Impact of the National Response: Mathematical Modeling and Analysis." *Mathematical Biosciences and Engineering* 6, no. 4 (2009): 779–813.
Rao, M. Govinda and Mita Choudhury. "Health Care Financing Reforms in India." *National Institute of Public Finance and Policy*. Accessed March 2012. http://www.nipfp.org.in/media/medialibrary/2013/04/wp_2012_100.pdf.
"Rape for Profit: Trafficking of Nepali Girls and Women to India's Brothels." *Human Rights Watch*. Last modified October 1995. http://www.hrw.org /reports/1995/India.htm.

"Report of The Health Survey and Development Committee." *Government of India*. Accessed May 12, 2014. http://nihfw.org/NDC/DocumentationServices/Reports/bhore%20Committee%20Report%20VOL-1%20.pdf.
"Report of the Working Group on Medical Education." *National Knowledge Commission*. Accessed May 12, 2010. http://www.knowledgecommission.gov.in/downloads/documents/wg_med.pdf.
"Resolution on NRHM." *National Rural Health Mission*. Last modified February 29, 2008. http://mohfw.nic.in/NRHM/RESOLUTIONon%20NRHM.htm.
"Restrictions on AIDS Activists in China." *Human Rights Watch*. Last modified June 2005. http://www.hrw.org/en/reports/2005/06/14/restrictions_aids_activists_china.
"Restrictions on AIDS NGOs in Asia." *Asia Catalysts*. Last modified December 1, 2009. http://www.asiacatalyst.org/news/restrictionsAIDSngos1209.pdf.
"Rising Powers: The Changing Geopolitical Landscape." *Mapping the Global Future: Report of the National Intelligence Council's 2020 Project, National Intelligence Council*. Accessed March 5, 2010. http://www.dni.gov/nic/NIC_globaltrend2020_s2.html.
Rollet, Vincent. "Taiwanese NGOs and HIV/AIDS: From the National to the Transnational." *China Perspectives* 60, (2005): 1–17.
Rotnem, Thomas E. and Tinaz Pavri. "The HIV/AIDS Pandemic in Comparative Perspective: The Cases of India and Russia." Paper presented at the Georgia Political Science Association, Conference Proceedings, 2006.
"Rural Health Care System in India." *Bulletin on Rural Health Statistics in India*. Last modified March 2008. http://www.mohfw.nic.in/Bulletin%20on%20RHS%20-%20March,%202008%20-%20PDF%20Version/Rural%20Health%20Care%20System%20in%20India.pdf.
Rushton, Simon. "AIDS and International Security in the United Nations System." *Health Policy and Planning* 25, no. 6 (2010): 495–504.
Rushton, Simon. "Securitizing HIV/AIDS: Pandemics, Politics and SCR 1308." Paper presented at the International Studies Association Convention, Chicago, 2007.
Rushton, Simon. "The Development of the HIV/AIDS and Security Discourse: The Role of CSOs." Paper presented at Peter Wall Institute's London Workshop on Civil Society Organizations and Global Health Governance, October 2007.
"Russian Government Commission." *Government of the Russian Federation*. Accessed August 30, 2010. http://www.government.ru/eng/gov/agencies/154/.
Ryan, Frank. *Virus X: Tracking the New Killer Plagues: Out of the Present and into the Future*. Boston: Little, Brown and Company, 1997.
Sahni, A. K., V. V. S. P. Prasad, and P. Seth. "Genomic Diversity of Human Immunodeficiency Virus Type-1 in India." *International Journal of STD and AIDS* 13, no. 2 (2002): 115–118.
Saich, Tony. *Governance and Politics of China*. Basingstoke: Palgrave Macmillan, 2004.
Salter, Mark B. "Securitization and Desecuritization: A Dramaturgical Analysis of the Canadian Air Transport Security Authority." *Journal of International Relations and Development* 11, no. 4 (2008): 321–349.

Salter, Mark B. "When Securitization Fails: The Hard Case of Counter-Terrorism Programs." In *Securitization Theory: How Security Problems Emerge and Dissolve*, edited by Thierry Balzacq, 116–132. London: Routledge, 2011.
Sarkar, S., N. Das, S. Panda, T. N. Naik, K. Sarkar, B.C. Singh, J. M. Ralte, S. M. Aier, and S. P. Tripathy. "Rapid Spread of HIV among Injecting Drug Users in North-Eastern States of India." *Bulletin on Narcotics* 45, no. 1 (1993): 91–105.
Seckinelgin, Hakan. *International Politics of HIV/AIDS: Global Disease—Local Pain*. London: Routledge, 2008.
"Securitization: What Makes Something a Security Threat." *Megalinks in Criminal Justice*. Last modified October 25, 2008. http://www.apsu.edu/oconnort/GSS2010/GSS2010lect01a.htm.
Selgelid, Michael J. and Christian Enemark. "Infectious Diseases, Security and Ethics: The Case of HIV/AIDS." *Bioethics* 22, no. 9 (2008): 457–465.
Seth, Pradeep. "The Situation of HIV/M. Tuberculosis Co-infection in India." *The Open Infectious Disease Journal* 5, Supplementary 1-M5 (2011): 51–59.
Settle, Edmund. "AIDS in China: An Annotated Chronology 1985–2003." *China AIDS Survey*. Last modified November 14, 2003. http://portal.unesco.org/education/en/file_download.php/82b973698fcdf215528d63d2b6796087AIDSchron_111603.pdf.
Shah, Duru, Safala Shroff, and Kedar Ganla. "HIV in Pregnancy in the City of Mumbai." *Bombay Hospital Journal*. Accessed May 5, 2012. http://bhj.org/journal/2000_4201_jan00/original_112.htm.
Sharma, Dinesh C. "India's Free Antiretroviral Program Gets Off to Slow Start." *The Lancet* 363, no. 9416 (2004): 1205.
Sharma, Mukta, Samiran Panda, Umesh Sharma, Haobam Nanao Singh, Charanjit Sharma, and Rajkumar Raju Singh. "Five Years of Needle Syringe Exchange in Manipur, India: Program and Contextual Issues." *International Journal of Drug Policy* 14, no. 5–6 (2003): 407–415.
Shen, Jie and Dong-bao Yu. "Governmental Policies on HIV Infection in China." *Cell Research* 15, no. 11–2 (2005): 903–907.
Sheng, Lei and Wu-kui Cao. "HIV/AIDS Epidemiology and Prevention in China." *Chinese Medical Journal* 121, no. 13 (2008): 1230–1236.
Shi, Lei Yu. "Health Care in China: A Rural-Urban Comparison after the Socioeconomic Reforms." *Bulletin of the World Health Organization* 71, no. 6 (1993): 723–736.
Shinde, Santosh, Setia Maninder Singh, Row-Kavi Ashok, Vivek Anand, and Hemangi Jerajani. "Male Sex Workers: Are We Ignoring a Risk Group in Mumbai, India?" *Indian Journal of Dermatology, Venereology and Leprology* 75, no. 1 (2009): 41–46.
Shnayerson, Michael and Mark J. Plotkin. *The Killers Within: The Deadly Rise of Drug-Resistant Bacteria*. New York: Little, Brown and Company, 2002.
Singh, T. N. and H. L. Singh. "HIV/AIDS Wasting Syndrome in Manipur—A Case Report." *Kathmandu University Medical Journal* 3, no. 4 (2005): 425–427.
Singhal, Arvind and Everett M. Rogers. *Combating AIDS: Communication Strategies in Action*. New Delhi: Sage Publications, 2003.

Sjöstedt, Roxanna. "Exploring the Construction of Threats: The Securitization of HIV/AIDS in Russia." *Security Dialogue* 39, no. 1 (2008): 7–29.
Sjöstedt, Roxanna. "Health Issues and Securitization: The Construction of HIV/AIDS as a US National Security Threat." In *Securitization Theory: How Security Problems Emerge and Dissolve*, edited by Thierry Balzacq, 150–169. London: Routledge, 2011.
Smallman-Raynor, Matthew R., and Andrew D. Cliff. *War Epidemics: An Historical Geography of Infectious Diseases in Military Conflict and Civil Strife, 1850–2000*. New York: Oxford University Press, 2004.
Smith, Julia H. and Alan Whiteside. "The History of AIDS Exceptionalism." *Journal of The International AIDS Society* 13, no. 47 (2010): 1–8.
Solomon, S., S. S. Solomon, and A. K. Ganesh. "AIDS in India." *Post Graduate Medical Journal* 82, no. 971 (2006): 545–547.
"South Africa's Top Twelve AIDS Dissidents." *Democratic Alliance*. Last modified August 9, 2010. http://www.da.org.za/docs/612/Top12AIDSDissidents_document.pdf.
"Speech by Executive Vice Minister of Health, Mr. Gao Qiang, at the HIV/AIDS High-Level Meeting of the UN General Assembly." *Permanent Mission of the People's Republic of China to the UN*. Last modified September 22, 2003. http://www.china-un.org/eng/lhghyywj/ldhy/previousga/58/t28511.htm.
"State Council Notice on Strengthening HIV/AIDS Prevention and Control." *NCAIDS, China CDC*. Last modified March 16, 2004. http://www.chinaaids.cn/n1971/n2301/n8034/32205.html.
Steinbrook, Robert. "HIV in India—A Complex Epidemic." *The New England Journal of Medicine* 356, no. 11 (2007): 1089–1093.
Sternberg, Steve. "In India, Sex Trade Fuels HIV's Spread." *USA Today*. Last modified February 24, 2005. http://www.usatoday.com/news/health/2005-02-23-aids-india-cover_x.htm.
Stones, William, and Saseendran Pallikadavath. "HIV and AIDS in India: Will the Next 20 Years Be Different?" *Harvard Health Policy Review* 7, no. 2 (2006): 112–124.
StØre, Jonas Gahr, Jonathan Welch, and Lincoln Chen. "Health and Security for a Global Century." In *Global Health Challenges for Human Security*, edited by Lincoln C. Chen, Jennifer Leaning, and Vasant Narasimhan, 67–84. Cambridge, MA: Global Equity Initiative, Asia Center, Harvard University, 2003.
Stritzel, Holger. "Towards a Theory of Securitization: Copenhagen and Beyond." *European Journal of International Relations* 13, no. 3 (2007): 357–383.
Suhrke, Astri. "Human Security and the Interests of States." *Security Dialogue* 30, no. 3 (1999): 265–276.
Sullivan, Sheena G. and Zun-you Wu. "Rapid Scale Up of Harm Reduction in China." *International Journal of Drug Policy* 18, no. 2 (2007): 118–128.
"Table 6: Command over Resources, The Rise of the South: Human Progress in a Diverse World." *United Nations Development Program*. Last modified March 14, 2013. http://www.undp.org/content/dam/undp/library/corporate/HDR/2013GlobalHDR/English/HDR2013%20Report%20English.pdf.

"Targeted Interventions under NACP-III: Core High Risk Groups." *National AIDS Control Organization, Government of India*. Last modified October 2007. http://www.nacoonline.org/upload/Policies%20&%20Guidelines/27,%20 NACP-III.pdf.

"Thailand's Response to HIV/AIDS: Progress and Challenges." *United Nations Development Program*. Accessed August 2, 2010. http://www.undp.or.th /download/HIV_AIDS_FullReport_ENG.pdf.

"The National AIDS Control Program (1, 2, 3)." *InfoChange News and Features*. Last modified March 2008. http://www.hivaidsonline.in/index.php/Response /the-national-aids-control-programme-1-2-3.html.

"The Paris Declaration." *ParisAIDS Summit*. Last modified December 1, 1994. http:// data.unaids.org/pub/externaldocument/2007/theparisdeclaration_en.pdf.

"The Top 10 Causes of Death." *World Health Organization*. Last modified May 2014. http://www.who.int/mediacentre/factsheets/fs310/en/.

Thiesmeyer, Lynn. "Gender, Public Health, and Human Security Policy in Asia." *United Nations: Division for the Advancement of Women*. Last modified October 28, 2005. http://www.un.org/womenwatch/daw/egm/enabling -environment2005/docs/EGM-WPD-EE-2005-EP_2_%20L_Thiesmeyer. pdf.

Thomas, Nicholas and William T. Tow. "The Utility of Human Security: Sovereignty and Humanitarian Intervention." *Security Dialogue* 33, no. 2 (2002): 177–192.

Thompson, Drew and Xiao-qing Lu. "China's Evolving Civil Society: From Environment to Health." *Woodrow Wilson International Center for Scholars*. Accessed February 15, 2012. http://208elmp02.blackmesh.com/sites/default /files/CEF_Feature.2.pdf.

Tickner, J. Ann. "Re-Visioning Security." In *International Relations Theory Today*, edited by Ken Booth and Steve Smith, 175–197. London: Polity Press, 1995.

Tovanabutra, Sodsai, Deborah L. Birx, and Francine E. McCutchan, "Molecular Epidemiology of HIV in Asia and the Pacific." In *AIDS in Asia*, edited by Lu Yi Chen and Max Essex, 181–206. New York: Kluwer Academic/Plenum Publishers, 2004.

Trombetta, Maria Julia. "Rethinking the Securitization of the Environment: Old Beliefs, New Insights." In *Securitization Theory: How Security Problems Emerge and Dissolve*, edited by Thierry Balzacq, 135–149. London: Routledge, 2011.

Twigg, Judyth. "HIV/AIDS in Russia: Commitment, Resources, Momentum, Challenges." *Center for Strategic and International Studies*. Last modified October 2007. http://csis.org/files/media/csis/pubs/071016_russiahivaids.pdf.

Ullman, Richard H. "Redefining Security." *International Security* 8, no. 1 (1983): 129–153.

"UN Security Council Resolution 1308 (2000) on the Responsibility of the Security Council in the Maintenance of International Peace and Security: HIV/AIDS and International Peace-Keeping Operations." *United Nation Security Council*. Last modified July 17, 2000. http://data.unaids.org/pub /BaseDocument/2000/20000717_un_scresolution_1308_en.pdf.

"UNAIDS Outlook Report 2010." *UNAIDS*. Last modified July 2010. http://data.unaids.org/pub/Outlook/2010/20100713_outlook_report_web_en.pdf.
"Understanding Vaccines." *National Institute of Allergy and Infectious Diseases, National Institutes of Health*. Last modified January 2008. http://www3.niaid.nih.gov/topics/vaccines/PDF/undvacc.pdf.
"UNGASS Country Progress Report 2010: India." *National AIDS Control Organization*. Last modified March 31, 2010. http://data.unaids.org/pub/Report/2010/india_2010_country_progress_report_en.pdf.
van Stuijvenberg, Pieter A. "Structural Adjustment in India—What About Poverty Alleviation?" In *Economic Reforms and Poverty Alleviation in India*, edited by C. H. Hanumantha Rao and Hans Linnemann, 31–89. New Delhi: Sage Publications, 1996.
"Varro, On Agriculture (1st century BCE)." *Catena: Digital Archive of Historic Gardens Landscapes*. Accessed April 11, 2012. http://catena.bgc.bard.edu/texts/varro.htm.
Vaughn, Jocelyn. "The Unlikely Securitizer: Humanitarian Organizations and the Securitization of Indistinctiveness." *Security Dialogue* 40, no. 3 (2009): 263–285.
Vieira, Marco Antonio. "The Securitization of the HIV/AIDS Epidemic as a Norm: A Contribution to Constructivist Scholarship on the Emergence and Diffusion of International Norms." *Brazilian Political Science Review* 1, no. 2 (2007): 137–181.
Vuori, Juha A. "A Timely Prophet? The Doomsday Clock as a Visualization of Securitization Moves with a Global Referent Object." *Security Dialogue* 41, no. 3 (2010): 255–277.
Vuori, Juha A. "Illocutionary Logic and Strands of Securitization: Applying the Theory of Securitization to the Study of Non-Democratic Political Orders." *European Journal of International Relations* 14, no. 1 (2008): 65–99.
Wæver, Ole. "Aberystwyth, Paris, Copenhagen: New 'Schools' in Security Theory and Their Origins between Core and Periphery." Paper presented at the annual meeting for the International Studies Association, Montreal, March 17–20, 2004.
Wæver, Ole. "Securitization: Taking Stock of a Research Program in Security Studies." Unpublished draft, 2003: 1–36.
Wæver, Ole. "Securitization and Desecuritization." In *On Security*, edited by Ronnie D. Lipschutz, 46–86. New York: Columbia University Press, 1995.
Wæver, Ole. "Securitizing Sectors? Reply to Eriksson." *Cooperation and Conflict* 34, no. 3 (1999): 334–340.
Wæver, Ole. "Security, Insecurity and Asecurity in the West European Non-War Community." In *Security Communities*, edited by Emanuel Adler and Michael N. Barnett, 69–118. Cambridge: Cambridge University Press, 1998.
Wæver, Ole. "The EU as a Security Actor: Reflections from a Pessimistic Constructivist on Post-Sovereign Security Orders." In *International Relations Theory and the Politics of European Integration*, edited by Morten Kelstrup and Michael C. Williams, 250–294. London: Routledge, 2000.

Wajda, Patricia K. "AIDS." In *A Comparative Perspective on Major Social Problems*, edited by Rita J. Simon, 201–244. Lanham, MD: Lexington Books, 2001.
Walt, Stephen M. "Rigor or Rigor Mortis? Rational Choice and Security Studies." In *Rational Choice and Security Studies: Stephen Walt and His Critics*, edited by Michael Edward Brown, Owen R. Coté, Sean M. Lynn-Jones, and Steven E. Miller, 1–44. London: The MIT Press, 2000.
Walt, Stephen M. "The Renaissance of Security Studies." *International Studies Quarterly* 35, no. 2 (1991): 211–240.
Walters, Mark Jerome. *Six Modern Plagues and How We Are Causing Them*. Washington DC: Island Press/Shearwater Books, 2003.
Wan, Yan-hai and Xiao-rong Li. "Consequences of a Stalled Response: Iatrogenic Epidemic among Blood Donors in Central China." In *Public Health and Human Rights: Evidence-Based Approaches*, edited by Chris Beyrer and Hank F. Pizer, 65–87. Baltimore: The Johns Hopkins University Press, 2007.
Wang, Gui-ying. "Gao Qiang Set Requirements for Future Response to HIV/AIDS in China." *NCAIDS/China CDC*. Accessed February 22, 2012. http://www.chinaaids.cn/n1971/n2091/111203.html.
Wang, Shao Guang. "Uneven Economic Development." In *Critical Issues in Contemporary China*, edited by Czeslaw Tubilewicz, 79–112. London: Routledge and Hong Kong: Open University of Hong Kong Press, 2006.
Wee, Sui-lee. "Cutting AIDS Funding to China a Big Mistake: UNAIDS." *Canada.com*. Last modified July 11, 2011. http://www2.canada.com/topics/lifestyle/parenting/story.html?id=5083992.
Wenzel, Friedemann, Fouad Bendimerad, and Ravi Sinha. "Megacities—Megarisks." *Natural Hazards* 42, no. 3 (2007): 481–491.
Whiteside, Alan, Alex de Waal, and Tsadkan Gebre-Tensae. "AIDS, Security and the Military in Africa: A Sober Appraisal." *African Affairs* 105, no. 419 (2006): 201–218.
Wilkinson, Claire. "The Copenhagen School on Tour in Kyrgyzstan: Is Securitization Theory Useable Outside Europe?" *Security Dialogue* 38, no. 1 (2007): 5–25.
"Will Balbir Pasha Get AIDS? Case Study: An Innovative Approach to Reduce HIV/AIDS Prevalence through Targeted Mass Media Communications in Mumbai, India." *Population Services International*. Last modified May 2003. http://pdf.usaid.gov/pdf_docs/PNADE789.pdf.
Williams, Michael C. "The Continuing Evolution of Securitization Theory." In *Securitization Theory: How Security Problems Emerge and Dissolve*, edited by Thierry Balzacq, 212–222. London: Routledge, 2011.
Williams, Michael C. "Words, Images, Enemies: Securitization and International Politics." *International Studies Quarterly* 47, no. 4 (2003): 511–531.
Wishnick, Elizabeth. "The Securitization of Chinese Migration to the Russian Far East: Rhetoric and Reality." In *Security and Migration in Asia: The Dynamics of Securitization*, edited by Melissa G. Curley and Siu-lun Wong, 83–99. London: Routledge, 2008.
Wolfensohn, James D. *Voice for the World's Poor: Selected Speeches and Writings of World Bank President James D. Wolfensohn*. Washington DC: The World Bank, 2005.

"World Malaria Report 2011." *World Health Organization.* Accessed April 24, 2011. http://www.who.int/malaria/world_malaria_report_2011/9789241564403_eng.pdf.
"World Report 2009—China." *Human Rights Watch.* Accessed September 24, 2009. http://www.hrw.org/sites/default/files/reports/wr2009_web.pdf.
Wu, Zun-you, Ke-ming Rou, and Hai-xia Cui. "The HIV/AIDS Epidemic in China: History, Current Strategies and Future Challenges." *AIDS Education and Prevention* 16, Supplementary A (2004): 7–17.
Wu, Zun-you, Sheena G. Sullivan, Yu Wang, Jane Rotheram-Borus Mary, and Roger Detels. "Evolution of China's Response to HIV/AIDS." *The Lancet* 369, no. 9562 (2007): 679–690.
Xiao, Yan, Sibylle Kristensen, Jiang-ping Sun, Lin Lu, and Sten H. Vermund. "Expansion of HIV/AIDS in China: Lessons from Yunnan Province." *Social Science and Medicine* 64, no. 3 (2007): 665–675.
Xien, Gui and Zhuang Ke. "AIDS in China." In *Emerging Infections in Asia*, edited by Yi-chen Lu, M. Essex, and Bryan Roberts, 143–162. New York: Springer, 2008.
Xu, Ying and Li-tao Zhao. "China's Rapidly Growing Non-Governmental Organizations." *EAI Background Brief No. 514.* Last modified March 25, 2010. http://www.eai.nus.edu.sg/BB514.pdf.
Xue, Bin. "HIV/AIDS Policy and Policy Evolution in China." *International Journal of STD and AIDS* 16, no. 7 (2005): 459–464.
"XV International AIDS Conference Ends with Leaders Calling for Increased Commitment to Fight HIV/AIDS Worldwide." *Kaiser Family Foundation.* Last modified July 16, 2004. http://dailyreports.kff.org/Daily-Reports/2004/July/16/dr00024798.aspx.
Yin, Wen-yuan and Zun-you Wu. "Challenges and Opportunities: The Expanded Government-Led HIV/AIDS Programs in China." *Virologica Sinica* 22, no. 6 (2007): 493–500.
Yip, Winnie and Ajay Mahal. "The Health Care Systems of China and India: Performance and Future Challenges." *Health Affairs* 27, no. 4 (2008): 921–932.
Yu, Dong-bao, Yves Souteyrand, Mazuwa A. Banda, Joan Kaufman, and Joseph H. Perriëns. "Investment in HIV/AIDS Programs: Does it Help Strengthen Health Systems in Developing Countries?" *Globalization and Health* 4, no. 8 (2008): 1–10.
Yu, Elena S. H., Qi-yi Xie, Kong-lai Zhang, Ping Lu, and Lillian L. Chan. "HIV Infection and AIDS in China, 1985 through 1994." *American Journal of Public Health* 86, no. 8 (1996): 1116–1122.
Zhang, Fu-jie, Jessica E. Haberer, Yu Wang, Yan Zhao, Ye Ma, De-cai Zhao, Lan Yu, and Eric P. Goosby. "The Chinese Free Antiretroviral Treatment Program: Challenges and Responses." *AIDS* 21, Supplementary 8 (2007): 143–148.
Zhang, Fu-jie, Zhi-hui Dou, Ye Ma, Yan Zhao, Zhong-fu Liu, Marc Bulterys, and Ray Y. Chen. "Five-Year Outcomes of the China National Free Antiretroviral Treatment Program." *Annals of Internal Medicine* 151, no. 4 (2009): 241–251.
Zhang, Gui-hong. "China's Peaceful Rise and Sino-Indian Relations." *China Report* 41, no. 2 (2005): 159–171.

Zhang, Heather Xiao-quan. "The Gathering Storm: AIDS Policy in China." *Journal of International Development* 16, no. 8 (2004): 1155–1168.

Zhang, Xiu-lan, Pierre Miège, and Yu-rong Zhang. "Decentralization of the Provision of Health Services to People Living with HIV/AIDS in Rural China: The Case of Three Counties." *Health Research Policy and Systems* 9, no. 9 (2011): 1–7.

Zhe, Dong and Phillips, Michael R. "Evolution of China's Health-Care System." *The Lancet* 372, no. 9651, (2008): 1715–1716.

Zheng, Xi-wen, Chun-qiao Tian, Kyung-hee Choi, Jia-peng Zhang, He-he Cheng, Xin-zhen Yang, Da-qin Li, Ji-sheng Lin, Shu-quan Qu, Xin-hua Sun, Thomas Hall, Jeff Mandel, and Norman Hearst. "Injecting Drug Use and HIV Infection in Southwest China." *AIDS* 8, no. 8 (1994): 1141–1147.

Zhou, Feng, Gerald F. Kominski, Han-zhu Qian, Jian-sheng Wang, Song Duan, Zhi-wei Guo, and Xin-ping Zhao. "Expenditure for the Care of HIV-Infected Patients in Rural Areas in China's Antiretroviral Therapy Programs." *BMC Medicine* 9, no. 6 (2011): 1–10.

Zimmerman, Barry E. and David J. Zimmerman. *Killer Germs: Microbes and Diseases That Threaten Humanity.* New York: McGraw-Hill, 2003.

"$25M for MSM and TG Communities in India." *International HIV/AIDS Alliance.* Last modified September 13, 2010. http://www.aidsalliance.org/NewsDetails.aspx?Id=687.

"2003: TAC and Civil Disobedience." *JournAIDS.* Accessed August 9, 2010. http://www.journaids.org/index.php/factsheets/the_politics_of_hivaids_in_south_africa/tac_and_civil_disobedience/.

"2005 Update on the HIV/AIDS Epidemic and Response in China." *Ministry of Health, People's Republic of China and Joint United Nations Program on HIV/AIDS, World Health Organization.* Last modified January 24, 2006. http://data.unaids.org/publications/External-Documents/rp_2005china estimation_25jan06_en.pdf.

2009/2010 China HIV/AIDS NGO Directory. People's Republic of China: National Centre for AIDS/STD Control and Prevention, China CDC and China HIV/AIDS Information Network, 2009.

"2011 Estimate for the HIV/AIDS Epidemic in China." *Ministry of Health, Joint United Nations Program on HIV/AIDS, World Health Organization.* Last modified November 2010. http://www.chinaids.org.cn/n1971/n2151/n777994.files/n777993.pdf.

"2012 China AIDS Response Progress Report." *Ministry of Health of the People's Republic of China.* Last modified March 31, 2012. http://www.unaids.org/en/dataanalysis/monitoringcountryprogress/progressreports/2012countries/ce_CN_Narrative_Report[1].pdf.

"2014 China AIDS Response Progress Report," *National Health and Family Commission of the People's Republic of China,* June 2014, accessed January 31, 2015, http://www.unaids.org/sites/default/files/documents/CHN_narrative_report_2014.pdf. 中国艾滋病传播途径以性传播为主 ["Sex Becomes the Main Route of HIV/AIDS Transmission in China."] *Docin.com.Inc.* Accessed February 20, 2012. http://www.docin.com/p-236465268.html.

"台爱滋病防治推动委员会成立 斥资2亿斗爱滋"[The Establishment of Taiwan Committee for the Promotion of AIDS Prevention and Treatment, with an Allocation of 2 Billions to Fight HIV/AIDS]. 北方网 *[enorth.com.cn]*. Last modified December 20, 2001. http://news.enorth.com.cn/system/2001/12/20/000222602.shtml.

张可 [Zhang, Ke.] 既往有偿献血人员HIV感染者自然史分析 ["The Natural History of HIV Infection among Paid Blood Donors in Henan Province."] *中国艾滋病性病* [*China Journal of AIDS and STD*] (2006年第12卷第4期) [12, no. 4 (2006)]: 291–293.

张福杰, 文毅, 于兰, 马烨, 潘捷, 赵燕 [Zhang, Fu-jie, Yi Wen, Lan Yu, Ye Ma, Jie Pan, and Yan Zhao.] 艾滋病的抗病毒治疗与我国的免费治疗现状 ["Antiretroviral Therapy for HIV/AIDS and Current Situation of China Free ARV Program."] *科技4747* [*Science and Technology Review*] (2005年第23卷第7期) [23, no. 7 (2005)]: 24–29.

李宁, 王哲, 孙定勇 [Li, Ning, Zhe Wang, and Ding-yong Sun.] 河南省艾滋病流行现状分析 ["Analysis of HIV/AIDS Epidemic in Henan Province."] *医药论坛杂志* [*Journal of Medical Forum*] (2007年第28卷第19期) [28, no. 19 (2007)]: 22–23.

昆明累计报告艾滋病1.5万余例 ["The Cumulative Reported Number of HIV/AIDS in Kunming is above 15,000."] *云南网* [*Yunnan Wang.*] (2010年12月2日) [Last modified December 2, 2010.] http://special.yunnan.cn/feature3/html/2010-12/02/content_1427519.htm.

国务院关于进一步加强艾滋病防治工作的通知 ["State Council Notice on Further Strengthening HIV/AIDS Prevention and Control."] *国发48号 [State Council Document No. 48.]* (二○一○年十二月三十一日) [Last modified December 31, 2010.] http://www.gov.cn/zwgk/2011-02/16/content_1804536.htm.

溫家寶: 全社會共同努力有效預防和控制艾滋病（全文）["Wen Jiabao: The Whole Community Work Together to Prevent and Control HIV/AIDS."] *中國中央電視臺* [*CCTV.*] (2004年7月10日) [Last modified July 10, 2004.] http://big5.cctv.com/gate/big5/apps.cctv.com/health/20040710/100150.shtml.

2007年国家艾滋病防治社会动员经费支持<目一览表 ["A Table Shows the Budget of HIV/AIDS Prevention and Treatment Supported through Social Mobilization Program in 2007."] *Docin.com.Inc*. Accessed February 20, 2012. http://www.docin.com/p-262618485.html.

2008年国家艾滋病防治社会动员经费支持<目一览表 ["A Table Shows the Budget of HIV/AIDS Prevention and Treatment Supported through Social Mobilization Program in 2008."] *Docin.com.Inc*. Accessed February 20, 2012. http://www.docin.com/p-31402759.html.

Index

1918 flu pandemic (Spanish flu), 2, 6

AIDS Awareness Group, 153
AIDS Healthcare Foundation—India Cares, 142, 153
AIDS Prevention Bill (India), proposed bill, 126, 128
audience acceptance. *See also* moral support; technical support
case studies. *See* audience acceptance of failed securitizing moves in India, case studies; audience acceptance of full securitizing moves in China, case studies
operationalization
   contribution of comparative case studies, "role of audience," 172
   lack of operationalization and differentiation and, 23, 24
   securitizer and audience involvement in the securitization process, reoperationalized, 162
policy evaluation, 33–5
policy formulation and decision-making stage, 33
securitizing actors, 19, 22
   audience involvement in securitization process, reoperationalized, 162
success of securitization, 5
threat framing, 168
audience acceptance of failed securitizing moves in India, case studies, 139–60
   analysis, 151–9
   comparison, 167–8
   overall acceptance levels and types of securitization, 170
   contributions of revised framework and comparative case studies, 171–4
   degree of success, 170–1
   failed HIV/AIDS securitizing moves in India, 169–70
   moral support, 148–50
   overview, 139–51
   results, failed HIV/AIDS securitization, 159–60, 167–70
   selected cities, 141–8
   technical support, 151–9
   trend identified, 167
audience acceptance of full securitizing moves in China, case studies, 97–121
   analysis, 109–15
   comparison, 167–8
   overall acceptance levels and types of securitization, 170
   contributions of revised framework and comparative case studies, 171–4
   degree of success, 170–1
   full HIV/AIDS securitizing moves in China, 168–9
   moral support, 109–11, 121
   level of, 105–6
   overview, 97–109
   results, 115–21
      false securitization, 120–1
      full HIV/AIDS securitization, 115–20, 121, 167–9
   selected cities, 99–105
   technical support, 112–15, 121
      factors hindering, 115–21
      government and individual organized HIV/AIDS-focused NGOs in China, 113, 114t

266   Index

audience acceptance—*Continued*
  grassroots NGOs, restrictive legal status of, 115–19
  level of, 106–9
  repression of HIV/AIDS-focused NGOs and activists, 119–20
  trend identified, 167
Austin, John Langshaw, 18, 21, 29
Austinian speech-act theory, 18, 21
avian influenza virus (H5N1), 6, 46

Balzacq, Thierry, 22, 172
Beijing (China)
  audience acceptance, level of acceptance toward full HIVAIDS securitizing move. *See* audience acceptance of full securitizing moves in China, case studies
  local understanding of full HIV/AIDS securitizing moves, 99–100
  overview of HIV/AIDS situations, 99
  benefits of securitization, 58–60
  budgets, maintain sustainable HIV/AIDS-related, 59–60
  stigmatization and discrimination, reduction of, 58–9
"Berlin patient" (Timothy Brown), 3
Bhanu, Vinod, 136, 142
Bhardwaj, Kajal, 149, 156
Bhore, Joseph, 67
Bhore Committee Report (also known as *The Report of the Health Survey and Development Committee*), 67
Bill and Melinda Gates Foundation, 63
bioterrorism threats, 47, 48
Black Death, comparisons to, 2, 6, 36
Blackwill, Robert, 130
branches of securitization, 32–3, 35–43, 165–6. *See also specific type of securitization*
Brazil, void failed securitization (1995–2011), 40–1
Brown, Timothy ("Berlin patient"), 3

budgetary allocation
  maintaining sustainable HIV/AIDS-related budgets, benefits of securitization, 59–60
  policy formulation and decision-making stage in health security analysis, 31
securitizing HIV/AIDS in China
  full securitizing move (from 2004 onward), 89
  performative securitizing move (1995–1999), 84–5, 86
  rhetorical securitizing move (2000–2003), 88
securitizing HIV/AIDS in India
  full securitizing move (2004–2009), 131
  performative securitizing move (1992–1997), 127–8
  rhetorical securitizing move (1998–2003), 38, 129
Buggineni, Padma, 135
bureaucratic resistance
  to full securitizing move (from 2004 onward), 92–5, 96
  performative securitizing move (1995–1999), 86
burn-out effect, 171
Bush, George W., 61
Buzan, Barry, 4, 11, 18–19, 21–2, 27, 33, 40, 57
  audience acceptance, 19, 22
  Copenhagen School of Securitization Theory, 4
  discourse analysis, 11
  emergency mode, 21–2
  goal of desecuritization, 39–40
  securitizing actors, choosing not securitize a challenge, 51
  speech acts, 18, 27
  valid securitization moves, 33

Caballero-Anthony, Mely, 47, 48
"California baby," 3
Calvary Counseling Centre, 147
Cardoso, Fernando H., 40
Catholic Relief Services, 146, 155

causal linkage between HIV/AIDS and
   security threats, differing
   scholarly opinions, 46
CD4 receptor, 51–2
Center for Legislative Research and
   Advocacy, 136
*Certain Regulations on the Monitoring and
   Control of AIDS* (China), 91
Chebbi, Amita, 135, 141, 153
Chen, Lincoln C., 48
Chen Shui-Bian, 36
Chen Zhu, 115
China CARES, 88
China Comprehensive AIDS
   Response Program (China
   CARES Program), 88
China-Bill Gates Project, 117
Chinese Academy of Preventive Medical
   Sciences, 80
Choudhury, Lincoln, 152
Ciută, Felix, 21
civil society groups, defined, 33–4
Cliff, Andrew D., 45
Clinton Foundation, 63, 137
cocktail therapy, 3, 54
Cohen, Marc, 171
combating HIV/AIDS, 54–7
   HIV/AIDS treatment, 54–5
   ignorance of people, 57
   social attitudes and behaviors
      regarding, 56–7
   spreading of HIV/AIDS, 56–7
   vaccine development,
      obstacles, 55–6
Commonwealth Games
   (India, 2009), 63
Confederation of Indian Industry (CII), 38
constructivism paradigm, 24
constructivist theory, 4–5
contributions of securitization, 19
Copenhagen School of Securitization
   Theory, 4–5, 18–25
   audience acceptance
      critical condition for successful
         securitization, 19
      securitization framework, internal
         problem within, 22–3

   contributions of securitization, 19
   securitization framework, internal
      problems, 20–5, 163–4
   applicability of securitization theory
      in non-Western context,
      shortcomings, 23–5
   audience acceptance, 22–3, 163–4
   black and white judgments, 24–5, 172
   constructivism paradigm, 24
   democratic assumptions, 23–4
   emergency mode and measures,
      21–2, 163
   Eurocentrism in securitization,
      20, 23, 43
   lack of operationalization and
      differentiation, 20, 24, 43
   operationalization of audience
      acceptance, 24
   speech acts, 20–1, 163
   technical and moral support, 22–3,
      163–4
   Westphalian straitjacket
      phenomenon, 23–4
speech acts
   Austinian speech-act theory, 18, 21
   bodily aspect of speech acts, 20–1
   illocutionary nature of speech acts,
      18, 21, 30, 163
   media restrictions, nondemocratic
      countries, 20
   securitization framework, internal
      problem within, 20–1
   security as, 18
corona virus, 46
countries with largest HIV/AIDS
   populations, 2
Crimean War, 45–6
Curley, Melissa G., 8, 23, 94, 118

Darwin, Charles, 4, 47
de Wilde, Jaap, 4, 18
deaths caused by, 51
Deng Xiaoping, 69, 72
desecuritization, 39–40
developed and developing countries, public
   spending on health, education,
   and military, 49–51

development of HIV/AIDS epidemic
  China, 79, 80–2, 95
    expansion phase (1995–present), 81–2
    introduction phase (1985–1988), 80, 95
    spreading phase (1989–1994), 80–1
  India, 123, 124–5, 138
    current epidemiological situation (2007–present), 125
    historical epidemiological situation (1986–2005), 124–5
    spreading, 124
differentiation, lack of. *See* lack of operationalization and differentiation
discourse analysis, 11
discovery of HIV/AIDS, 52–4
discrimination. *See* stigmatization and discrimination
Drèze, Jean, 71

Easton, David, 25–6
economic development of India and China, 8–9
Elbe, Stefan, 46, 58
emergency mode/measures. *See also* budgetary allocation; legislation amendment and formulation; policy measures and institutional arrangement
  Copenhagen School of Securitization Theory
    securitization framework, internal problems, 21–2, 163
    emergency and nonemergency, distinction, 30–1, 32
    lack of operationalization and differentiation and, 21
    policy formulation and decision-making stage in health security analysis, 30–3, 43, 164
    positive and negative speech acts, 32
  securitizing HIV/AIDS in China
    failed securitizing move (1985–1994), 83–4
    full securitizing move (from 2004 onward), 89–92, 94, 96
    performative securitizing move (1995–1999), 84–6, 92–4

    rhetorical securitizing move (2000–2003), 87–8
  securitizing HIV/AIDS in India
    fading-out of full HIV/AIDS securitizing moves (2010 onward), reaction to non-emergency mode, 135
    failed securitizing move (1986–1991), 126–7
    full securitizing move (2004–2009), 130–2
    performative securitizing move (1992–1997), 127–8
    rhetorical securitizing move (1998–2003), 38, 128–30
  securitizing moves matrix, 32
  self-referential practice, securitization theory shortcomings, 6
emerging and reemerging infectious diseases (ERIDs), 47, 48, 51
emerging issues
  China, bureaucratic resistance to full securitizing moves, 92–5, 96
  India, fading-out of full HIV/AIDS securitizing moves (2010 onward), 133–8
    budgetary allocations to HIV/AIDS interventions, augmenting, 134
    financial expenditures of the Indian government and external agencies on NACPs, 136, 137t
    health budget allocated to NRHM and HIV/AIDS (2005–2011), 134
    HIV/AIDS Bill, resistance to pass, 133, 139–40, 156–7
    international or agency funding, 136–8
    non-emergency mode, reaction to, 135
    strategic reasons for drawback, 136–8
Emmers, Ralf, 23
Eriksson, Johan, 27
Erwin, Alec, 42
Eurocentrism in securitization, 6, 8, 161, 174
  securitization framework, internal problems, 20, 23, 43

INDEX

The Evangelical Fellowship of India
  Commission Relief, 141, 153
Executive Yuan (the executive branch of
  China), 36–7

fading-out of full HIV/AIDS
  securitizing moves (2010
    onward), 133–8
  budgetary allocations to
    HIV/AIDS interventions,
    augmenting, 134
  financial expenditures of the Indian
    government and external
    agencies on NACPs, 136, 137t
  health budget allocated to
    NRHM and HIV/AIDS
    (2005–2011), 134
  HIV/AIDS Bill, resistance to pass, 133,
    139–40, 156–7
  international or agency funding,
    136–8
  non-emergency mode, reaction to, 135
  strategic reasons for drawback, 136–8
failed securitization
  case studies. See audience acceptance
    of failed securitizing moves in
    India, case studies
  China, failed securitizing move
    (1985–1994), 82–4
    emergency measures, 83–4
    legislation or formulation, 83–4
    policy measures and institutional
      arrangement, 83
    positive speech, 84
  defined, 32, 42, 165
  India, failed securitizing move
    (1986–1991), 126–7
    emergency measures, 126–7
    legislation amendment and
      formulation, 126–7
    policy measures and institutional
      arrangement, 126–7
    positive speech acts, 126
  South Africa, failed securitized move
    (1999–2008), 41–2
  void failed securitization
    Brazil, void failed securitization
      (1995–2011), 40–1
    defined, 41, 165

false securitization
  China, false securitization
    (1985–1997), 42–3, 120–1
  defined, 43
Family Health International AIDS Institute
  (U.S.), 6, 124–5, 136–7
Fanci, Anthony, 56
feedback loop, 25, 26, 28f, 173–4
first indigenous recorded infections
  China, 1, 42, 80, 85, 100, 102
  India, 1, 124, 126, 138, 143
first recorded diagnosis (U.S.),
  52–3, 63
Floyd, Rita, 23, 172
Ford Foundation, 63
"foreigner disease" (China), 42, 82
Four Free and One Care Policy (China),
  90, 91, 92
framing. See threat framing
full securitization
  case studies. See audience
    acceptance of full
    securitizing moves in
    China, case studies
  China, full securitizing move
    (from 2004 onward), 88–92
    budgetary allocation, 89
    bureaucratic resistance to,
      92–5, 96
    emergency measures, 89–92, 94, 96
    legislation amendment and
      formulation, 89, 90–2
    policy measures and institutional
      arrangement, 89–90
    positive speech acts, 89, 96
  defined, 32, 35, 165
  India, full securitizing move
    (2004–2009), 130–2
    budgetary allocation, 131
    emergency measures, 130–2
    legislation amendment and
      formulation, 132
    policy measures and institutional
      arrangement, 131–2
  Thailand, full securitization
    (1991–1995), 35–6
  void full securitization, defined,
    36, 165
"functionally cured," 3

Gaikwad, Timothy, 152
Gallo, Robert, 53
Gandhi, Rajiv, 69
Gandhi, Sonia, 131
Gangte, Loon, 135
Gao Qi, 93
Gao Qiang, 87–8, 112
Gao Yaojie, 120
Garrett, Lousie, 2
Gates, Bill, 130
 China-Bill Gates Project, 117
Gauri, Varun, 7
Gay Related Immunodeficiency
  Disease (GRID), 1–2, 53
GFATM. *See* Global Fund to Fight HIV/
  AIDS, Tuberculosis, and Malaria
  (GFATM)
Global Fund to Fight HIV/AIDS,
  Tuberculosis, and Malaria
  (GFATM)
 audience acceptance of securitizing
   moves, 168–70, 172
 China CARES, launch, 88
 Country Coordinating Mechanism (CCM)
   (China), 61–2, 108, 113, 119
 development of, 61
 development of HIV/AIDS related NGOs,
   China, 34, 112–13, 115, 118–21
 generally, 12
 influence on HIV/AIDS securitization,
   60–2
 requirements for recipient countries, 61–2
 Round 2, 158
 Round 3, 113
 Round 4, 113, 158
 Round 5, 113
 Round 6, 113, 158–9
 Round 7, 158
 Round 9, 158–9, 170, 172
global funding, pattern shift, 62–3
Golden Triangle, 10, 81, 102
Gore, Al, 4, 60
governmental approach to
  HIV/AIDS problem, 9
government-organized nongovernmental
  organizations (GONGOs)
  (China), 116, 118–19
Gulf War, 69

H5N1 avian influenza virus, 6, 46
Hansen, Lene, 20–1, 30, 163
health security analysis. *See* securitization
health security and HIV/AIDS, 45–64
 causal linkage between HIV/AIDS
   and security threats, differing
   scholarly opinions, 46
 combating HIV/AIDS, 54–7
 health-security linkages, 48–51
 HIV/AIDS securitized, 46
  (*See also* United Nations
  Security Council (UNSC)
  Resolution 1308)
 securitization of HIV/AIDS,
   national level in China and
   India, 57–60
health-security linkages, 48–51
 causal linkage between HIV/AIDS
   and security threats, differing
   scholarly opinions, 46
 developed and developing countries,
   public spending on health,
   education, and military, 49–51
 emerging and reemerging infectious
   diseases (ERIDs), 47, 48, 51
 government prioritization of public
   health policy, 49–52
 HIV/AIDS securitized, 46 (*See also*
   United Nations Security Council
   (UNSC) Resolution 1308)
 logic of securitization, 49
 public health expenditures, developing
   countries, 49–51
hemophiliac patients, 53, 57, 80
Herington, Jonathan, 8, 23
HIV/AIDS, disease specifics
 combating HIV/AIDS, 54–7
  HIV/AIDS treatment, 54–5
  human attitudes and behaviors
    regarding, 56–7
  ignorance of people, 57
  social attitudes and behaviors
    regarding, 56–7
  spreading of HIV/AIDS, 56–7
  vaccine development, obstacles, 55–6
 countries with largest HIV/AIDS
   populations, 2
 deaths caused by, 51

INDEX

development of HIV/AIDS epidemic
  China, 79, 80–2, 95
    expansion phase (1995–present), 81–2
    introduction phase (1985–1988), 80, 95
    spreading phase (1989–1994), 80–1
  India, 123, 124–5, 138
    current epidemiological situation (2007–present), 125
    historical epidemiological situation (1986–2005), 124–5
    spreading, 124
  discovery of, 52–4
  facts and statistics, generally, 2, 6–7, 51
  first indigenous recorded infections
    China, 1, 42, 80, 85, 100, 102
    India, 1, 124, 126, 138, 143
  first recorded diagnosis (U.S.), 52–3, 63
  "functionally cured" of, 3
  historic background of disease, 1–3, 6–7, 52–4
  host cells, 51–2, 54, 56
  human attitudes and behaviors regarding, 56–7
  ignorance of people, 57
  infections since 1981, 51
  misperceptions of HIV/AIDS, 1–2
  social attitudes and behaviors regarding, 56–7
  South Africa, population with HIV/AIDS, statistics, 2
  spreading of HIV/AIDS, 56–7
    China, spreading phase (1989–1994), 80–1
    India, 124
  successfully cured of, 3
  T cells, 2, 51–2, 53
  virology of, 51–2
HIV/AIDS Bill (India), resistance to pass, 133, 139–40, 156–7
HIV/AIDS securitized, 46. *See also* United Nations Security Council (UNSC) Resolution 1308
homosexuality, legalization of
  China, 101
  India, 156

host cells, 51–2, 54, 56
Howlett, Michael, 25–6
HTVL (Human T cell lymphottropic virus), 51, 53
Hu Jintao, 87
human security, 16, 17. *See also* health-security linkages
  components of, 17, 48
Human T cell lymphottropic virus (HTVL), 51, 53
Huysmans, Jef, 16, 29

identifying the type of problem presented by HIV/AIDS, 2–4
illocutionary acts/illocutionary speech acts. *See* speech acts
Imphal (India)
  audience acceptance, level of acceptance toward failed HIVAIDS securitizing moves. *See* audience acceptance of failed securitizing moves in India, case studies
  local understanding of failed HIV/AIDS securitizing moves, 147
  overview of the HIV/AIDS situation, 144–7
India
  health-security linkages
    developed and developing countries, public spending on health, education, and military, 49–50
  HIV/AIDS securitization under Prime Minister Vajpayee (1998–2003), 38
India, void rhetorical securitization (1998–2003), 38, 128–30
India Cares, AIDS Healthcare Foundation, 142, 153
Indian Business Trust for HIV/AIDS (IBT), 38
Indian HIV/AIDS Alliance, 159
Indian Penal Code, Section 377, 132
infectious diseases, generally. *See also* HIV/AIDS, disease specifics
  background, 45–6
  bioterrorism threats, 47–8
  emerging and reemerging infectious diseases (ERIDs), 47, 48, 51

infectious diseases—*Continued*
  framed as threats, 48–51
  killing power of diseases *vs.*
    physical weapons, 46
  microbes and people, 46–8
  securitization *vs.* normal political
    response, 51
  institutional arrangement. *See* policy
    measures and institutional
    arrangement
  institutionalization of securitization.
    See performance securitization
Integrated Biological Behavioral
  Assessments (IBBA)
  surveys, 124
International AIDS Summit, 84
International Development Association
  (IDA) of the World Bank,
  129, 137
International HIV/AIDS Alliance, 135
International Monetary Fund (IMF),
  69–70, 72
intersubjectivity, 5, 18, 23, 34, 111
Iqbal, Javed Mohammad, 31

Jiang Zemin, 42, 86–7
Joshi, Murli Manohar, 130

Kapila, Uma, 7
Karlen, Arno, 57
Kavi, Ashok Row, 143
Kazatchkine, Michel, 152–3
Kunming (China)
  audience acceptance, level of acceptance
    toward full HIVAIDS
    securitizing move. *See* audience
    acceptance of full securitizing
    moves in China, case studies
  local understanding of full HIV/AIDS
    securitizing moves, 103–4
  overview of HIV/AIDS
    situations, 102–3

lack of operationalization and
  differentiation, 161, 164,
  166, 174
audience acceptance and, 23, 24
emergency measures and, 21

securitization framework, internal
  problems, 20, 24, 43
self-referential practice, securitization
  theory shortcomings, 6
Lamptey, Peter, 6
LAV (lymph-associated virus), 53
Law of Infectious Diseases Prevention and
  Control of 1989
  (China), 84
Law on Communicable Diseases Prevention
  and Control (China), 90
legislation amendment and formulation
  policy formulation and decision-making
    stage in health security analysis,
    31–2
securitizing actors, 32–3
securitizing HIV/AIDS in China
  failed securitizing move
    (1985–1994), 83–4
  full securitizing move (from 2004
    onward), 89, 90–2
  performative securitizing move
    (1995–1999), 85–6
securitizing HIV/AIDS in India
  failed securitizing move (1986–1991),
    126–7
  full securitizing move (2004–2009), 132
  performative securitizing
    move (1992–1997), 128
  rhetorical securitizing move
    (1998–2003), 38, 129
Leivon, Amun, 147
"lenti-property," 54–5, 63
lentivirus, 51
Li Peng, 42–3
Lieberman, Evan S., 7
Lin Oi-chu, 111, 113
logic of securitization, 49
Lu, Xiao-qing, 118
lymph-associated virus (LAV), 53

Mahal, Ajay, 72
Malaria, 105–6, 109–10, 127.
  See also Global Fund to Fight
  HIV/AIDS, Tuberculosis,
  and Malaria (GFATM)
lack of stigma as compared to
  HIV/AIDS, 110

INDEX

Mao Zedong, 66, 68
Mapping the Global Future : Report of the National Intelligence Council's 2020 Project, 8
Mbeki, Thabo, 41–2
McDonald, Matt, 20
McInnes, Colin, 7, 24, 32, 164–5
measles, 47
Médecins Sans Frontières (MSF) (Doctors without Borders, France), 62
media restrictions, nondemocratic countries, 20
medical problem, identifying HIV/AIDS as, 2–3
Meinya, Thokchom, 136
Meng Lin, 119
methicillin-resistant Staphylococcus aureus (MRSA), 47
microbes
   antibiotics, resistance to and improper usage of, 47
   bioterrrorism threats, 47–8
   historical background and acceptance of, 45
   human behavior, 47
   human immune systems, 47
   and people, 46–8
   reemergence of "ancient diseases," contributing factors, 47
   role in wars and war like events, 45–6
   vaccination policies, reduced compliance, 47
Ministry of Health and Family Welfare (MoHFW), 127, 131–2, 158
misperceptions of HIV/AIDS, 1–2
"Mississippi baby," 3
Mlambo-Ngcuka, Phumzile, 41
modernization, 10
Möller, Frank, 20
Montagnier, Luc, 53
Mookherjee, S. B., 38
moral support
   China, 109–11, 121
   level of moral support, 105–6
   health security analysis, policy evaluation, 35
   India, level of moral support, 148–50

securitization framework, internal problems, 22–3, 163–4
MRSA (methicillin-resistant Staphylococcus aureus), 47
Mukherjee, Anuradha, 149
Mukherjee, Gopal, 125, 136, 149
Mukti Sadan Foundation, 144
Mumbai (India)
   audience acceptance, level of acceptance toward failed HIVAIDS securitizing moves. *See* audience acceptance of failed securitizing moves in India, case studies
   local understanding of failed HIV/AIDS securitizing moves, 144
   overview of the HIV/AIDS situation, 142–4

Nabeel, M. K., 132, 141, 152, 157
NACO. *See* National AIDS Control Organization (NACO)
NACP. *See* National HIV/AIDS Control Programme (NACP) (India)
Nandy, Subinay, 92
National AIDS Committee (China), 83
National AIDS Committee (India), 127
National AIDS Committee (Thailand), 35
National AIDS Control Organization (NACO)
   administration of, 132, 135, 147, 150–1
   division of India into groups, 124
   granted special powers by government, 142
   NACP programs, implementation of, 127–8
   PR eligibility, 158
National Centre in HIV Epidemiology and Clinical Research, 171
National HIV/AIDS Control Programme (NACP) (India)
   convergence with NRHM, 134–6, 138–9, 154–5, 168
   financial expenditures of Indian government and external agencies on NACPs, 136, 137t
   future, stand-alone NACPs, 138–9, 154, 168
   launch of, 127

National HIV/AIDS—*Continued*
Medium-Term Plan, 85, 127
phases
  NACP-I, 127–8, 137t
  NACP-II, 129
  NACP-III, 134, 147, 151, 157, 169–70
  NACP-IV
    development of, 12, 133, 136, 168, 170
    priority states, 155
  programs by, NACO implementation of, 127–8
National Institute of Allergy and Infectious Diseases (NIAID), 47, 56
National Institute of Health, 55
national level securitization of HIV/AIDS, 57–60
  benefits of securitization, 58–60
    budgets, maintain sustainable HIV/AIDS-related, 59–60
    stigma and discrimination, reduction of, 58–9
  global funding, pattern shift, 62–3
  international institutions and other countries, influences of, 60–3
  normative dangers of securitization, 58
  normative influences, 60–1
  not securitizing HIV/AIDS, reasons supporting, 57–8
  technical influences, 61–2
National Rural Health Mission (NRHM) (India)
  budgetary allocation, 134
  fading-out of full HIV/AIDS securitizing moves (2010 onward), 133–6, 138
  NACP, convergence with, 134–6, 138–9, 154–5, 168
  program, generally, 133–5
The Naz Foundation (India) Trust, 132, 149, 156
New Delhi (India)
  audience acceptance, level of acceptance toward failed HIVAIDS securitizing moves. *See* audience acceptance of failed securitizing moves in India, case studies

local understanding of failed HIV/AIDS securitizing moves, 141–2
overview of the HIV/AIDS situation, 141
NGO respondents. *See* headings *under audience acceptance*
Nigeria
  population with HIV/AIDS, statistics, 2

Olympics (China, 2007–2008), 20, 63, 119
On Agriculture (Marcus Terentius Varro), 45
operationalization
  audience acceptance
    contribution of comparative case studies, "role of audience," 172
    lack of operationalization and differentiation and, 23, 24
    securitizer and audience involvement in the securitization process, reoperationalized, 162
  lack of operationalization and differentiation, 161, 164, 166, 174
  audience acceptance and, 23, 24
  emergency measures and, 21
  securitization framework, internal problems, 20, 24, 43
  self-referential practice, securitization theory shortcomings, 6
Orbinski, James, 49
origin of name "AIDS," 2. *See also* Gay Related Immunodeficiency Disease (GRID)
original securitization, 18, 34, 174

Panyarachun, Anand, 35–6
Paris Declaration, 84
PCP (Pneumocystis carinii pneumonia), 52–3
Peking Union College Hospital, 1
PEPFAR (President's Emergency Plan for AIDS Relief), 61, 137t
performance securitization
  China, performative securitizing move (1995–1999), 84–6, 96
  budgetary allocation, 84–5, 86

bureaucratic resistance, 86
emergency measures, 84–6
legislation amendment and
  formulation, 85–6
policy measures and institutional
  arrangement, 85–6, 92–4
positive speech acts, 86
defined, 39–40, 165
India, performative securitizing move
  (1992–1997), 127–8
budgetary allocation, 127–8
emergency measures, 127–8
legislation amendment and
  formulation, 128
policy measures and institutional
  arrangement, 127–8
positive speech acts, 128
void performance securitization
defined, 39, 165
Russia, void performance
  securitization (2006–2011),
  38–40
performance securitization, defined,
  39–40, 165
Perl, Anthony, 25
pertussis (whooping cough), 47
Pneumocystis carinii pneumonia (PCP),
  52–3
policy evaluation. *See also* policy
  evaluation case studies,
  typology of securitization
policy formulation and
  decision-making stage, 27–33
revised securitization framework, 33–5,
  162–6
synthesizing policy process model
  and the securitization
  process, 25–6
policy evaluation case studies, typology of
  securitization, 35–43
Brazil, void failed securitization
  (1995–2011), 40–1
China, false securitization
  (1985–1997), 42–3
India, void rhetorical securitization
  (1998–2003), 38, 128–30
Russia, void performance securitization
  (2006–2011), 38–40

South Africa, failed securitized move
  (1999–2008), 41–2
Taiwan, rhetorical securitization
  (2001–2008), 36–7
Thailand, full securitization
  (1991–1995), 35–6
policy formulation and decision-making
  stage in health security
  analysis, 27–33
audience acceptance, 33
Austinian speech-act theory, 18, 21
emergency mode/measures, political
  reaction, 30–3, 43, 164
budgetary allocation, 31
emergency and nonemergency,
  distinction, 30–1, 32
legislation amendment or
  formulation, 31–2
policy measures and institutional
  arrangement, 31
positive and negative speech acts, 32
securitizing moves matrix, 32
external conditions, 27–9
internal conditions, 29–30
speech acts, 27, 33
policy measures and institutional
  arrangement
policy formulation and
  decision-making stage in health
  security analysis, 31
securitizing HIV/AIDS in China
failed securitizing move
  (1985–1994), 83
full securitizing move (from 2004
  onward), 89–90
performative securitizing move
  (1995–1999), 85–6, 92–4
rhetorical securitizing move
  (2000–2003), 88
securitizing HIV/AIDS in India
failed securitizing move
  (1986–1991), 126–7
full securitizing move
  (2004–2009), 131–2
performative securitizing move
  (1992–1997), 127–8
rhetorical securitizing move
  (1998–2003), 38, 128–9

276　Index

post-reform systems of public health care, collapse of, 71–6
  decentralization and privatization, 73–5
  health priority setting and level of spending, 71–3
  implications for HIV/AIDS in China and India, 75–6
President's Emergency Plan for AIDS Relief (PEPFAR), 61, 137t
public health care systems in China and India, 65–77
  economic reforms, 69–70
  post-reform systems of public health care, collapse of, 71–6
  decentralization and privatization, 73–5
  health priority setting and level of spending, 71–3
  implications for HIV/AIDS in China and India, 75–6
  pre-reform systems of public health care in China and India, 66–8
  universal access to public health care, 68
  urban–rural economic inequalities and disparities, 70–1
public health problem, identifying HIV/AIDS as, 3
Putin, Vladimir, 38–40

Rai, Mohammad A., 59
Ramesh, M., 25
Ramiah, Ilavenil, 31, 86
Regulations Concerning the Monitoring and Control of AIDS (China), 83–4
The Report of the Health Survey and Development Committee (also known as *Bhore Committee Report)*, 67
Report of the National Intelligence Council's 2020 Project, Mapping the Global Future, 8
research program, overview, 9–11
Resolution 1308. *See* United Nations Security Council (UNSC) Resolution 1308
retrovirus, generally, 51, 53
revised securitization framework
  contributions of, 171–4

public policy domain, advanced applicability of securitization process in, 173–4
  remedied major shortcomings in single framework, 171–2
  study of securitization in non-western or nondemocratic contexts and implications to regime types, exploration of, 173
  criteria, 26–7, 28f, 162
  differentiated core elements, 163–4
  policy evaluation, 33–5, 162–6
  securitizer and audience involvement, reoperationalized, 162
  securitizing actors, 27, 162, 163, 166, 174–5
  theoretical revision, typology of securitization, 162–6
  types of securitizing moves, 164
  typology of securitization, 164–6
rhetorical securitization
  China, rhetorical securitizing move (2000–2003), 86–8, 96
    budgetary allocation, 88
    emergency measures, 87, 88
    policy measures and institutional arrangement, 88
    positive speech acts, 86–8
  defined, 32, 37, 165
  India, rhetorical securitizing move (1998–2003), 38, 128–30
    budgetary allocation, 38, 129
    emergency measures, 38, 128–30
    legislation amendment and formulation, 38, 129
    policy measures and institutional arrangement, 38, 128–9
    positive speech acts, 38, 128–9
  Taiwan, rhetorical securitization (2001–2008), 36–7
  void rhetorical securitization
    defined, 38, 165
    India, void rhetorical securitization (1998–2003), 38, 128–30
Rollet, Vincent, 37
Rushton, Simon, 7, 24, 31–2, 34, 164–5

INDEX 277

Russia
  antiretroviral treatment (ART), 39
  void performance securitization
    (2006–2011), 38–40

Sahu, Sujit Kumar, 136, 141, 153
Salter, Mark B., 22
Samraj, S., 125, 127, 135
SARS (severe acute respiratory syndrome),
    46, 87, 100, 106, 112
Schwartlande, Bernhard, 92
securitization, 26–35
  beginning of HIV/AIDS
    securitization, 4
  benefits of securitization, 58–60
  budgets, maintain sustainable
    HIV/AIDS-related, 59–60
  stigmatization and discrimination,
    reduction of, 58–9
  branches of securitization, 32–3, 35–43,
    165–6 (*See also specific type of
    securitization*)
  concept defined under International
    Relations (IR), 4
  constructivist theory and, 4–5
  contributions of securitization, 19
  Copenhagen School of Securitization
    Theory, 4–5, 18–25
  framework, internal problems, 20–5,
    163–4
    applicability of securitization theory
      in non-Western context,
      shortcomings, 23–5
    audience acceptance, 22–3, 163–4
    black and white judgments, 24–5, 172
    constructivism paradigm, 24
    democratic assumptions, 23–4
    emergency mode and measures, 21–2,
      163
    Eurocentrism in securitization, 20,
      23, 43
    lack of operationalization and
      differentiation, 20, 24, 43
    operationalization of audience
      acceptance, 24
    speech acts, 20–1, 163
    technical and moral support, 22–3,
      163–4

  Westphalian straitjacket phenomenon,
    23–4
  framework, revised. *See revised
    securitization framework*
  national level securitization of
    HIV/AIDS, 57–60
  origination of concept, 4–6
  policy evaluation, 33–5
  policy evaluation case studies, typology
    of securitization, 35–43
  policy formulation and
    decision-making stage, 27–33
  Resolution 1308. *See United Nations
    Security Council (UNSC)
    Resolution 1308*
  revised securitization framework. *See
    revised securitization framework*
  self-referential practice, shortcomings,
    5–6
  synthesizing policy process
    model and the securitization
    process, 25–6
  theory, 4–6
  threat framing. *See threat framing*
  typology of securitization criteria,
    main conditions, 26–7, 162,
    164–6
securitizers. *See securitizing actors*
securitizing actors
  audience acceptance, 19, 22
  bureaucratic resistance to full
    securitization, 95
  choosing not securitize a
    challenge, 51
  contribution of securitization, 19
  legislation amendment and formulation,
    32–3
  nature of security act, 27
  policy formulation, 27
    external conditions, 27–8
    internal conditions, 29–30
  revised securitization framework, 27,
    162–3, 166, 174–5
  securitization framework, internal
    problems, 21
  securitization process, 23, 165
  threat framing, 5, 18, 51
securitizing agents. *See securitizing actors*

securitizing HIV/AIDS in China, 79–96
  bureaucratic resistance to full
    securitizing moves, 92–5, 96
  securitizing move, policy development,
    82–92, 95–6
  failed securitizing move (1985–1994),
    82–4
  full securitizing move (from 2004
    onward), 88–92
  performative securitizing move
    (1995–1999), 84–6, 96
  rhetorical securitizing move
    (2000–2003), 86–8, 96
securitizing HIV/AIDS in India, 123–38
  fading-out of full HIV/AIDS
    securitizing moves (2010
    onward), 133–8
  securitizing move, policy development,
    126–32
  failed securitizing move (1986–1991),
    126–7
  full securitizing move (2004–2009),
    130–2
  performative securitizing move
    (1992–1997), 127–8
  rhetorical securitizing move
    (1998–2003), 38, 128–30
security, generally
  defined, 15
  human security, 16, 17
  military and non-military threat, 17
  rethinking security, 16–17
  as underdeveloped concept, 15
  wideners *vs.* traditionalists concept of
    security, 15–16
security issue, identifying HIV/AIDS
  as, 3–4
self-referential practice, 5–6
Sen, Amartya, 71
severe acute respiratory syndrome (SARS),
  46, 87, 100, 106, 112
Shanghai (China)
  audience acceptance, level of acceptance
    toward full HIVAIDS
    securitizing move. *See*
    audience acceptance of full
    securitizing moves in
    China, case studies

local understanding of full HIV/AIDS
  securitizing moves, 101
overview of HIV/AIDS situations, 100–1
Sidibe, Michel, 62
silent security dilemma, 163
Simian Immunodeficiency Virus (SIV), 54
Singh, K. Priyokumar, 146, 155
Singh, Manmohan, 131
Singh, R. K. Gyanandra, 146, 147, 155
Sinha, Shatrughan, 130
SIV (Simian Immunodeficiency Virus), 54
Sjöstedt, Roxanna, 21
Smallman-Raynor, Matthew R., 45
smallpox, 47, 55
soft security threat, 7
Solution Exchange AIDS Community of
  UNAIDS India Office, 141,
  152, 157
South Africa
  failed securitized move (1999–2008), 41–2
  population with HIV/AIDS, statistics, 2
Spanish flu (1918 flu pandemic), 2, 6
speech acts
  audience acceptance in China, case
    studies, positive speech acts
    by Chinese leaders, 97
  by securitizers, 111
  Austinian speech-act theory, 18, 21
  bodily aspect of speech acts, 20–1
  facilitating conditions, 27
  illocutionary nature of speech acts, 18,
    21, 30, 163
  media restrictions, nondemocratic
    countries, 20
  policy formulation and decision-making
    stage in health security analysis,
    27, 33
  positive and negative speech acts, 32
  securitization framework, internal
    problems, 20–1, 163
  securitizing HIV/AIDS in China
    failed securitizing move (1985–1994), 84
    full securitizing move (from 2004
      onward), 89, 96
    performative securitizing move
      (1995–1999), 86
    rhetorical securitizing move
      (2000–2003), 86–8

INDEX   279

securitizing HIV/AIDS in India
   failed securitizing move
     (1986–1991), 126
   performative securitizing move
     (1992–1997), 128
   rhetorical securitizing move
     (1998–2003), 38, 128–9
security as, 18
self-referential practice, securitization
   theory shortcomings, 6
threat framing via speech acts, 51 (*See
   also* United Nations Security
   Council (UNSC) Resolution
   1308)
*State Council Notice on Further
   Strengthening HIV/AIDS
   Prevention and Control*
   (China), 89
*State Council Notice on Strengthening HIV/
   AIDS Prevention and Control*
   (China), 88–9
Stewart, William, 47
stigmatization and discrimination
   acts of humiliation against drug-users,
     China, 93–4
   audience acceptance, case studies
     China, 106, 110–11, 121, 168
     India, 145, 149, 153–4
   decrease in prevention due to, 101
   lack of knowledge by general
     public, 1, 57, 111
   misperceptions of HIV/AIDS, 1–2
   pessimistic outlook on resolution due to, 3
   reduction of, benefit of securitization,
     58–9, 91
   social attitudes and behaviors regarding,
     56–7
   threat framing, avoidance, 39
successfully cured, 3
"superbug," 47
Swaraj, Sushma, 127, 130
Swine Influenza A H1N1, 47, 135

T cells, 2, 51–2, 53
Taiwan, rhetorical securitization
   (2001–2008), 36–7
Tamiflu-resistant H1N1, 47
Tandel, Umesh, 144

technical support
   China, 112–15, 121
   factors hindering, 115–21
   government and individual organized
     HIV/AIDS-focused NGOs in
     China, 113, 114t
   grassroots NGOs, restrictive legal
     status of, 115–19
   level of technical support, 106–9
   repression of HIV/AIDS-focused
     NGOs and activists, 119–20
   India, 151–6, 156–9
   level of technical support, 150–1
   policy evaluation, health security
     analysis, 35
   securitization framework, internal
     problems, 22–3, 163–4
terminology, origin of name "AIDS,"
   2. *See also* Gay Related
   Immunodeficiency Disease
   (GRID)
Thai Business Coalition on AIDS (TBCA), 36
Thailand, full securitization (1991–1995),
   35–6
Thompson, Drew, 118
threat framing
   audience acceptance, 168
   avoidance of, 39
   feedback loop, securitizers and, 174
   intersubjectivity, 34, 111
   process of, 4–5
   securitizing actors, 5, 18, 51
   via speech acts, 51 (*See also* United
     Nations Security Council
     (UNSC) Resolution 1308)
traditionalists *vs.* wideners, concept
   of security, 15–16
Tshabalala-Msimang, Manto, 41–2
Tuberculosis (TB), 105–6, 109–10. *See
   also* Global Fund to Fight HIV/
   AIDS, Tuberculosis, and Malaria
   (GFATM)
   lack of stigma as compared to HIV/
     AIDS, 110

United Nations
   declaration of commitment on HIV/
     AIDS, 61

280 INDEX

United Nations—*Continued*
  political declarations on HIV/AIDS, 61
  Solution Exchange AIDS Community of UNAIDS India Office, 141, 152, 157
  UNAIDS (China), 92
  UNAIDS (India), 132, 141, 150, 152, 157
United Nations Development Program (UNDP), 17
1994 United Nations Development Program Report: New Dimensions of Human Security, 17, 48
United Nations Security Council (UNSC) Resolution 1308, 4, 6–7, 46, 60–3
United Progressive Alliance (UPA), 8
United States Agency for International Development (USAID), 129, 137
universal access to public health care, 68
Upadhyaya, Pallavi, 142, 153
urban–rural economic inequalities and disparities, 70–1

Vajpayee, Atal Bihari, 38, 128–30
Varro, Marcus Terentius
  (On Agriculture), 45
Vatsysyan, Siddhartha, 153
Vaughn, Jocelyn, 22, 24
Viravaidya, Mechai, 29
virology of HIV/AIDS, 51–2
void failed securitization
  Brazil, void failed securitization (1995–2011), 40–1
  defined, 41, 165
void full securitization, defined, 36, 165
void performance securitization
  defined, 39, 165
  Russia, void performance securitization (2006–2011), 38–40
void rhetorical securitization
  defined, 38, 165
  India, void rhetorical securitization (1998–2003), 38, 128–30
Vuori, Juha A., 24, 165

Wæver, Ole
  audience acceptance, 19, 22, 33
  contributions of securitization, 19
  Copenhagen School of Securitization Theory, 4
  deliberated study of specific securitizing moves, 32, 164
  discourse analysis, 11
  emergency mode/measures, 21–2, 31–2
  goal of desecuritization, 39–40
  operation of politics, 23
  securitization theory, internal problems, 24–5
  securitizing actors, choosing not securitize a challenge, 51
  speech acts, 18, 27
  valid securitization moves, 33
  Westphalian straitjacket phenomenon, 23–4
Walt, Stephen M., 9, 16–17
Wang Longde, 112
Wang Yanhai, 120
war epidemics, impact of, 45–6
Wen Jiabao, 87–8, 91
Westphalian straitjacket phenomenon, 23–4
whooping cough (pertussis), 47
wideners *vs.* traditionalists concept of security, 15–16
Wilkinson, Claire, 20
Williams, Michael C., 20, 31
Wilson, David, 171
World Bank, 8, 61, 70, 127, 128
  International Development Association (IDA) of the World Bank, 129, 137
World Health Organization (WHO), 48, 49, 61, 82, 137
Wu Yi, 88, 89, 112

Yin Li, 112
Yip Wen-yuan, 72

Zeng Yi, 80
Zhang Kaining, 103–4

The manufacturer's authorised representative in the EU is Springer Nature Customer Service Centre GmbH, Europaplatz 3, 69115 Heidelberg, Germany. If you have any concerns regarding our products, please contact ProductSafety@springernature.com

Printed and bound by CPI Group (UK) Ltd, Croydon, CR0 4YY

24/03/2026

02077827-0001